Dental Implants, Part I: Reconstruction

Editor

OLE T. JENSEN

ORAL AND MAXILLOFACIAL SURGERY CLINICS OF NORTH AMERICA

www.oralmaxsurgery.theclinics.com

Consulting Editor
RUI P. FERNANDES

May 2019 • Volume 31 • Number 2

ELSEVIER

1600 John F. Kennedy Boulevard • Suite 1800 • Philadelphia, Pennsylvania, 19103-2899

http://www.oralmaxsurgery.theclinics.com

ORAL AND MAXILLOFACIAL SURGERY CLINICS OF NORTH AMERICA Volume 31, Number 2
May 2019 ISSN 1042-3699, ISBN-13: 978-0-323-67827-8

Editor: John Vassallo; j.vassallo@elsevier.com
Developmental Editor: Laura Fisher

Oral and Maxillofacial Surgery Clinics of North America (ISSN 1042-3699) is published quarterly by Elsevier Inc., 360 Park Avenue South, New York, NY 10010-1710. Months of issue are February, May, August, and November. Business and Editorial Offices: 1600 John F. Kennedy Blvd., Suite 1800, Philadelphia, PA 19103-2899. Periodicals postage paid at New York, NY and additional mailing offices. Subscription prices are $401.00 per year for US individuals, $720.00 per year for US institutions, $100.00 per year for US students and residents, $474.00 per year for Canadian individuals, $863.00 per year for Canadian institutions, $520.00 per year for international individuals, $863.00 per year for international institutions and $235.00 per year for Canadian and foreign students/residents. To receive student/resident rate, orders must be accompanied by name or affiliated institution, date of term, and the *signature* of program/residency coordinator on institution letterhead. Orders will be billed at individual rate until proof of status is received. Foreign air speed delivery is included in all *Clinics* subscription prices. All prices are subject to change without notice. **POSTMASTER:** Send address changes to *Oral and Maxillofacial Surgery Clinics of North America,* Elsevier Periodicals **Customer Service, 11830 Westline Industrial Drive, St. Louis, MO 63146. Tel: 1-800-654-2452 (U.S. and Canada); 314-447-8871 (outside U.S. and Canada). Fax: 314-447-8029. E-mail: journals customerservice-usa@elsevier.com (for print support); journalsonlinesupport-usa@elsevier.com (for online support).**

Reprints. For copies of 100 or more, of articles in this publication, please contact the Commercial Reprints Department, Elsevier Inc., 360 Park Avenue South, New York, NY 10010-1710. Tel.: 212-633-3874; Fax: 212-633-3820; Email: reprints@elsevier.com.

Oral and Maxillofacial Surgery Clinics of North America is covered in *MEDLINE/PubMed (Index Medicus)*, *Science Citation Index Expanded (SciSearch®)*, *Journal Citation Reports/Science Edition*, and *Current Contents®/Clinical Medicine.*

Printed in the United States of America.

Contributors

CONSULTING EDITOR

RUI P. FERNANDES, MD, DMD, FACS, FRCS(Ed)
Clinical Professor and Chief, Division of Head and Neck Surgery, Departments of Oral and Maxillofacial Surgery, Neurosurgery, and Orthopaedic Surgery and Rehabilitation, University of Florida Health Science Center, University of Florida College of Medicine, Jacksonville, Florida, USA

EDITOR

OLE T. JENSEN, DDS, MS
Adjunct Professor, Department of Oral and Maxillofacial Surgery, University of Utah, School of Dentistry, Salt Lake City, Utah, USA

AUTHORS

TARA L. AGHALOO, DDS, MD, PhD
Professor, Section of Oral and Maxillofacial Surgery, Division of Diagnostic and Surgical Sciences, UCLA School of Dentistry, Los Angeles, California, USA

MICHAEL S. BLOCK, DMD
Private Practice, Metairie, Louisiana, USA

MARCO BRINDIS, DDS
Assistant Professor, Louisiana State University, School of Dentistry, New Orleans, Louisiana, USA

VISHTASB BROUMAND, DMD, MD
Oral and Maxillofacial Surgery Private Practice, Phoenix, Arizona, USA; Adjunct Assistant Clinical Professor, Department of Oral and Maxillofacial Surgery, University of Florida College of Dentistry, Gainesville, Florida, USA

LESLEY DAVID, DDS, DOMFS, FRCDC
Staff Surgeon, Trillium Health Partners and Mount Sinai Hospital, Clinical Instructor, Oral and Maxillofacial Surgery, University of Toronto, Private Practice, Toronto, Canada

RUBÉN DAVÓ, MD, PhD
Head of Oral and Maxillofacial Surgery, Department of Implantology and Maxillofacial Surgery, Medimar International Hospital, Alicante, Spain

MARK DURHAM, DMD
Assistant Professor, Section Head, Prosthodontics, University of Utah, School of Dentistry, Salt Lake City, Utah, USA

NICHOLAS EGBERT, DDS, MSD
Assistant Professor, General Practice Residency, Prosthodontist, University of Utah, School of Dentistry, Salt Lake City, Utah, USA

PIETRO FERRARIS, MD
Private Practitioner of Dentistry, Alessandria, Italy

GHALI E. GHALI, DDS, MD, FACS, FRCS(Ed)
Jack W. Gamble Professor and Chairman, Division of Head and Neck Oncology and Microvascular Reconstructive Surgery, Department of Oral and Maxillofacial Surgery/Head and Neck Surgery, Chancellor, Louisiana State University Health Sciences Center, Shreveport, Louisiana, USA

DANNY HADAYA, DDS
PhD Candidate, UCLA School of Dentistry, Los Angeles, California, USA

LESLIE R. HALPERN, DDS, MD, PhD, MPH, FACS
Professor, Section Head, Oral and Maxillofacial Surgery, University of Utah, School of Dentistry, Salt Lake City, Utah, USA

JOHN F. ERIC HAMRICK, DMD
Private Periodontal Practice, Associate Clinical Professor, Department of Periodontics, Medical University of Southern Carolina, School of Dentistry, Greenville, South Carolina, USA

ALAN S. HERFORD, DDS, MD, FACS
Professor and Chair, Department of Oral and Maxillofacial Surgery, Loma Linda University School of Dentistry, Loma Linda, California, USA

OLE T. JENSEN, DDS, MS
Adjunct Professor, Department of Oral and Maxillofacial Surgery, University of Utah, School of Dentistry, Salt Lake City, Utah, USA

PAUL JUNG, DDS
Research Intern, Department of Oral and Maxillofacial Surgery, Loma Linda University School of Dentistry, Loma Linda, California, USA

KELLY S. KENNEDY, DDS, MS, FACS
Associate Professor and Residency Program Director, Division of Oral and Maxillofacial Surgery and Dental Anesthesiology, The Ohio State University College of Dentistry, Columbus, Ohio, USA

DONGSOO D. KIM, DMD, MD, FACS
Edwards and Freda Green Endowed Professor and Chief, Division of Head and Neck Oncology and Microvascular Reconstructive Surgery, Department of Oral and Maxillofacial Surgery/Head and Neck Surgery, Louisiana State University Health Science Center, Shreveport, Louisiana, USA

PETER E. LARSEN, DDS, FACS
The Larry J. Peterson Endowed Professor and Chair of Oral and Maxillofacial Surgery and Dental Anesthesiology, The Ohio State University College of Dentistry, Columbus, Ohio, USA

PATRICK J. LOUIS, DDS, MD
Professor and Residency Training Program Director, Vice Chair for Academic Affairs, Department of Oral and Maxillofacial Surgery, The University of Alabama at Birmingham, School of Dentistry, Birmingham, Alabama, USA

ISAAC LOWE, MPH, DDS
Resident, Department of Oral and Maxillofacial Surgery, Loma Linda University School of Dentistry, Loma Linda, California, USA

ALBERTO MONJE, DDS, MS
Department of Periodontology, Universitat Internacional de Catalunya, Barcelona, Spain; CICOM-Monje Periodontics Institute, Badajoz, Spain

FEDERICO NICOLI, MD, PhD
Center for Clinical Ethics, Insubria University, Varese, Italy; Clinical Ethics Services "Teresa Camplani Foundation" Domus Salutis Clinic Brescia, Brescia, Italy

GIOVANNI NICOLI, MD
Private Practitioner of Maxillofacial Surgery, Brescia, Italy

STAVAN Y. PATEL, DDS, MD
Fellow, Division of Head and Neck Oncology and Microvascular Reconstructive Surgery, Department of Oral and Maxillofacial Surgery/Head and Neck Surgery, Louisiana State University Health Sciences Center, Shreveport, Louisiana, USA

SIMONE PIVA, MD
Department of Anesthesia, Critical Care and Emergency, Spedali Civili University Hospital, Brescia, Italy

ADI RACHMIEL, DMD, PhD
Head, Department of Oral and Maxillofacial Surgery, Rambam Medical Care Center, Associate Clinical Professor, Ruth and Bruce Rappaport Faculty of Medicine, Technion-Israel Institute of Technology, Haifa, Israel

DEKEL SHILO, DMD, PhD
Department of Oral and Maxillofacial Surgery, Rambam Medical Care Center, Ruth and Bruce Rappaport Faculty of Medicine, Technion-Israel Institute of Technology, Haifa, Israel

SOMSAK SITTITAVORNWONG, DDS, DMD, MS
Professor, Department of Oral and Maxillofacial Surgery, The University of Alabama at Birmingham, School of Dentistry, Birmingham, Alabama, USA

R. JOHN TANNYHILL III, DDS, MD, FACS
Assistant Visiting Surgeon, Department of Oral and Maxillofacial Surgery, Massachusetts General Hospital, Instructor in Oral and Maxillofacial Surgery, Harvard School of Dental Medicine, Boston, Massachusetts, USA

ETHAN TENCATI, BTech, ME
Dental Student, UCLA School of Dentistry, Los Angeles, California, USA

LEN TOLSTUNOV, DDS, DMD
Oral and Maxillofacial Surgery Private Practice, Associate Clinical Professor, Oral and Maxillofacial Surgery, University of the Pacific, School of Dentistry, Assistant Clinical Professor, Oral and Maxillofacial Surgery, University of California, San Francisco, School of Dentistry, San Francisco, California, USA

MARIA J. TROULIS, DDS, MSc, FACS
Chair and Visiting Surgeon, Department of Oral and Maxillofacial Surgery, Massachusetts General Hospital, Walter C. Guralnick Professor of Oral and Maxillofacial Surgery and Chair of the Department of Oral and Maxillofacial Surgery, Harvard School of Dental Medicine, Boston, Massachusetts, USA

ISTVAN A. URBAN, DMD, MD, PhD
Graduate Implant Dentistry, Loma Linda University, Loma Linda, California, USA; Urban Regeneration Institute, Budapest, Hungary

Contents

Surgical Algorithm for Alveolar Bone Augmentation in Implant Dentistry   155

Len Tolstunov

> Replacement of failing and ailing natural teeth with dental implants has become a mainstream treatment option since the discovery of osseointegration by P.-I. Brå-nemark in the 1960s. The techniques and the variety of methods for alveolar bone reconstruction have evolved to address a restoratively driven approach in implant dentistry. Modern 3D cone-bean computed tomography has helped with the diagnosis and treatment of bone deficiencies to idealize implant positioning. This article focuses on bone augmentation techniques, classified into horizontal and vertical ridge augmentation, and discusses block grafting, guided bone regeneration particulate grafting, distraction osteogenesis, and ridge-split expansion procedures.

Bone Augmentation Techniques for Horizontal and Vertical Alveolar Ridge Deficiency in Oral Implantology   163

Len Tolstunov, John F. Eric Hamrick, Vishtasb Broumand, Dekel Shilo, and Adi Rachmiel

> Bone deficiency is the major obstacle in implant dentistry. Guided bone regeneration (GBR) with particulate bone and barrier membranes has been the primary surgical technique used to regenerate alveolar bone for dental implant therapy. This proced-ure has been used in implant dentistry for more than 30 years and continues to be developed and refined for more predictable surgical outcomes. This article reviews GBR and alternative ride expansion procedures and reviews the use of various par-ticulate graft materials. Alveolar distraction osteogenesis, used as an augmentation technique, is also presented.

Biomimetic Enhancement of Bone Graft Reconstruction   193

Tara L. Aghaloo, Ethan Tencati, and Danny Hadaya

> With aging populations and increasing oral rehabilitation, use of dental implants for oral reconstruction is increasing. Adequate hard/soft tissue are required to support use of titanium implants. Bone augmentation is sometimes a necessary procedure to supplement existing alveolar bone. With a wide variety of biomaterials available for clinical use, we focus on the enhancement of bone graft materials, targeting new technologies with potential clinical use. Clinical indications supported by research studies are provided for platelet-rich fibrin, various growth factors, and newly emerging scaffolds. Interestingly, modified biomaterials are being developed and have potential clinical use as more data become available.

Implant Therapy in Alveolar Cleft Sites   207

R. John Tannyhill III and Maria J. Troulis

> Dental implant therapy in the non-cleft patient is familiar to most oral and maxillofa-cial surgeons. Understanding the differences in surgical treatment planning in the cleft patient versus the non-cleft patient is the key to highly functional and esthetic

long-term outcomes. CBCT and computer-assisted planning, as well as improved technology in grafting and implant materials, result in excellent outcomes. Communication with the restorative team remains of paramount importance in planning treatment.

Algorithms for predictable outcomes, or checklists in health care, have been widely supported due to their highly effective outcomes. This article shares "algorithmic roadmaps" to restore single-tooth, partially edentulous, and fully edentulous complex dental implant cases in the patient population. A review of the current literature is presented to provide systematic assessments followed by criteria in a checklist format that allows the surgeon and restorative dentist to determine whether a removable or fixed implant prosthesis is the best patient option. Several cases have been chosen to illustrate the algorithms the authors used to provide an optimized prognosis for surgical/restorative success.

The replacement of one tooth using one implant involves a set of unique criteria for long-term success. Successful therapy should be based on long-term function and health of the adjacent tissues. Sections of this article examine these critical criteria that when working together can result in successful long-term tooth replacement.

Maxillofacial subunit reconstruction using vascularized fibula free flap and endosseous implants is a complex and exciting topic. Use of this technique has profoundly improved patients' function, form, and quality of life. This article outlines the goals and requirements of reconstruction and patient selection. Current data are examined and issues related to flap selection, irradiation, primary versus secondary implant placement, timing and type of implants, use of virtual surgical planning, soft-tissue management, and prosthesis selection fabrication are discussed. Careful planning, communication, and collaboration between reconstructive surgeons and prosthodontists are critical in achieving optimal and stable long-term outcomes.

Four zygomatic implants may be used in patients with severe maxillary atrophy for rehabilitation with a fixed or removable prosthesis. Immediate loading is also typically performed, providing patients with a less invasive and more efficient solution for rehabilitation. Options for immediate loading are presented. The indications, contraindications, procedure, and complications are reviewed. Appropriate treatment planning and work-up are highlighted, as they are required for success in conjunction with advanced surgical skill. Scientific evidence, although lacking in quantity, suggests that the quad zygoma approach offers a predictable solution for the challenge of severe maxillary atrophy; high implant survival rates are noted.

autograft placement. The patients were subsequently treated with 8 implants placed in the molar, bicuspid, and canine regions for complete arch ceramo-metal fixed restorations. Anterior emergence profile esthetics was obtained in 2 patients who had high smile lines. Following final restoration, no maxillary relapse was evident, and no implants were lost. Implant bone levels were stable, although 2 implants had 3 mm of bone loss over the 12-year follow-up period.

Extra-Long Nasal Wall–Directed Dental Implants for Maxillary Complete Arch Immediate Function: A Pilot Study

Giovanni Nicoli, Simone Piva, Pietro Ferraris, Federico Nicoli, and Ole T. Jensen

Immediate loading of maxillary denture prostheses in the context of severe bone atrophy is complicated by posterior implant placement, sometimes requiring a complex surgical approach as zygomatic or pterygoid implants. To overcome this complexity, the authors developed an extra-long (20–24 mm) 24-degree angulated platform. It was tested on 33 patients, with 24 patients immediately loaded (72.7%) for a total of 115 implants (46% nasal). All delayed loading implants osseointegrated. Eight bilateral and six unilateral sinus grafts were performed. There were no complications during the follow-up period.

ORAL AND MAXILLOFACIAL SURGERY CLINICS OF NORTH AMERICA

SERIES OF RELATED INTEREST

Atlas of the Oral and Maxillofacial Surgery Clinics
www.oralmaxsurgeryatlas.theclinics.com

Dental Clinics
www.dental.theclinics.com

THE CLINICS ARE NOW AVAILABLE ONLINE!
Access your subscription at:
www.theclinics.com

ORAL AND MAXILLOFACIAL SURGERY
CLINICS OF NORTH AMERICA

FORTHCOMING ISSUES

August 2019
Dental Implants, Part II: Computer Technology
Ole T. Jensen, Editor

November 2019
Advances in Oral and Maxillofacial Surgery
Jose M. Marchena, Jonathon S. Jundt, and Jonathan W. Shum, Editors

February 2020
Orthodontics for the Oral and Maxillofacial Surgery Patient
Michael R. Markiewicz, Veerasathpurush Allareddy, and Michael Miloro, Editors

RECENT ISSUES

February 2019
The Head and Neck Cancer Patient: Neoplasm Management
Zvonimir L. Milas and Thomas D. Shellenberger, Editors

November 2018
The Head and Neck Cancer Patient: Perioperative Care and Assessment
Zvonimir L. Milas and Thomas D. Shellenberger, Editors

August 2018
Current Controversies in the Management of Temporomandibular Disorders
Daniel M. Laskin and Shravan Kumar Renapurkar, Editors

SERIES OF RELATED INTEREST

Atlas of the Oral and Maxillofacial Surgery Clinics
www.oralmaxsurgeryatlas.theclinics.com

Dental Clinics
www.dental.theclinics.com

Preface

Orthoalveolar Form: The Future State of Alveolar Tissue Engineering

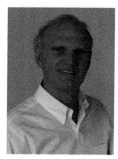

Ole T. Jensen, DDS, MS
Editor

The current state-of-the-art and science for alveolar reconstruction remains tied to the biological principle of engraftment and subsequent maintenance remodeling within the mechanostat of function as it relates to dental implants. The use of titanium implant devices screwed into replacement hard tissue architecture defines successful outcome, but bone grafts in themselves do not. The current state-of-the-art is a mechanical paradigm that argues that a bone graft may well not matter, that osseointegration takes priority to success of a graft, and therefore, alveolar reconstruction. Seldom is recovery of *orthoalveolar form*, that is to say, establishment of anatomic alveolar bone mass that is in arch relation alignment, considered the ultimate measure of success in the literature. In fact, when success of a bone graft, as it might relate to alveolar form, is discussed, the context is one of "emergence profile" of the device, "ridge-lap" of the prosthesis, or implant-associated "papillary height." Therefore, one could pose a question: How much longer will alveolar bone grafting serve an ancillary role while prosthetics, including the implant device componentry, play the primary role toward reconstructing a patient to function?

Imagine a future where titanium devices are not present at all, but that instead, alveolar reconstruction is the *prima solution*—the main event that is prescribed, engineered, and developmentally brought to pass, the prosthetic solution a priority no more.

Ole T. Jensen, DDS, MS
Department of Oral and Maxillofacial Surgery
University of Utah
School of Dentistry
530 Wakara Way
Salt Lake City, UT 84108, USA

E-mail address:
oletjensen@icloud.com

Oral Maxillofacial Surg Clin N Am 31 (2019) xiii
https://doi.org/10.1016/j.coms.2019.02.001
1042-3699/19/© 2019 Published by Elsevier Inc.

Surgical Algorithm for Alveolar Bone Augmentation in Implant Dentistry

Len Tolstunov, DDS, DMD[a,b,c,*]

KEYWORDS

- Dental implantation • Bone augmentation • Surgical algorithm • Cone-beam computed tomography
- Ridge-split • Block graft • Distraction osteogenesis • Guided bone regeneration

KEY POINTS

- Replacement of falling and ailing natural teeth with dental implants has become an alternative treatment option since the discovery of osseointegration by Dr. Brånemark in the early 1960s.
- A surgical-restorative team approach is the best way to evaluate and devise a treatment plan for an implant patient.
- Use of modern 3D CBCT imaging technology helps to diagnose and treat bone deficiency and idealize implant positioning.
- Surgical algorithm can help to determine the best bone augmentation technique for a particular patient in a systematic manner.
- Bone augmentation procedures can be classified on the base of their degree of vascularization that defines their biologic rationale.

INTRODUCTION

Replacement of failing or ailing natural teeth with dental implants has become an alternative treatment option since the discovery of osseointegration by P.-I. Brånemark in the early 1960s.[1–4] Since the early 1980s, surgical-restorative treatment with dental implants become mainstream dentistry.[5,6] Originally surgically driven, the definition of success was an actual osseointegration of titanium implant screw without regard to prosthetics and occlusion. Later, the restoratively driven concept became prevalent with placement of implants linked to proper function and occlusion.[7–10] With time, both surgical and restorative colleagues had to find a common understanding to place implants in the alveolar ridge that would provide functional implant restorations. Techniques and a variety of methods of alveolar bone reconstruction have slowly developed to accommodate the restorative necessity of proper implant placement. A team approach is the best way to evaluate and devise a treatment plan for an implant patient. Use of modern 3D cone-beam computed tomography (CBCT) imaging technology helps to diagnose and treat bone deficiency and idealize implant positioning.

Alveolar bone grafting can be divided into ridge preservation and ridge augmentation.

Ridge preservation (prophylactic approach) involves hard and soft-tissue grafting procedures that intend to preserve the existing ridge volume

Disclosure: The author has nothing to disclose.
[a] Oral and Maxillofacial Surgery Private Practice, San Francisco, CA, USA; [b] Oral and Maxillofacial Surgery, University of the Pacific, School of Dentistry, San Francisco, CA, USA; [c] Oral and Maxillofacial Surgery, University of California San Francisco, School of Dentistry, San Francisco, CA, USA
* 1 Daniel Burnham Court, Suite 366C, San Francisco, CA 94109, USA.
E-mail address: Tolstunov@yahoo.com

Oral Maxillofacial Surg Clin N Am 31 (2019) 155–161
https://doi.org/10.1016/j.coms.2019.01.001
1042-3699/19/© 2019 Elsevier Inc. All rights reserved.

within its bony envelope; they are usually performed at the time of tooth extraction with the goal of minimizing tissue loss after the tooth loss. This surgical approach tends to mostly involve an interpositional or inlay bone grafting with a bone material (routinely, a particulate graft) placed in between the walls of a fresh (postextraction) tooth socket. Ridge preservation using guided bone regeneration (GBR) and guided tissue regeneration (GTR) techniques helps to decrease or eliminate larger surgical bone augmentation procedures.[11,12] An accepted objective after successful grafting is to place a restoratively driven dental implant(s) 3 to 6 months later into mature bony housing. Immediate implantation is possible if primary implant stability can be achieved.[13,14] Although complete prevention of bone collapse with ridge preservation techniques is challenging, the objective here is to minimize it as much as possible.[15–17]

Ridge augmentation (treatment approach) involves hard and soft-tissue grafting procedures that intend to increase (augment) the alveolar ridge volume beyond the existing skeletal envelope; they are usually performed at the edentulous state of a collapsed or deficient alveolar ridge. This surgical approach can involve an onlay (external) or inlay (internal) technique of bone grafting, as well as distraction methods. An accepted objective after successful grafting is to place a restoratively driven dental implant(s) 4 to 6 months later into a mature bony housing. Immediate implantation, in some cases, is possible, if primary implant stability can be achieved.[18] Overcorrection in bone augmentation is often deliberate, knowing the tendency of bone to remodel with some degree of relapse and resorption over time.[19,20]

This article focuses on bone augmentation techniques, which can mainly be classified into horizontal bone augmentation (HBA) and vertical (volumetric) bone augmentation (VBA).

SURGICAL ALGORITHM FOR ALVEOLAR BONE AUGMENTATION

A rationale for a particular bone augmentation procedure in oral implantology originates from the very beginning—the patient's consultation—using clinical and radiographic data. The patient's complaints (symptoms) as well as objective signs of the oral condition lead to a diagnosis and treatment plan. The surgeon's knowledge, skills, and preferences will ultimately dictate the particular bone augmentation technique used.

Ten specific treatment questions (Qs) outlined below can help a surgeon to follow a targeted surgical algorithm to determine the best bone augmentation technique for a particular patient in a logical manner (**Fig. 1**).

Surgical algorithm based on 10 systematic diagnostic questions

Q1: Does the patient lack function of mastication or have esthetic compromise caused by a missing tooth or teeth in the particular area of the jaw?

Example: when a missing tooth would not compromise the function of mastication such as a missing second maxillary molar or mandibular incisor, there may be no discernible lack of function or esthetics.

- If the answer is "Yes", the next question is:

Q2: What would be the most efficient and long-lasting method to improve function, esthetics, and comfort for this patient:

- With restorative means only or through a
- Surgical-restorative approach?

  Example: a fixed bridge would become a favorable treatment if both abutment teeth have crowns and advanced bone loss is present in the pontic region, dictating an extensive vertical ridge augmentation.

  o If the answer is surgical-restorative approach (implant), the next question is:

Q3: Does the patient have sufficient bone stock (foundation) to accommodate an endosseous implant (implants) for the restorative goal selected (eg, single implant crown, 2- to 3-unit implant bridge, full-arch implant rehabilitation)? Use of CBCT scan is encouraged at this stage but not mandatory.

- If the answer is "No", that is, there is bone deficiency present, the next question is

Q4: Does the patient have mainly a horizontal bone defect (HBD), a vertical bone defect (VBD), or a composite bone defect (HDB/VDB)? Clinical and 3D radiographic evaluation with CBCT images can help to answer this question and determine the need for an HBA, a VBA, or both.

- Now, it is important to determine the degree of bone deficiency (horizontal or vertical).

Q5H and *Q5V*: Determine the severity (mild, moderate, severe) of the alveolar ridge deficiency. This can be determined based on the need to accommodate typical root-form dental implant of 4 mm diameter (D) and 10 mm length (L) (4 × 10). Both 2D and 3D imaging is important.

Alveolar Bone Classification by Deficiency (ABCD) (Tolstunov classification):

HBD (WIDTH compromise): types

   0. No HBD is present

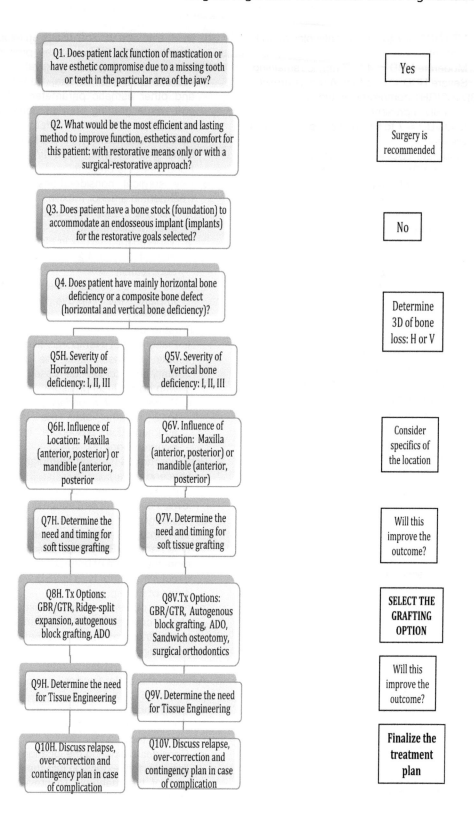

Fig. 1. 10-point surgical algorithm of implant-driven alveolar bone reconstruction in oral implantology.

I. Mild HBD = 7 to 9 mm of alveolar width is present
II. Moderate HBD = 4 to 7 mm is remaining
III. Severe HBD = less than 4 mm is present

VBD (HEIGHT compromise): types
0. No VBD is present
I. Mild VBD = 7 to 9 mm of alveolar height is present
II. Moderate VBD = 4 to 7 mm is remaining
III. Severe VBD = less than 4 mm is present

Variants of alveolar bone loss:
1. Patient has mainly *horizontal* bone deficiency (I, II, or III),
2. Patient has mainly *vertical* bone deficiency (I, II, or III),
3. Patient has a *combination* bone defect: I/I or II/I, or III/III, etc., where the first number indicates horizontal deficiency and the second, vertical.

Example: If a patient's posterior maxillary ridge has 6 mm of edentulous ridge width and 8 mm of alveolar height from the alveolar crest to the sinus floor, this will be type II/I bone defect according to Tolstunov ABCD classification. It means that a surgeon should concentrate mainly on correction of the HBD (from 6 mm to 10 mm) and also improve bone height in a staged or simultaneous fashion trying to achieve 10 x 10 stock of bone.

After determining the bone defect (its dimension and extent), one can proceed to the next algorithmic questions (Q6 and Q7) before making a decision on a particular bone-grafting technique (Q8, Q9, and Q10).

Q6H and *Q6V*: Think about the location, that is, how a particular location of the alveolar ridge would influence or modify the selected diagnosis and treatment plan. Pay attention to the following:

1. Anterior maxilla (incisor, canine, and first premolar):
   a. Evaluate labial cortical plate deficiency (horizontal collapse is very common) and the extent of HBD versus VBD
   b. Determine exacerbating history of:
      i. Apicoectomy(ies) where one would expect periapical bone loss
      ii. Traumatic accident(s) where one would expect horizontal bone loss with scarring and associated vascular compromise
      iii. Pathologic lesion(s) where one would expect a large defect after excision
   c. Consider bone-grafting methods including particulate GBR, block, or alveolar distraction osteogenesis (ADO).

d. Next, evaluate the soft-tissue envelope and esthetic profile including the presence of keratinized gingiva, gingival biotype, esthetic score, smile line, transition line, and other esthetic parameters. Consider soft tissue grafting prior to bone grafting when type III/III bone defect (Tolstunov ABCD classification) is present or after bone grafting when type II/II or smaller bone defect is present.
e. Key surgical considerations for implant treatment in anterior maxilla:
   i. Using a staged approach with delayed implant placement
   ii. Tapered internal hex implants with diameter of 3.5 to 4.2 mm, placed 3 mm subcrestally
   iii. 3+ mm of buccal bone in front of the implant will improve longevity and success
f. Prosthetics:
   i. Placement of a temporary fixed or removable prosthesis after the surgery (eg, Maryland bridge or Essex appliance) with no occlusal pressure
   ii. Placement of a *definitive* prosthesis 8 to12 months after the initial bone augmentation procedure into a fully matured bone

2. Posterior maxilla (second premolar, first molar, and second molar):
   a. Type 3 and 4 bone (poor bone density) that lowers overall implant success
   b. Maxillary sinus pneumatization often requires VBA through the crestal or indirect sinus lift for type I and II VBD (ABCD classification) with more than 4 mm of bone present or lateral or direct sinus lift for type III VBD with less than 4 mm of bone present
   c. For the posterior zone of mastication, one should consider 1 implant per missing tooth and splinting of implant restorations,
   d. Avoid single implants in the second molar position (highest failure rate)

3. Anterior mandible (incisor, canine, and first premolar):
   a. Often horizontal bone deficiency is present
   b. Consider 2 implants to support 3 to 6 missing teeth
   c. Consider evaluating the location of the sublingual artery extension into the symphyseal part of the mandible to prevent vascular injury and a potential for severe bleeding

4. Posterior mandible (second premolar, first molar, and second molar):
   a. Consider an inferior alveolar nerve proximity of 3 mm to be an adequate safety zone

b. Combination bone defect (HBD + VBD) with a staged surgical approach

c. For this zone of mastication, 2 to 3 implants are ideal for 3 to 4 missing teeth

d. Avoid single implants in the second molar position

5. Full Arch:

a. Fixed or removable full-arch implant rehabilitation choices are based on quality of remaining dentition (if present), remaining bone stock, patient's systemic condition and desires, and surgical-restorative team experience

b. All-On-4, zygomatic, and pterygoid implant approaches with either delayed or immediate prosthetics are alternative treatment options that require an advanced surgical and restorative training for success

Q7H and *Q7V*: Determine the need for soft-tissue grafting (quantity and quality of soft-tissue envelope) that can be done before or after the bone grafting and implant treatment using, for example, free palatal graft or connective tissue graft

• If the answer is "No," bone deficiency treatment is the priority. The next question is:

Q8H and *Q8V*: What would be the most predictable and least invasive method of HBA or VBA that would enable placement of implant(s) with a lasting function, esthetics, and comfort?

• Suggested surgical treatment options for HBD based on Tolstunov ABCD classification:

1. GBR/GTR with a particulate graft for types I and II HBD

2. Ridge-split expansion procedure (RSEP) with a particulate graft for types I and II HBD

3. Autogenous block bone (ABB) graft for types II and III HBD

• Suggested surgical treatment options for VBD based on Tolstunov ABCD classification:

1. Surgical orthodontics (forced eruption) for type I VBD

2. GBR/GTR with a particulate graft and Ti-reinforced membrane or Ti-mesh (protected GBR) for types I, II and III VBD

3. ABB graft for types II and III VBD

4. Segmental sandwich osteotomy (SSO) with a particulate or block graft for types II and III VBD

5. Alveolar distraction osteogenesis (ADO) procedure for types II and III VBD

Q9H and *Q9V*: At this point, the need for biomimetics for advanced tissue engineering such as for use in the treatment of complex reconstructive cases, large bone defects, or compromised immune response/compromised healing

history, or both, consider the use of bone morphogenetic protein-2, platelet-rich plasma, platelet-rich fibrin, and bone marrow aspirate to enhance bone regeneration and/or bone growth.

Q10H and *Q10V*: Consider a contingency plan in cases of complication and loss of a graft. Consider the possibility of relapse of each bone-grafting procedure. Consider overcorrection.

When both a surgeon and restorative implant practitioner follow this surgical algorithm, he or she would have very few unanswered questions before selecting the best bone augmentation technique for each particular case of alveolar bone defect as related to implant dentistry (see **Fig. 1**).

BIOLOGIC RATIONALE OF A SURGICAL PROCEDURE: BONE AUGMENTATION

Although many key surgical principles, such as stabilization of bone fragments, fixation of the jaws, space maintenance, and proper wound closure, are important for success, vitality of bone segments seems to be the key surgical principle. Continuous adequate vascularization to bone fragments and grafts is exceedingly important and relies on central (centrifugal or endosteal) and peripheral (centripetal or periosteal) blood supply. Many surgical procedures can be classified by this principle as having higher or lower biologic rationale (BR).[21]

Vascularized bone free flap is a bone augmentation procedure with instant revascularization of tissues by means of a microvascular anastomosis. Among many distant bone free flaps, reconstruction of large mandibular defects with free fibular osteocutaneous flap is often selected for patients with cancer. Establishment of a central anastomosis with a recipient artery leads to full reperfusion of transferred bone and soft tissues (**Table 1**).

ADO is performed for mostly vertically deficient alveolar ridges. The vitality of the osteotomized (transport) bone segment is preserved from 2 vascular sources: endosteal (through the slow separation of fragments at a distraction rate of about 1-mm per day) and peripheral (through the intact and slow-stretching mucoperiosteal flaps). This technique provides an uninterrupted vascular supply important for bone healing that starts with woven (embryonic) bone formation and progresses to lamellar (mature) bone. The BR of the ADO is very high and may only be considered slightly behind the microvascular flap (see **Table 1**).

The RSEP is used for horizontal ridge augmentation. It is an excellent example of pedicled

Table 1
Stratification of bone augmentation procedures by their biologic rationale (BR) (vascularization)

Surgical Techniques	Biologic Rationale (1 to 5 Stars)	Vascularization (Type)	Revascularization (Reperfusion)
Free bone-soft tissue flap transfer	*****	Central (reperfusion)	Optimal to all transferred donor tissues
Distraction osteogenesis	****	Periosteal and endosteal preserved for mobilized bone segments	Optimal, dual (endosteal and periosteal), uninterrupted
Ridge-split expansion, pedicled sandwich osteotomy, ridge preservation, tunnel technique, sinus lift	***	Periosteal for mobilized bone segment and endosteal for inlay bone graft	Optimal periosteal but some loss of endosteal vascularity to the fractured bone segment
Autogenous onlay block bone graft, Ti-mesh or Tent-pole with nonresorbable membrane	**	Plasmatic imbibition (endosteal)	Slow endosteal reperfusion, delayed or missing periosteal source
Cortical tenting (cortical bone block tented over a defect filled with particulate material)	*	Plasmatic imbibition to particulate graft (endosteal), none (initially) to tented cortical block bone	Detached block bone undergoes delayed, partial, and poor revascularization

*****, outstanding vascularization is realized during and after the surgical procedure, BR = 5; ****, excellent vascularization is achieved during and after the surgical procedure, BR = 4; ***, good vascularization is attained during and after the surgical procedure, BR = 3; **, marginal vascularization is realized during and after the surgical procedure, BR = 2; *, poor vascularization is achieved during and after the surgical procedure, BR = 1.

From Tolstunov L. Biologic rationale of a surgical procedure: bone augmentation. J Oral Maxillofac Surg 2018;76(5):915; with permission.

segmental osteotomy[22,23] with optimal vascularization preserved throughout the entire procedure. Continuous blood supply is provided through the peripheral source of intact periosteum attached to the mobilized bone segment, as well as central endosteal source from the trabecular bone feeding the interpositional (inlay) particulate bone graft placed between bone segments. Loss of endosteal vascularity to the subfractured bone segment is the only temporary drawback and is usually well compensated by the peripheral source in the osteoperiosteal flap. Pedicled sandwich osteotomy is a modification of the alveolar split that is used for vertical ridge augmentation, and has the same robust vascularization basis. Postextraction ridge preservation through GBR, tunnel technique, and sinus lift are other methods of internal bone grafting with a particulate graft placed into a 2-to-4 wall defect (socket, collapsed alveolar ridge, or subantral pocket) that is protected and well vascularized with both endosteal and periosteal sources (see **Table 1**).

ABB grafting (extraoral or intraoral) is performed for mainly horizontally deficient alveolar ridges. This is an onlay bone block graft that is separated from its original source of vascularization (donor site) and transferred to the collapsed alveolar ridge. Vitality of transferred graft is temporarily interrupted. It is also not consistently restored. The early route of nurture for the free donor block bone is from the recipient site by plasmatic imbibition from the endosteum via the formation of "vascular sprouts,"[24] which is a slow reperfusion process from the underlying bone that provides marginal vascularization of the grafted bone during the early bone healing. The graft initially undergoes bone resorption followed by a cycle of bone modeling and remodeling leading to a delayed bone formation. With regard to the periosteal source of vitality for a block graft, detached periosteum eventually revascularizes the bone block from the periphery 2 to 4 weeks later, a delayed contribution to overall bone healing.

Ti-mesh and Tent-pole bone augmentation methods used with non-resorbable dense polytetrafluoroethylene (d-PTFE) membrane techniques are other methods of protected onlay bone augmentation having a single endosteal source of blood supply. Frequent exposure and infection of these devices are common as the body attempts to rid itself of the "foreign body" and re-establish missing periosteal vascularization to feed the particulate graft underneath. Because of the missing or delayed periosteal or endosteal source of blood supply, the BR of ABB and Ti-reinforced graft success can be modest (see **Table 1**).

It seems that success of segmental bone osteotomies and bone-grafting procedures depends profoundly on initial revascularization from 2 primary sources of blood supply, endosteal (central) and periosteal (peripheral). Early vitality of osteotomized bone segments is critically important for early bone healing initiated as bone modeling, which forms a callus of woven bone matrix followed later by bone remodeling and maturation. Late-term bone loss or resorption is associated with interruption of vascularization during different stages of bone and implant reconstruction.

The BR of any surgical procedure is defined by the quality of vascularization and preservation of blood supply throughout the surgery. This determines the success of bone and soft-tissue healing and the ultimate success of a surgical technique. Surgical practitioners should always attempt to select a procedure with the utmost potential for physiologic healing, with the highest BR.

REFERENCES

1. Branemark PI, Adell R, Breine U, et al. Intra-osseous anchorage of dental prostheses. I. Experimental studies. Scand J Plast Reconstr Surg 1969;3:81–100.
2. Adell R, Hansson BO, Branemark PI, et al. Intra-osseous anchorage of dental prostheses. II. Review of clinical approaches. Scand J Plast Reconstr Surg 1970;4:119–34.
3. Branemark PI, Breine U, Hallen O, et al. Repair of defects in mandible. Scand J Plast Reconstr Surg 1970;4:2100–8.
4. Adell R, Lekholm U, Rockler B, et al. A 15-year study of osseointegrated implants in the treatment of the edentulous jaw. Int J Oral Surg 1981;10:6387–416.
5. Attard NJ, Zarb GA. Long-term treatment outcomes in edentulous patients with implant overdentures: the Toronto study. Int J Prosthodont 2004;17:4425–33.
6. Attard NJ, Zarb GA. Long-term treatment outcomes in edentulous patients with implant-fixed prostheses: the Toronto study. Int J Prosthodont 2004;17:4417–24.
7. Sones AD. Complications with osseointegrated implants. J Prosthet Dent 1989;62:5581–5.
8. Tinsley D, Watson CJ, Preston AJ. Implant complications and failures: the fixed prosthesis. Dent Update 2002;29:9456–60.
9. Watson CJ, Tinsley D, Sharma S. Implant complications and failures: the complete overdenture. Dent Update 2001;28:5234–8, 240.
10. Watson CJ, Tinsley D, Sharma S. Implant complications and failures: the single-tooth restoration. Dent Update 2000;27:135–8, 40, 42.
11. Mellonig JT, Triplett RG. Guided tissue regeneration and endosseous dental implants. Int J Periodontics Restorative Dent 1993;13:2108–19.
12. Tomlin EM, Nelson SJ, Rossmann JA. Ridge preservation for implant therapy: a review of the literature. Open Dent J 2014;8:66–76.
13. Masaki C, Nakamoto T, Mukaibo T, et al. Strategies for alveolar ridge reconstruction and preservation for implant therapy. J Prosthodont Res 2015;59:4220–8.
14. Zeren KJ. Minimally invasive extraction and immediate implant placement: the preservation of esthetics. Int J Periodontics Restorative Dent 2006;26:2171–81.
15. Buser D, Chappuis V, Belser UC, et al. Implant placement post extraction in esthetic single tooth sites: when immediate, when early, when late? Periodontol 2000 2017;73:84–102.
16. Buser D, Halbritter S, Hart C, et al. Early implant placement with simultaneous guided bone regeneration following single-tooth extraction in the esthetic zone: 12-month results of a prospective study with 20 consecutive patients. J Periodontol 2009;80:1152–62.
17. Raes S, Eghbali A, Chappuis V, et al. A long-term prospective cohort study on immediately restored single tooth implants inserted in extraction sockets and healed ridges: CBCT analyses, soft tissue alterations, aesthetic ratings, and patient-reported outcomes. Clin Implant Dent Relat Res 2018;20(4):522–30.
18. Cortese A, Pantaleo G, Amato M, et al. Ridge expansion by flapless split crest and immediate implant placement: evolution of the technique. J Craniofac Surg 2016;27:2e123–8.
19. Chappuis V, Cavusoglu Y, Buser D, et al. Lateral ridge augmentation using autogenous block grafts and guided bone regeneration: a 10-year prospective case series study. Clin Implant Dent Relat Res 2017;19:185–96.
20. Chiapasco M, Abati S, Romeo E, et al. Clinical outcome of autogenous bone blocks or guided bone regeneration with e-PTFE membranes for the reconstruction of narrow edentulous ridges. Clin Oral Implants Res 1999;10:4278–88.
21. Ewers R, Tomasetti B, Ghali G, et al. A new biologic classification of bone augmentation. In: Jensen OT, editor. The osteoperiosteal flap: a simplified approach to alveolar bone reconstruction. Chicago: Quintessence Publishing; 2010. p. 19–42.
22. Bell WH. Revascularization and bone healing after anterior maxillary osteotomy: a study using adult rhesus monkeys. J Oral Surg 1969;27:4249–55.
23. Bell WH, Levy BM. Revascularization and bone healing after anterior mandibular osteotomy. J Oral Surg 1970;28:3196–203.
24. De Marco AC, Jardini MA, Lima LP. Revascularization of autogenous block grafts with or without an e-PTFE membrane. Int J Oral Maxillofac Implants 2005;20:6867–74.

Bone Augmentation Techniques for Horizontal and Vertical Alveolar Ridge Deficiency in Oral Implantology

Len Tolstunov, DDS, DMD[a,b,c,*],
John F. Eric Hamrick, DMD[d,e],
Vishtasb Broumand, DMD, MD[f,g], Dekel Shilo, DMD, PhD[h,i,j],
Adi Rachmiel, DMD, PhD[h,i,j]

KEYWORDS

- Guided bone regeneration • Alveolar ridge split • Block grafting • Osteoperiosteal flap
- Distraction osteogenesis • Bone augmentation • Ridge expansion

KEY POINTS

- This article helps the understanding of the basic principles of different jawbone augmentation techniques.
- This article identifies which type of alveolar bone defects require what type of augmentation.
- This article describes staging, instrumentation, and materials necessary for each grafting technique.
- This article helps in the understanding of the risks, benefits, alternatives, and complications of each technique.

INTRODUCTION

A variety of traumatic events cause alveolar bone loss. These traumatic events include tooth loss, sinus pneumatization, periodontal disease, facial and dentoalveolar trauma, odontogenic and nonodontogenic cysts and tumors, oral pathologic lesions, and many other conditions. Alveolar bone grafting can be divided into ridge preservation (RP) and ridge augmentation (RA). These 2 methods are designed to prevent or correct bone deficiency: to maintain or re-create the necessary bone stock for dental implant placement.

Ridge Preservation

RP is accomplished with socket grafting procedures that intend to preserve the existing ridge volume *within* its bony envelope; they are usually performed at the time of tooth extraction with an

Disclosure: The authors have nothing to disclose.
[a] Oral and Maxillofacial Surgery Private Practice, San Francisco, CA, USA; [b] Oral and Maxillofacial Surgery, University of the Pacific, School of Dentistry, San Francisco, CA, USA; [c] Oral and Maxillofacial Surgery, University of California San Francisco, School of Dentistry, San Francisco, CA, USA; [d] Private Periodontal Practice, Greenville, SC, USA; [e] Department of Periodontics, Medical University of Southern Carolina, School of Dentistry, Greenville, SC, USA; [f] Oral and Maxillofacial Surgery Private Practice, Phoenix, AZ, USA; [g] Department of Oral and Maxillofacial Surgery, University of Florida College of Dentistry, Gainesville, FL, USA; [h] Department of Oral and Maxillofacial Surgery, Rambam Medical Care Center, Haifa, Israel; [i] Ruth and Bruce Rappaport Faculty of Medicine, Technion-Israel Institute of Technology, Haifa, Israel; [j] Rambam Health Care Campus, 8 Ha'Aliyah Street, PO Box 9602, Haifa 3109601, Israel
* Corresponding author. 1 Daniel Burnham Court, Suite 366C, San Francisco, CA 94109, USA.
E-mail address: tolstunov@yahoo.com

Oral Maxillofacial Surg Clin N Am 31 (2019) 163–191
https://doi.org/10.1016/j.coms.2019.01.005
1042-3699/19/© 2019 Elsevier Inc. All rights reserved.

"inlay" particulate graft with the goal to minimize tissue loss after tooth loss. Although complete prevention of bone collapse with the RP techniques is challenging, the objective is to minimize volumetric loss as much as possible.[1–3]

Ridge Augmentation

RA is accomplished using both hard and soft tissue grafting procedures that intend to augment the alveolar ridge volume *beyond* the existing skeletal envelope; they are usually performed at the edentulous site of a deficient alveolar ridge. This surgical approach can involve either onlay or inlay grafting and may include the alveolar distraction method.

In this article, the authors discuss bone *augmentation* techniques and classify them into horizontal bone augmentation (HBA) and vertical bone augmentation (VBA).

Although there are a large variety of alveolar RA techniques with various degrees of success,[4] in this article, the authors concentrate on the HBA and VBA using guided bone regeneration (GBR), autogenous block grafting, alveolar ridge split expansion, and alveolar distraction osteogenesis (ADO).

ALVEOLAR RIDGE-SPLIT EXPANSION TECHNIQUE

The alveolar ridge-split expansion procedure (RSEP) is intended for horizontal alveolar ridge deficiency by means of splitting the existing narrow ridge and expanding it to accommodate placement of dental implants. The procedure is based on the use of interpositional grafting using particulate graft material that is placed in an inlay fashion into the surgically widened ridge. Names that are associated with this procedure are *expansion*, *widening*, *spreading*, and *osteoperiosteal flap*. They imply the specifics of the technique, an end result of the ridge splitting, or the type of flap that is used for this procedure.[5]

RSEP is not a new procedure. Dr W. Bell studied and documented the rationale for segmental jaw osteotomies in the late 1960s based on their vitality through vascularized osteoperiosteal flaps.[6–8] Drs Simion, Pikos, and Scipioni in the 1990s described the specifics of the "split-crest technique and guided tissue regeneration."[9–11] Other practitioners and researchers advanced the knowledge of the 1- and 2-stage, partial- and full-thickness flap approaches of the edentulous ridge expansion, their successes, and failures.[12–16]

The indication for the procedure, as mentioned above, is horizontal bone loss usually from resorption. *Resorption* implies diminished bone volume

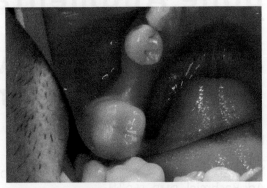

Fig. 1. Collapse of the buccal cortical plate and resulting horizontal (width) deficiency of the alveolar ridge. (*From* Tolstunov L. Diagnosis and treatment planning. In: Tolstunov L, editor. Horizontal alveolar ridge augmentation in implant dentistry: a surgical manual. Hoboken, NJ: John Wiley & Sons; 2016. p. 173–84; with permission.)

effecting both cortical and trabecular bone manifesting as a net reduction of the trabecular compartment due to loss of the dental root and its related function. This buccal cortical plate collapse leads to a decreased buccal prominence or width of the alveolar ridge (**Fig. 1**). The alveolar split repositions the collapsed cortical plate facially, creating intra-alveolar space for a particulate graft. An actual split occurs through the trabecular space. A 3- to 5-mm ridge is the most common indication for the procedure. Although practitioners may attempt to apply this technique for a 2- to 3-mm width, this is folly. Immediate implant is commonly used, although delayed implant placement is safer and more predictable. Cone beam computed tomography (CBCT) images give a surgeon an in-depth analysis of the 3-dimensional anatomy of the alveolar ridge before surgery (**Fig. 2**).

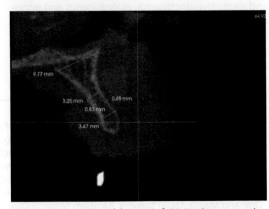

Fig. 2. Cross-sectional image of CBCT demonstrating alveolar width deficiency. (*From* Tolstunov L. Diagnosis and treatment planning. In: Tolstunov L, editor. Horizontal alveolar ridge augmentation in implant dentistry: a surgical manual. Hoboken, NJ: John Wiley & Sons; 2016. p. 173–84; with permission.)

"Book" Flap
(greenstick-fracture)

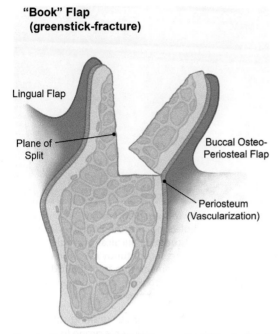

Lingual Flap

Plane of
Split

Buccal Osteo-
Periosteal Flap

Periosteum
(Vascularization)

"Island" Flap
(fracture-displacement)

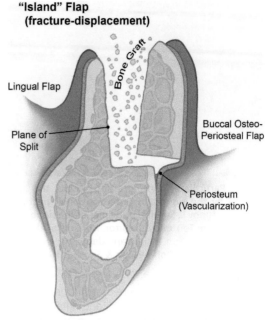

Lingual Flap

Plane of
Split

Buccal Osteo-
Periosteal Flap

Periosteum
(Vascularization)

Fig. 3. The ridge-split technique called "Book flap." (*From* Tolstunov L. Surgical principles of the ridge-split procedure. In: Tolstunov L, editor. Horizontal alveolar ridge augmentation in implant dentistry: a surgical manual. Hoboken: John Wiley & Sons; 2016. p. 185–91; with permission.)

Fig. 5. The ridge-split technique called "Island flap." (*From* Tolstunov L. Surgical principles of the ridge-split procedure. In: Tolstunov L, editor. Horizontal alveolar ridge augmentation in implant dentistry: a surgical manual. Hoboken: John Wiley & Sons; 2016. p. 185–91; with permission.)

Description of the Technique

The flap that is being repositioned facially usually includes buccal cortical plate with some trabecular bone. Therefore, a combined hard-soft tissue flap that provides vascularization for the fractured osteotomized segment is termed an osteoperiosteal flap.[5]

There are 2 main ways to reposition a buccal osteoperiosteal flap. The most common is the greenstick outfracture from basal bone with the buccal segment movement similar to a hinge or a book opening on its binder, therefore, the designation of the term the outfractured alveolar split or a "book flap" (**Figs. 3** and **4**). The second method of alveolar splitting is used to reposition the buccal plate even more facially requiring separation of bony connection to allow for a bigger horizontal advancement termed an island osteoperiosteal flap or I-flap for short (**Figs. 5** and **6**).[17–19] In either case, a particulate

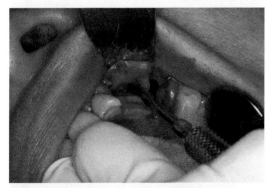

Fig. 4. Clinical intraoperative photograph of the ridge-split technique called "Book flap." (*From* Tolstunov L. Surgical principles of the ridge-split procedure. In: Tolstunov L, editor. Horizontal alveolar ridge augmentation in implant dentistry: a surgical manual. Hoboken: John Wiley & Sons; 2016. p. 185–91; with permission.)

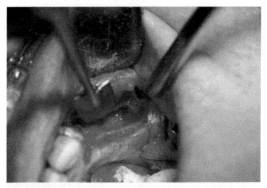

Fig. 6. Clinical intraoperative photograph of the ridge-split technique called "Island flap." (*From* Tolstunov L. Surgical principles of the ridge-split procedure. In: Tolstunov L, editor. Horizontal alveolar ridge augmentation in implant dentistry: a surgical manual. Hoboken: John Wiley & Sons; 2016. p. 185–91; with permission.)

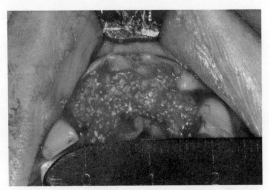

Fig. 7. Particulate bone grafting inside the gap created by the ridge-split (interpositional grafting). (*From* Tolstunov L. Surgical principles of the ridge-split procedure. In: Tolstunov L, editor. Horizontal alveolar ridge augmentation in implant dentistry: a surgical manual. Hoboken: John Wiley & Sons; 2016. p. 185–91; with permission.)

graft of choice is then positioned into the created gap between repositioned buccal and intact lingual (palatal) cortical bone fragments as an interpositional graft. This technique is analogous to the *RP procedure following tooth extraction*. In both cases, it is an *inlay* graft placed either inside a 3- or 4-wall socket or 2-wall bony gap created by the split ridge procedure (see **Fig. 6**; **Figs. 7** and **8**). Therefore, physiologically, bone healing of the interpositional particulate graft is similar and in both cases occurs though the endosteal and periosteal sources of vascularization. In most cases, primary wound closure is not necessary, and healing by secondary intention preserves attached gingiva and the depth of vestibule (see **Fig. 8**; **Figs. 9** and **10**).

Maxilla and mandible are different in a sense of rigidity or density of bone. Bone density may not be important for a block bone graft that is fixated on top of the ridge (onlay or external grafting) but

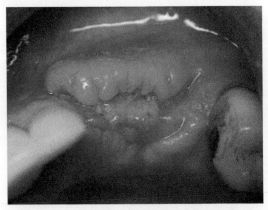

Fig. 9. Healing by secondary intention: 2-month postoperative vestibule and attached gingiva are preserved. (*From* Tolstunov L. Surgical principles of the ridge-split procedure. In: Tolstunov L, editor. Horizontal alveolar ridge augmentation in implant dentistry: a surgical manual. Hoboken: John Wiley & Sons; 2016. p. 185–91; with permission.)

is essential for the internal grafting of RSEP. Mandibular bone being denser is prone to fractures rather than maxillary bone that is more malleable and tends to improve with bone compression. That is why maxillary RSEP is often done in a single stage (osteotomies-split-expansion-grafting) and mandibular RSEP frequently requires a 2-stage approach (stage 1: osteotomies followed by the stage 2: split-expansion-grafting). It is often said that *osteo-condensation* occurs with maxillary RSEP (similar to a crestal sinus lift) and *osteo-mobilization* occurs with mandibular RSEP. Implants can be placed at the same time but more predictably are positioned at a separate stage 4 to 6 months later after healing of the augmented bone.

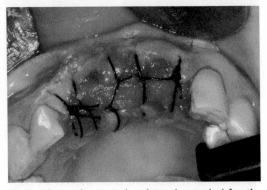

Fig. 8. Closure by secondary intention typical for the ridge-split and similar to the RP procedure after tooth extraction. (*From* Tolstunov L. Surgical principles of the ridge-split procedure. In: Tolstunov L, editor. Horizontal alveolar ridge augmentation in implant dentistry: a surgical manual. Hoboken: John Wiley & Sons; 2016. p. 185–91; with permission.)

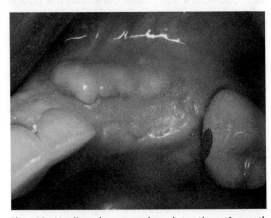

Fig. 10. Healing by secondary intention: 4-month postoperative preservation of the soft tissue envelope. (*From* Tolstunov L. Surgical principles of the ridge-split procedure. In: Tolstunov L, editor. Horizontal alveolar ridge augmentation in implant dentistry: a surgical manual. Hoboken: John Wiley & Sons; 2016. p. 185–91; with permission.)

RSEP requires special instrumentation (as any surgical technique) that usually consists of sharp chisel osteotomes and/or spreaders of progressive size, mallet, microsaw, or thin burs (**Fig. 11**). Piezoelectric instrumentation is another way to place small osteotomy cuts. These bone cuts are also often called corticotomies because they are placed through the cortical bone only. Maxillary bone being more pliable conventionally does not require many bony cuts. In later discussion, the authors present 2 cases of mandibular 2-stage and maxillary single-stage RSEP.

Mandibular Ridge-Split Expansion Procedure

Mandibular RSEP is often done in 2 stages due to denser bone. The first stage (stage 1) consists of creating "window" corticotomies in the indicated area (similar to a bony window of a lateral sinus lift procedure). The second stage (stage 2) is done 4 weeks later and consists of the actual split along the lines of the corticotomies, followed by expansion and then grafting with particulate graft material inserted into the gap, and followed

by a closure after guided tissue regeneration (GTR) membrane placement with the intention of secondary healing. The lingual mucosa in the mandible can alternatively be advanced to close over the split-gap using primary wound closure. Stage 2 is performed only after about 4 weeks to allow for the previously reflected mucoperiosteal soft tissue flap to readhere and heal back to the bone to provide an important source of peripheral (periosteal) vascularization for the osteoperiosteal flap created at stage 2. Although implants can be placed at the same time, primary stability may be difficult to achieve, so it is often done at a separate stage 4 months later into a fully healed ridge.

Case Report

A 60-year-old healthy woman presented with a narrow mandibular alveolar ridge in the second premolar–first molar region (**Fig. 12**). The RSEP included removal of the retained first premolar and staged approach for the expansion of the ridge in the region.

At stage 1, after extraction of the bicuspid, the full-thickness flap was reflected and 4 window corticotomies were placed from the canine to the second molar in the area where the future implants would be positioned (see **Fig. 12**; **Fig. 13**). These typical ridge-split corticotomies consisted of crestal, apical, and 2 slightly divergent vertical ones (**Figs. 14** and **15**). In some cases of softer mandibular bone (type 2–3), 3 corticotomies can be done, skipping the apical one. The flap was then repositioned, and the wound was closed with resorbable sutures (4-0 chromic gut).

Stage 2 was done 4 weeks later to allow soft tissue adhesion to the buccal bony cortex. It is

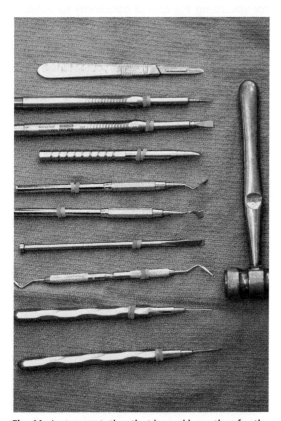

Fig. 11. Instrumentation that is used by author for the RSEP. (*From* Tolstunov L. Mandibular two-stage alveolar ridge-split procedure. In: Tolstunov L, editor. Horizontal alveolar ridge augmentation in implant dentistry: a surgical manual. Hoboken: John Wiley & Sons; 2016. p. 192–9; with permission.)

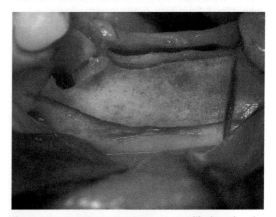

Fig. 12. Case report 1: narrow mandibular alveolar ridge in the second premolar–first molar region. (*From* Tolstunov L. Mandibular two-stage alveolar ridge-split procedure. In: Tolstunov L, editor. Horizontal alveolar ridge augmentation in implant dentistry: a surgical manual. Hoboken: John Wiley & Sons; 2016. p. 192–9; with permission.)

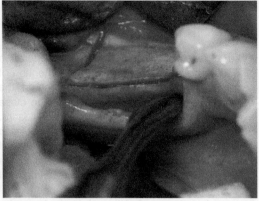

Fig. 13. Stage 1: 4 window corticotomies placed from the canine to the second molar in the area where the future implants will be placed. (*From* Tolstunov L. Mandibular two-stage alveolar ridge-split procedure. In: Tolstunov L, editor. Horizontal alveolar ridge augmentation in implant dentistry: a surgical manual. Hoboken: John Wiley & Sons; 2016. p. 192–9; with permission.)

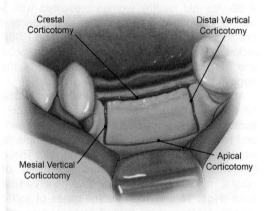

Fig. 14. Schematic representation of the typical *mandibular* 4-window corticotomies done during the stage 1 RSEP (crestal, apical, and 2 vertical). (*From* Tolstunov L. Mandibular two-stage alveolar ridge-split procedure. In: Tolstunov L, editor. Horizontal alveolar ridge augmentation in implant dentistry: a surgical manual. Hoboken: John Wiley & Sons; 2016. p. 192–9; with permission.)

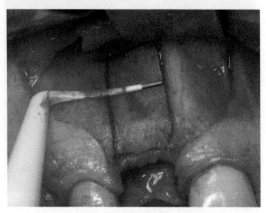

Fig. 15. Clinical intraoperative photograph of the typical mandibular 4-window corticotomies done during the stage 1 RSEP (crestal, apical, and 2 vertical). (*From* Tolstunov L. Mandibular two-stage alveolar ridge-split procedure. In: Tolstunov L, editor. Horizontal alveolar ridge augmentation in implant dentistry: a surgical manual. Hoboken: John Wiley & Sons; 2016. p. 192–9; with permission.)

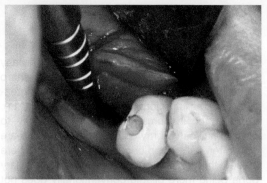

Fig. 16. Clinical intraoperative photograph of the stage 1 RSEP when consecutive enlarging chisel osteotomes are used in a progressive manner by tapping into the depth of the crestal groove to initiate and then widen the split. (*From* Tolstunov L. Mandibular two-stage alveolar ridge-split procedure. In: Tolstunov L, editor. Horizontal alveolar ridge augmentation in implant dentistry: a surgical manual. Hoboken: John Wiley & Sons; 2016. p. 192–9; with permission.)

important to be extremely careful with the healed buccal flap and reflect it sparingly, just on the top of the ridge, leaving the crest of the ridge barely visible but the buccal surface of the bone covered with the attached soft tissue to preserve vascularization. This limited flap reflection allows for visualizing the crestal osteotomy for initiation of the definitive alveolar split. The bone is already "weakened" at the previous stage; now it is time to fracture it along the window osteotomies. Consecutive enlarging chisel osteotomes were used in a progressive manner by tapping into the depth of the crestal groove to initiate and then widen the split (**Fig. 16**). The buccal plate was mobilized and repositioned laterally (**Fig. 17**). Inlay Puros corticocancellous allograft was used (Puros; Zimmer Dental Inc, Carlsbad, CA, USA), and Teflon nonresorbable GTR membrane (Kendall Curity, Tyco Healthcare, Mansfield, MA, USA)

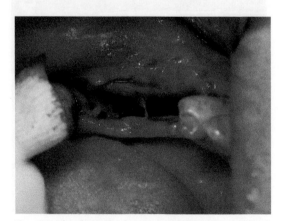

Fig. 17. The buccal plate is mobilized and repositioned laterally creating the bone gap for the particulate graft. (*From* Tolstunov L. Mandibular two-stage alveolar ridge-split procedure. In: Tolstunov L, editor. Horizontal alveolar ridge augmentation in implant dentistry: a surgical manual. Hoboken: John Wiley & Sons; 2016. p. 192–9; with permission.)

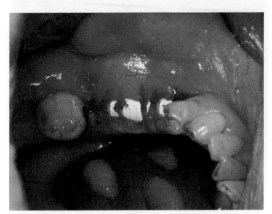

Fig. 18. Inlay Puros corticocancellous allograft and Teflon nonresorbable GTR membrane are used during the stage 2 of RSEP. Healing by secondary intention (chromic gut sutures). (*From* Tolstunov L. Mandibular two-stage alveolar ridge-split procedure. In: Tolstunov L, editor. Horizontal alveolar ridge augmentation in implant dentistry: a surgical manual. Hoboken: John Wiley & Sons; 2016. p. 192–9; with permission.)

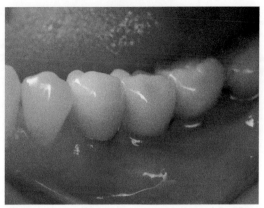

Fig. 20. Restorative stage: 3 separate PFM implant-supported crowns placed 6 months after the implant surgery. (*From* Tolstunov L. Mandibular two-stage alveolar ridge-split procedure. In: Tolstunov L, editor. Horizontal alveolar ridge augmentation in implant dentistry: a surgical manual. Hoboken: John Wiley & Sons; 2016. p. 192–9; with permission.)

was used to cover and protect the graft (**Fig. 18**). Healing by secondary intention was done with chromic gut sutures securing the repositioned buccal flap. Three implants were placed 6 months later (Replace Select implants; Nobel BioCare, Yorba Linda, CA, USA) (**Fig. 19**). After osseointegration, they were restored 6 months later with 3 separate porcelain fused to metal (PFM) implant-supported crowns to a fully functional occlusion (**Figs. 20** and **21**).

Maxillary Ridge-Split Expansion Procedure

Maxillary RSEP can be viewed as a simplified mandibular procedure due to a softer and more pliable bony envelope of type 3 to 4 bone. Although a staged approach is occasionally done

in denser bone, a single-stage approach is often used. Soft bone of a maxillary alveolar ridge allows split, expansion, graft, and, sometimes, implant placement at the same time. Only crestal and small initial vertical corticotomies are often needed to help to propagate the split of the buccal portion of bone away from the palatal cortex (**Fig. 22**). Progressive chisel osteotomes, similar to the stage 2 of the mandibular RSEP, then lead to luxation and greenstick outfracture of the buccal cortical plate to form a gap or a "socket" that is filled with a particulate bone material and covered with a resorbable GTR membrane. Piezoelectric instrumentation can also be used for a thinner bone cut. Secondary healing of the wound is preferred.

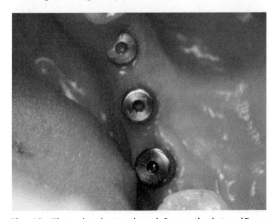

Fig. 19. Three implants placed 6 months later. (*From* Tolstunov L. Mandibular two-stage alveolar ridge-split procedure. In: Tolstunov L, editor. Horizontal alveolar ridge augmentation in implant dentistry: a surgical manual. Hoboken: John Wiley & Sons; 2016. p. 192–9; with permission.)

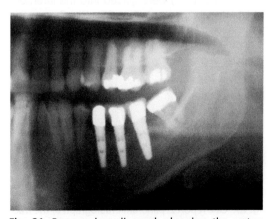

Fig. 21. Panoramic radiograph showing the restorative stage with 3 PFM implant-supported crowns. (*From* Tolstunov L. Mandibular two-stage alveolar ridge-split procedure. In: Tolstunov L, editor. Horizontal alveolar ridge augmentation in implant dentistry: a surgical manual. Hoboken: John Wiley & Sons; 2016. p. 192–9; with permission.)

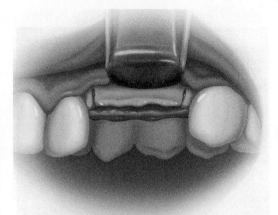

Fig. 22. Schematic representation of the typical maxillary corticotomies done during the stage 1 RSEP (crestal and 2 mini vertical). (*From* Tolstunov L. Maxillary single-stage alveolar ridge-split procedure. In: Tolstunov L, editor. Horizontal alveolar ridge augmentation in implant dentistry: a surgical manual. Hoboken: John Wiley & Sons; 2016. p. 200–6; with permission.)

Case Report

An 82-year-old healthy woman presented with severe alveolar ridge width deficiency and fractured cuspid in the upper right posterior quadrant (**Fig. 23**). After clinical and radiographic evaluation, the treatment plan was proposed and consisted of atraumatic extraction of the fractured canine and RSEP with possible immediate implant placement. After extraction of the canine, the thin ridge was visualized and approached with thin chisel osteotomes (**Fig. 24**). After careful buccal plate fracture and repositioning, 2 implant osteotomies were done, and both implants were inserted engaging the apical basal bone (good primary stability, 20-Ncm torque). Two Zimmer Biomet 3i 4-mm internal hex "Certain" implants (Biomet 3i, Palm Beach Gardens, FL, USA) were placed into the intercortical bony environment (**Fig. 25**). Bio-Oss xenograft (Geistlich Pharma, North America Inc, Princeton, NJ, USA) was used to fill the gap;

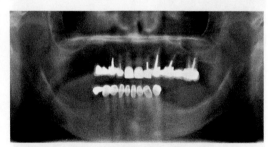

Fig. 23. Case report 2: panoramic radiograph of the fractured cuspid and severe alveolar ridge width deficiency in the upper right posterior quadrant. (*From* Tolstunov L. Maxillary single-stage alveolar ridge-split procedure. In: Tolstunov L, editor. Horizontal alveolar ridge augmentation in implant dentistry: a surgical manual. Hoboken: John Wiley & Sons; 2016. p. 200–6; with permission.)

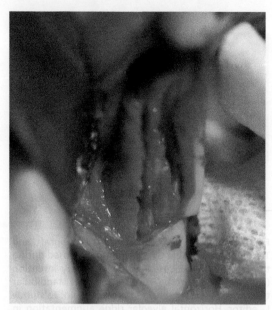

Fig. 24. Intraoperative photograph of the 3-mm-width alveolar ridge and the crestal corticotomy. (*From* Tolstunov L. Maxillary single-stage alveolar ridge-split procedure. In: Tolstunov L, editor. Horizontal alveolar ridge augmentation in implant dentistry: a surgical manual. Hoboken: John Wiley & Sons; 2016. p. 200–6; with permission.)

primary closure was achieved (**Fig. 26**). The restorative stage was completed after a year of healing and consisted of a splinted PFM implant-supported bridge placed into a stable group function occlusion (**Figs. 27** and **28**).

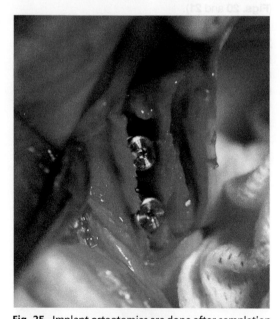

Fig. 25. Implant osteotomies are done after completion of the RSEP and 2 implants inserted. (*From* Tolstunov L. Maxillary single-stage alveolar ridge-split procedure. In: Tolstunov L, editor. Horizontal alveolar ridge augmentation in implant dentistry: a surgical manual. Hoboken: John Wiley & Sons; 2016. p. 200–6; with permission.)

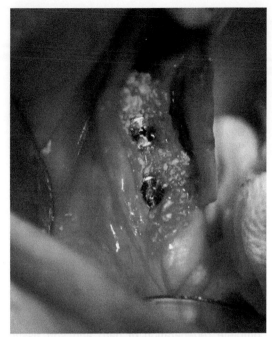

Fig. 26. Interpositional particulate bone graft is placed to fill the gaps between buccal and palatal cortical plates and implants. (*From* Tolstunov L. Maxillary single-stage alveolar ridge-split procedure. In: Tolstunov L, editor. Horizontal alveolar ridge augmentation in implant dentistry: a surgical manual. Hoboken: John Wiley & Sons; 2016. p. 200–6; with permission.)

Complications

Complications of RSEP are usually technically driven. They can be related to improper oblique splitting of the ridge causing only the part (not the whole) of the buccal crest to be fractured off, compromising an implant placement in a single-stage maxillary RSEP. In mandibular RSEP, the osteotomized ridge ("buccal window") can be

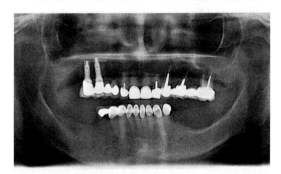

Fig. 27. Panoramic radiograph of the restorative stage completed after a year of healing and consisting of splinted 2-implant supported PFM bridge. (*From* Tolstunov L. Maxillary single-stage alveolar ridge-split procedure. In: Tolstunov L, editor. Horizontal alveolar ridge augmentation in implant dentistry: a surgical manual. Hoboken: John Wiley & Sons; 2016. p. 200–6; with permission.)

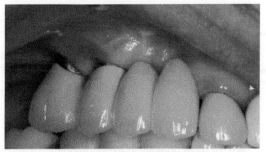

Fig. 28. The completion of the restorative stage: splinted 2-implant supported PFM bridge. (*From* Tolstunov L. Maxillary single-stage alveolar ridge-split procedure. In: Tolstunov L, editor. Horizontal alveolar ridge augmentation in implant dentistry: a surgical manual. Hoboken: John Wiley & Sons; 2016. p. 200–6; with permission.)

inadvertently completely separated from the basal bone. If this happens, it becomes a "free graft" that is totally devascularized. It needs to be fixated back to the donor site with screws, and it should be allowed to heal for 4 months before approaching the ridge again. RSEP in the lower premolar region has to be done carefully, paying attention to the mental nerve. Five millimeters of space between the apical osteotomy and the top portion of the mental foramen should be intact to prevent injury to the mental nerve.

It is important to keep at least 2 (or better, 3) millimeters of bone on the facial side of an implant placed either at the time of RSEP or later. Additional bone grafting might be needed to satisfy this condition. Immediate implant insertion *without* primary stability can lead to an implant failure. Unstable implants need to be removed, and the ridge needs to heal before a new bone grafting/implant procedure. Infection of the grafted site is rare but can happen and needs to be treated with graft debridement and antibiotics. Other complications are infrequent.

Summary

RSEP is primarily designed for HBA with the goal to increase the alveolar width through interpositional grafting by splitting the ridge and repositioning the facial cortical plate. This technique is done in a similar fashion to postextraction RP with internal grafting using particulate graft. It appears to be a physiologic surgical technique to reposition the collapsed cortical plate back to its preextraction position and place a dental implant intercortically within the trabecular space. In mandibular osteotomies, implants are usually placed in a delayed fashion. Maxillary implants can be placed immediately, if apical bone is present and good primary stability can be achieved.

RSEP is a technique-sensitive procedure (training and skills are important) that tends to have a higher success rate in ridges with 4 to

5 mm of alveolar width present, especially in anterior maxilla and posterior mandible.

To improve the outcome and avoid complications, the authors suggest following the following surgical principles:

1. Adequate surgical training
2. Careful patient selection, avoiding patients who smoke, have poor oral hygiene, are noncompliant, or have unrealistic expectations
3. Ideally use 2 to 3 edentulous tooth spaces for RSEP
4. Select a slow resorbable particulate bone-grafting material and mix it with autogenous bone and, possibly, biomimetics, like platelet-rich fibrin (PRF)
5. Overcorrect by widening the ridge up to 10 mm or more in anticipation of bone remodeling
6. Use a staged approach with delayed rather than immediate implant insertion
7. Select tapered and smaller-diameter (but longer) implants with good primary implant stability (torque = 30+ NCm)
8. Pay attention to the preservation of attached buccal gingival tissue throughout the case. Soft tissue grafting is optional in cases of deficiency of keratinized gingiva on the facial aspect of the ridge

GUIDED BONE REGENERATION WITH PARTICULATE BONE GRAFT
Introduction

When deciding about the type of bone grafting technique that should be used for any given patient needing implant therapy, at least 3 key factors must be considered, as follows:

1. The health of the patient, both oral and systemic
2. The size and morphology of the bone defect
3. The final prosthetic treatment plan for the patient

Before beginning any elective bone graft procedure for a patient, any oral disease or infection must be treated (ie, periodontal or endodontic) and stabilized. Patients who are systemically healthy and without serious medical limitations are candidates for more extensive bone grafting procedures.

In the case of GBR, medically fragile patients are often better treated with bioabsorbable barriers and particulate allograft[20,21] because this approach requires less surgical time with less potential postsurgical morbidity.

Defect morphology plays a significant role in decision making with GBR. Horizontal defects with natural space-maintaining shape are predictably treated with absorbable barriers and particulate bone allograft.[22,23] Vertical alveolar ridge defects with a lack of natural space-maintenance shape are better treated with nonresorbable barriers (titanium [Ti] mesh or membrane with Ti reinforcement), and a 50:50 mixture of autogenous bone chips and xenograft.[4,24] In some cases, where the vertical component is less than 5 mm, allograft can be used in the graft mixture.

The final prosthetic treatment plan must be known before choosing the appropriate GBR technique. This knowledge is particularly important in the esthetic zone where vertical and horizontal defects are encountered, prosthetic treatment planing is critical. If a fixed hybrid prosthesis is planned, reduction of bone height may be necessary, and augmentation of width may be all that is needed. If the treatment plan calls for a traditional fixed ceramic restoration, complete regeneration of hard and soft tissue will be necessary for a successful esthetic outcome.

Fig. 29 describes a basic algorithmic approach with GBR.

Basic Principles of Guided Bone Regeneration

Successful GBR follows the so-called PASS principles, as follows[25] (**Fig. 30**):

1. *Primary wound closure*
2. *Angiogenesis*
3. *Space maintenance*
4. *Stability of the wound*

Description of Technique

Incision and flap designs vary slightly, depending on the location of the defect in the oral cavity. A description of a technique for managing a defect in the posterior mandible is described in later discussion.

Technique

A midcrestal incision is made across the length of the defect, and vertical releasing incisions on the buccal are made 1 to 2 teeth away from the site being treated. In the case of a posterior edentulous site, a hockey-stick incision toward the buccal, just anterior to the retromolar pad, is extended 4 mm past the mucogingival junction. If a vertical alveolar defect is present, a small lingual vertical incision is made 1 tooth forward of the defect (usually the premolar area) being treated, slightly beyond the mucogingival junction.

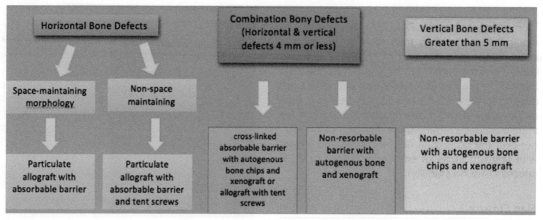

Fig. 29. GBR flow chart for the treatment of horizontal and vertical bone defects.

Flap Elevation and Site Preparation

Full-thickness mucoperiosteal flap elevation is completed at least 5 mm beyond the defect being treated. Careful removal of any residual soft tissue is completed, and decortication with a small round bur through the cortical bone into the bone marrow is accomplished to initiate angiogenesis.[26]

Harvesting of Bone

When treating larger alveolar defects with a significant vertical component, use of autogenous bone chips is vital.[27] The mandibular ramus buccal shelf is the primary donor site. Bone scrapers or trephines are used to accomplish this step. Where bone cores are harvested, they are particulated with a bone mill.

Flap Release

Buccal flap release is accomplished by making an incision with a new 15 or 15c blade, just through the periosteum, near the base of the flap. This incision connects the mesial and distal vertical incisions. This incision is modified to avoid damage to the mental nerve by going in a more coronal direction above the nerve. A more superficial incision is recommended, using blunt instrumentation to begin separating the elastic fibers in the flap. Flap elevation on the lingual is limited by the location of the mylohyoid muscle. More anteriorly, the back of a 15 blade may be used to separate the periosteum, and with blunt instrumentation, the elastic fibers are further separated. Posteriorly, blunt instrumentation only is recommended to avoid potential lingual nerve trauma. Blunt scissors can be advanced into the elastic fibers and opened to further release the buccal flap. The above will allow tension-free closure over the graft.

Barrier Fixation

The authors' preference when using a nonresorbable barrier is dense Ti-polytetrafluoroethylene

PASS Figure 2

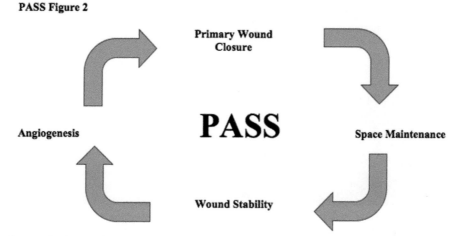

Fig. 30. Diagram for basic principles in GBR.

(PTFE) (Cytoplast Ti-250 PL; Osteogenics Biomedical, Lubbock, TX, USA). It is easier to manipulate and shape than titanium mesh, and when removed at the end of healing, separates easily from the underlying regenerated bone. The titanium in the barrier usually provides adequate support to eliminate the need for tent screws. Barrier mobility during healing will have a negative impact on bone regeneration. Fixation of the barrier over the bone graft on the buccal and lingual with titanium tacks or screws is critical to GBR success (wound stability).

Flap Closure

Flap closure is completed by closure in the 2 layers. The first layer (connective tissue) is closed with horizontal mattress sutures placed several millimeters away from the incision line. Interrupted sutures are used to close the incision line above the mattress sutures. This technique allows for flap eversion and intimate contact of the connective tissue below the incision line. PTFE sutures are used for flap closure.

Case Report 1

This case involves the treatment of a maxillary right first molar site that had bone loss from a periodontitis-endodontic infection (**Fig. 31**). Extraction of the maxillary right third molar and the maxillary right first molar was completed, with socket grafting done in the maxillary right first

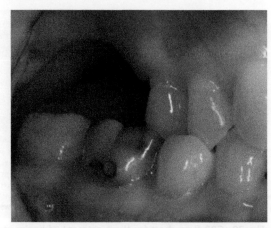

Fig. 32. Advanced vertical ridge defect after removal of the hopeless maxillary right first molar and third molar.

molar site. **Fig. 32** shows the resulting alveolar ridge defect after 12 weeks of healing.

Fig. 33 illustrates the use of a lateral window sinus bone graft, combined with the placement of a vertical tenting screw for graft support. A 50:50 mixture of autogenous bone and bovine xenograft, Bio-Oss (Geistlich Pharma North America, Inc), was placed into the defect and a well-adapted porcine collagen membrane was placed over the bone graft (Ossix Plus membrane; OraPharma, Bridgewater, NJ, USA). Primary wound closure was completed with 5.0 PTFE sutures (**Figs. 34–36**). **Figs. 37** and **38** demonstrate the healed vertical augmentation at 6 months, and 2 implants were placed. Final restorations were placed approximately 5 months after implant placement

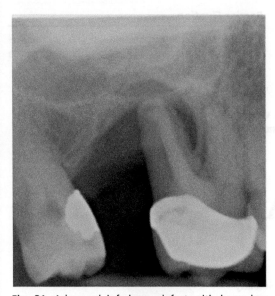

Fig. 31. Advanced infrabony defect with bone loss beyond the apex of the distal root of maxillary right first molar.

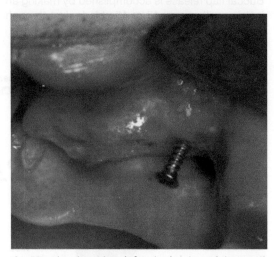

Fig. 33. Alveolar ridge defect in the sites of the maxillary right first and second molars; note the tenting screw used to support the GBR procedure.

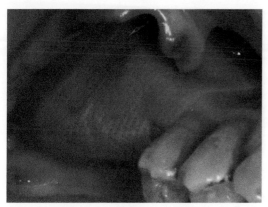

Fig. 34. Ossix Plus membrane positioned over the bone graft before the wound closure.

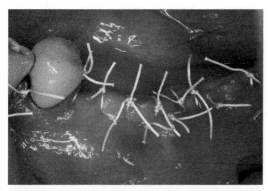

Fig. 35. Primary closure of the GBR site with PTFE sutures.

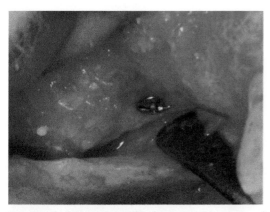

Fig. 36. Healed bone graft after several months of healing; note the vertical bone regeneration with the use of an absorbable barrier membrane.

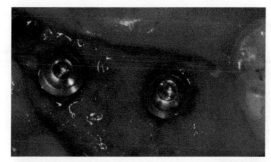

Fig. 37. Implant fixtures placed in the maxillary right first and second molar sites.

(**Fig. 39**). Final radiograph of restored implants is shown in **Fig. 40**.

Case Report 2

A significant vertical osseous defect in the mandibular left second molar site with the adjacent endodontically failing mandibular right first molar was noted (**Figs. 41** and **42**). A titanium-reinforced PTFE membrane was fixed lingually with bone tacks, and the bone graft was placed (**Figs. 43** and **44**). The membrane was secured buccally with bone screws. An additional porcine collagen membrane was placed over the graft site, and primary closure was completed (**Figs. 45–47**). The site was reentered at 7 months; the membrane removed, and 2 fixtures were installed (**Figs. 48** and **49**).

Complications

Early membrane exposure as a result of incision-line opening will result in less bone regeneration.[9] Even in the absence of incision-line opening, post-surgical infection of the surgical site will result in GBR failure. Absorbable membranes undergo rapid enzymatic degradation and less bone regeneration when prematurely exposed, but generally do not lend to postsurgical infection. When using d-PTFE (Cytoplast), early exposure of the

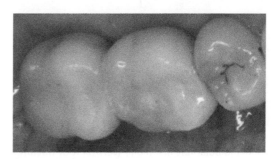

Fig. 38. Final restorations.

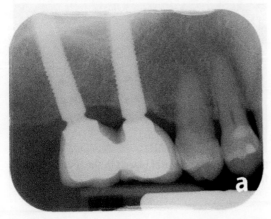

Fig. 39. Three-year follow-up radiograph of the implants.

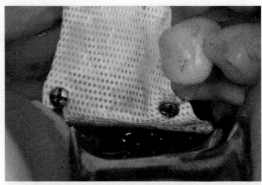

Fig. 42. Titanium-reinforced Cytoplast membrane initially fixated on the lingual side before the graft placement with fixation screws.

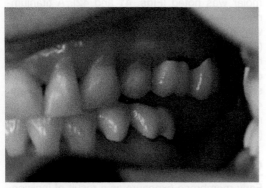

Fig. 40. Mandibular left first and second molar area; note the advanced vertical bone defect in the mandibular left second molar site.

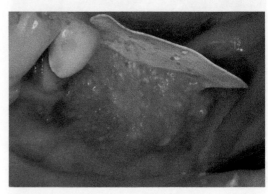

Fig. 43. Composite bone graft placement under the membrane.

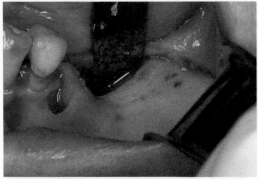

Fig. 41. Alveolar bone defect following extraction of the mandibular left first molar (vertical root fracture) and vertical bone defect in the second molar site.

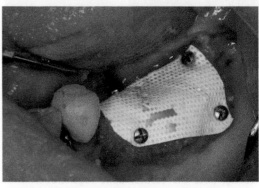

Fig. 44. Final fixation of membrane with bone screws.

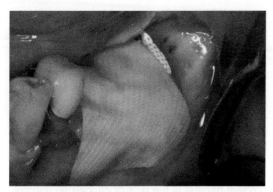

Fig. 45. Ossix Plus membrane placed over PTFE membrane to completely cover the bone graft.

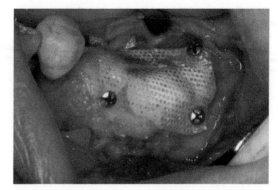

Fig. 47. Surgical exposure of the membrane before implant placement; note the significant gain in alveolar bone height.

membrane will result in bacterial contamination and infection. Because the pore size of the membrane restricts bacteria from penetrating through the membrane, bacterial contamination around the membrane edges will occur over time. Once exposed, it is recommended to remove the membrane within 4 weeks of exposure. The use of a chlorhexidine-based mouth rinse combined with the use of a broad-spectrum antibiotic may help reduce this potential complication. However, the best defense against early membrane exposure and resulting bone loss is excellent flap release and tension-free closure, combined with membrane stabilization.

Summary

GBR using barrier membranes and particulate bone grafts is a predictable technique for bone augmentation in implant dentistry. Careful treatment planning will help determine whether a bioabsorbable or nonresorbable barrier is appropriate. If the PASS principles[25] are carefully followed, predictable results are expected.

AUTOGENOUS ONLAY BLOCK BONE GRAFTING
Introduction

Alveolar horizontal and vertical defects of the mandible and maxilla have driven the use of autogenous bone harvest sites and advancement of grafting techniques in the clinical practice of dental rehabilitation with endosseous implants.[28]

In bone grafting, autogenous bone has long proved to be the gold standard, but rapid developments in the understanding of bone physiology and growth have led to near equal if not superior results with no autogenous harvest required.[29] Although many of the alternatives to autogenous bone grafting have proven to be quite technique sensitive, the tried and true methods of block graft harvesting and subsequent RA will be covered here in detail.

Nonvascular block bone harvests are discussed, including anterior and posterior ilium, mandibular ramus and chin, and cranium.[30] Selection of graft sites and their appropriate indications are discussed as well as caveats and various pitfalls in harvesting are presented.[31]

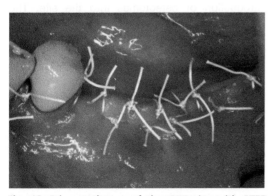

Fig. 46. Primary closure of the GBR site with PTFE sutures.

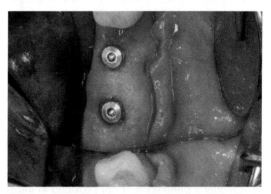

Fig. 48. Implants placed in the healed GBR site in preparation for final implant restorations.

Description of Technique, Donor Sites, Indications, Contraindications, and Complications

Intraoral harvest from mandibular ramus

When a small area of augmentation in a vertical or horizontal dimension is desired, the ramus is an obvious choice of mostly cortical bone stock. The amount of bone that can be harvested depends on the overall shape of the patient's mandible and the location of the mandibular canal. Average graft size ranges from 1 to 2 cm in length and about 1 cm in height. A CBCT scanner can aid significantly in planning these surgeries because of the ability to appropriately identify not only the height but also the buccolingual position of the inferior alveolar canal in relation to the desired graft site. The benefits of this procedure are the proximity of the graft harvest site to the recipient site, low rate of postoperative complications, and familiarity with the anatomy associated with the procedure.[32] In contrast, the downsides of ramus harvest include a relatively small availability of bone and the potential for inferior alveolar nerve (IAN) injury and associated lip numbness following the procedure.

The surgical technique for a ramus block graft harvest entails an approach very similar to the removal of full bone-impacted wisdom tooth or the approach to a sagittal ramus osteotomy. The surgical incision can be a sulcular design in the presence of adjacent teeth and include a distal release or can be placed laterally over the external oblique ridge in a vertical design. In the case of a thin mandibular ramus, exposure of the lingual cortex to gauge thickness may be beneficial. The graft should not extend more than half the width of the mandibular ramus. Osteotomy can be performed in 2 fashions: reciprocating saw or by using numbers 701 or 702 burs. These osteotomies should be performed through the cortex only especially as the vertical cuts are being made because the IAN may be in close proximity in this region. The authors prefer to use a round bur at the inferior aspect of the block to weaken but not fully perforate the cortex and thus allow for outfracture without significant risk of nerve injury. Once the block begins to mobilize, it can be outfractured with an osteotome. The donor site edges should be smoothed with a bur or bone file, and the site should be irrigated and closed primarily with a resorbable suture. Patients can follow up in 1 to 2 weeks, and saline mouth rinses may aid in healing. Postoperative antibiotics may be given based on practitioner's preference, if not provided in intravenous form during the procedure.

Intraoral harvest from the chin

An additional site of intraoral bone stock is the symphysis that yields a block of cortex with minimal cancellous marrow.[32] In the case of the symphysis, graft dimensions rarely extend beyond 2 cm in vertical height and 6 cm in width when extended across the midline. This block can be divided into 2 segments for bilateral applications. The benefits to this site of bone harvest include location within the oral cavity with the lack of a perceived donor site and a bone stock with a natural curvature. The potential downside of the symphyseal harvest is the lack of cancellous marrow, the possibility of postoperative anterior teeth numbness, mental nerve injury, and the relatively small bone stock available. Contraindications to use of the symphysis for bone harvest include previous radiation, excessive vertical bone loss from age or other preexisting conditions, and the presence of an alloplastic chin implant.

In approaching the symphyseal bone harvest, local anesthesia can be obtained with bilateral mental nerve blocks and vestibular infiltration for hemostasis. The incision is placed approximately 1 cm below the mucogingival junction from the distal of 1 canine to the other. This incision will protect not only the mental nerve, which is typically apical to the second molar, but also the labial branch of the mental nerve, which lies just deep to the mucosa in this region. Upon identification of the labial branch laterally, the incision can be deepened down to periosteum. The mentalis muscle will be reflected inferiorly, ensuring to leave the attachment of the mental tubercles because failure to preserve this attachment can lead to the chin ptosis. The superior tissues should also be reflected enough to visualize dental root form and possibly the root apices through the thin buccal cortex. Beginning approximately 0.5 cm apical to the root tips of the incisors, the outline of the graft can be completed with a 701 or 702 bur. This cut should be performed at a slight angle to allow for introduction of osteotomes into the site. The outline can be completed remaining at least 5 mm anterior to the mental foramen if the dissection has been carried posterior to this extent and 1 cm above the inferior border. Alternative cutting instruments include the reciprocating saw or a piezoelectric knife. After the cut has been sufficiently taken through the outer cortex, fine straight osteotomes can be used to wedge out the bone blocks. Once the grafts have been harvested, the defect can be left alone or an allogeneic graft material may be used per the surgeon's preference. Closure should be completed in layers, taking care to reapproximate the mentalis muscle. A chin pressure dressing such as used for a genioplasty can be used in the postoperative setting to limit postoperative edema or hematoma. Other than paresthesia, which can occur, although usually only transiently, and ecchymosis, rare complications following this procedure can include hematoma, wound dehiscence, infection, and mandibular fracture.

Extraoral harvest: posterior iliac crest

The posterior iliac crest (PIC) has long been one of the most common and plentiful sources of autogenous bone for use in oral and maxillofacial surgery. It has been demonstrated that 100 to 150 mL of corticocancellous bone can be safely harvested from this region due to uniform thickness of the PIC. When compared with other harvest sites, the major advantage of the PIC is that it only involves the primary reflection of 1 muscle, the gluteus maximus, which is not primary to ambulation.[33] Many consider the PIC the gold standard in quantity and quality of bone graft material.[34] The bone stock available in the posterior ilium has been found to be highly osteogenic, osteoinductive, and osteoconductive. Because of the complex anatomy immediately approximating this region, it is critical for the surgeon to know the anatomy of the posterior iliac region. There are nearly zero exclusion criteria when considering the PIC bone graft, with only several relative contraindications or cautions: severely osteoporotic individuals, previous hip replacements, retained hardware from previous femur fracture. The only known absolute contraindication to the authors' knowledge is the confirmed presence of pelvic metastasis in the setting of metastatic disease. With the use of proper surgical technique, the morbidity is minimal, and the bone stock is unmatched for bone grafting.[35]

Extraoral harvest: anterior iliac crest

The anterior iliac crest (AIC) has long been considered a mainstay of autogenous bone harvest for the oral and maxillofacial surgeon.[36] A source of cortical bone of up to 5 × 5 cm and 30 to 50 mL of uncompressed cancellous marrow can be harvested from this site. The AIC has a plethora of osteoprogenitor cells, which allows for favorable bone growth as well as rapid revascularization. The AIC has been shown to have the highest cancellous bone-to-cortical bone ratio. Unlike the posterior hip with its superior bone quantity, the anterior iliac crest bone graft (AICBG) requires minimal repositioning for harvest. The nerves that course in this area are all sensory cutaneous and not essential to gait. The most common complications associated with AICBG harvest are seroma formation, bruising, and gait disturbance associated with disturbance of the tensor fascia lata. As mentioned, major complications have been reported in small numbers to include fracture of the ilium, perforation of the peritoneum and/or bowel, infection, and sensory nerve damage. One must maintain the cartilaginous cap in children; therefore, during the harvest, the surgeon must either split or maintain it.

Calvarial bone harvest

When a curvilinear bone graft is required with little to no cancellous bone, the split or full-thickness calvarial bone should remain high on the list of bone stock available. Harvested from the parietal region, posterior to the pinna, where the calvarium is thickest, and a full-thickness graft on average can yield 7 to 8 mm of width.[37] The bone from this region has shown exceptional resistance to resorption once implanted compared with other autogenous sources.[38] Because of the native curvature of the calvarium in 2 dimensions, grafts from this region can fit perfectly into orbital floor defects, zygomatic fractures, and other curved structures of the craniofacial region and even to cover large buccal wall defects around dental implants.[39] The only significant anatomic structures of interest are the superficial temporary artery, which can be ligated when encountered, and the superior sagittal sinus, which should be avoided by remaining 1 to 2 cm away from the sagittal suture as the sinus usually extends 5 mm to each side of midline. Once adequately loosened, the graft can be delivered and put on the operating room table for further manipulation. The defect itself can be filled with bone cement or in larger harvests covered by a titanium mesh. Once hemostasis has been achieved, closure should be completed in 3 layers. A drain is rarely indicated. A pressure dressing using fluffs, Kerlix, and Coban in a Barton pressure bandage fashion can dress the area. In the postoperative setting, the patient is monitored neurologically for 24 hours. Skin staples are left in place for a minimum of 7 days. If drains are placed, they should be removed as soon as drainage has decreased to less than 10 ml in 24 hours. The more common complications include alopecia near the incision line and hematoma formation. Other complications, although rare, may present when the inner table is perforated, including cerebrospinal fluid leak, extradural hematoma, and direct intracerebral trauma.

Advantages and disadvantages

Autogenous block grafting is considered the "gold standard" for regeneration of bone for atrophic jaws. The graft should be stabilized on the recipient bed by fixation screws or with simultaneous placement of dental implants. During the healing period, grafted bone is gradually replaced by new regenerate, and it depends on revascularization from the recipient site.[40] Therefore, perforation of recipient site is recommended to enhance angiogenesis and provide osteogenic cells.[9] There is an advantage to using block grafting for simultaneous reconstruction of horizontal and vertical defects. In addition, higher primary stability is achieved when dental implants are placed in block graft–augmented ridges in comparison to GBR techniques.[41]

Block bone grafting also allows 3-dimensional reconstruction of defects with complicated morphology. The main disadvantage of autogenous block grafting is donor site morbidity and technical limitations.[42] In addition, one may see increased graft resorption and limited amount of bone gain. Block graft surgery may also be time consuming because of 2 operative sites. Commercial allogeneic or xenogeneic blocks have been developed as an alternative but remain unproven long term, although successful clinical application of these materials has been reported in the literature.[43–45]

Late-term bone resorption is the main challenge in autogenous block grafting. AIC showed a range resorption between 20% and 92% in 10-year follow-up.[46,47] Lateral ramus as intraoral donor site showed 17.4% of bone resorption after 4 to 6 months of bone grafting.[48] Membrane usage showed better results in the amount of bone gain when used in vertical defects.[49]

Prolonged treatment time, soft tissue complications, graft failure, and donor site morbidity categorize onlay block bone grafting as a technique-sensitive procedure. Excessive soft tissue tension in the recipient site may lead to graft exposure, excessive bone resorption, and peri-implantitis in the cases of immediate implant placement; therefore, simultaneous placement of implants might not lessen overall treatment time, whereas using a graft before implant therapy, complications, such as graft exposure, infection, and graft failure, do not result in implant failure.[50]

Case Reports

Mandibular ramus graft

A representative case treated by ramus grafting in the area of a central incisor with simultaneous

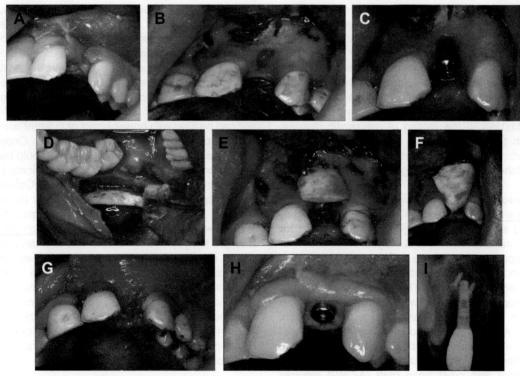

Fig. 49. Anterior maxillary defect with missing central incisor (*A*). Osteotomy with immediate implant placement and onlay bone grafting from lateral ramus (*B–E*). Implant site covered with allogeneic Dura and primary closure (*F–G*). Healed graft and restoration after 6 months (*H, I*). (*From* Broumand V, Khojateh A, Green III, JM. Vertical alveolar ridge augmentation with autogenous block grafts in implant dentistry. In: Tolstunov L, editor. Horizontal alveolar ridge augmentation in implant dentistry: a surgical manual. Hoboken: John Wiley & Sons; 2016. p. 274–307; with permission.)

implant placement is illustrated by the photographs and diagrams in **Fig. 49**. The patient had a large anterior maxillary defect with a missing central incisor that underwent onlay bone grafting from the lateral ramus with immediate implant placement. The grafted site was covered with allogeneic dura mater as a barrier membrane.[51] The patient had a healed graft and restoration after a period of 6 months.

Chin graft
A representation of chin harvesting is illustrated by the photographs and diagrams in **Fig. 50**.

Posterior iliac graft harvest
Representation of PIC harvesting is illustrated by the photographs and diagrams, and important anatomic landmarks are illustrated as well in **Fig. 51**. The patient lost the anterior maxillary teeth due to a motor vehicle accident along with the entire alveolar segment.

Anterior iliac graft harvest
Representation of AIC harvesting is illustrated by the photographs and diagrams; important anatomic landmarks are illustrated as well in **Fig. 52**. The patient had an isolated vertical and horizontal maxillary defect at the time of grafting and had an implant retained restoration 12 months later with stable vertical and horizontal augmentation.

Bone graft harvest from the calvarium
Photographs and diagrams illustrate representation of cranial bone harvesting, and important anatomic landmarks are illustrated as well in **Fig. 53**.

Case report
The representative case treated by AIC bone grafting for horizontal and vertical RA is shown (**Fig. 54**). A 65-year-old woman with a severely resorbed knife-edge maxillary anterior ridge underwent reconstruction with autogenous AIC block grafting and cortical fixation screws. The patient had severe maxillary atrophy due to long-standing edentulism wearing complete maxillary denture since the age of 15. The patient underwent reconstruction with placement of mandibular first and later maxillary implants after vertical and horizontal reconstruction.

Summary
An oral and maxillofacial surgeon is commonly faced with the task of hard tissue reconstruction for the following indications: benign and cancer ablated defects, extensive craniofacial fracture repair, and jaw bone atrophy with associated dental implant rehabilitation.[52] Reconstruction of hard tissue defects in the oral and maxillofacial region has made use of recent technological advances and tissue engineering (TE). Horizontal and especially *vertical* RAs have always posed a challenge even to the skilled surgeon. Although cancellous cellular marrow transfer still represents the gold standard for successful grafting and bone formation in oral and maxillofacial reconstruction, the use of many novel techniques and advances in science has lessened the need for autogenous grafting with decreased morbidity and operating room time and cost.[53] Implant osseointegration is determined

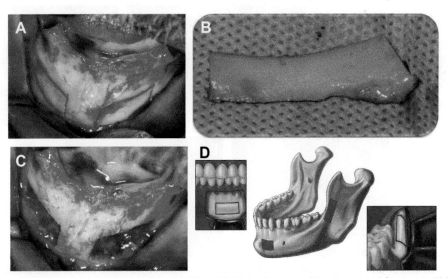

Fig. 50. Bone harvest site from the anterior mandible (*A*). Onlay bone grafting harvested from mandible (*B*). Remaining defect after harvest (*C*). Multiple harvest sites (*D*). (*From* Broumand V, Khojateh A, Green III, JM. Vertical alveolar ridge augmentation with autogenous block grafts in implant dentistry. In: Tolstunov L, editor. Horizontal alveolar ridge augmentation in implant dentistry: a surgical manual. Hoboken: John Wiley & Sons; 2016. p. 274–307; with permission.)

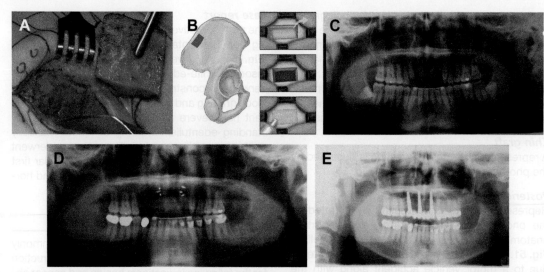

Fig. 51. PIC block graft (*A, B*) applied to anterior maxilla with fixation screws to gain width and height (*C, D*) and reconstructed with dental implants 9 months later (*E*). The patient had originally lost the anterior maxillary teeth due to a motor vehicle accident along with the entire alveolar segment. (*From* Broumand V, Khojateh A, Green III, JM. Vertical alveolar ridge augmentation with autogenous block grafts in implant dentistry. In: Tolstunov L, editor. Horizontal alveolar ridge augmentation in implant dentistry: a surgical manual. Hoboken: John Wiley & Sons; 2016. p. 274–307; with permission.)

by the de novo bone regeneration at the bone-implant surface.[54] Ideal osseointegration takes place in native bone with cortical components and trabecular vascular and marrow components. Predictable osseointegration also takes place with autogenous grafts that heal by osteoconduction and osteoinduction as well as with guided and engineered de novo regenerated bone.[55]

ALVEOLAR DISTRACTION OSTEOGENESIS

Dental implants have had tremendous success in the past 2 decades and have become synonymous for reconstructive dentistry in partial or fully edentulous patients, showing long-term survival.[56] Nevertheless, they require adequate bone volume for proper placement.

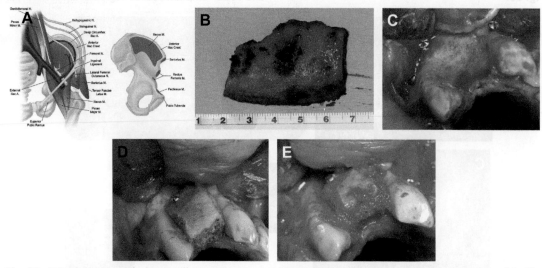

Fig. 52. AIC schematic and pictures illustrating sensory nerves in the region with muscle attachments (*A*). Iliac crest with cortical bone and cancellous marrow (*B*). Maxillary defect at the time of grafting and 12 months later with stable vertical and horizontal augmentation (*C–E*). (*From* Broumand V, Khojateh A, Green III, JM. Vertical alveolar ridge augmentation with autogenous block grafts in implant dentistry. In: Tolstunov L, editor. Horizontal alveolar ridge augmentation in implant dentistry: a surgical manual. Hoboken: John Wiley & Sons; 2016. p. 274–307; with permission.)

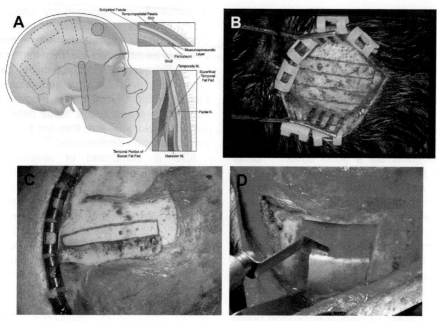

Fig. 53. Layers of scalp and position of the facial nerve and numerous acceptable locations for cranial bone harvest (*A*). Numerous blocks of cranial bone harvest for dentofacial or craniofacial reconstruction (*B*). Harvest of strut of bone for nasal reconstruction (*C*). Harvest of large cranial block with oscillating saw (*D*). (*From* Broumand V, Khojateh A, Green III, JM. Vertical alveolar ridge augmentation with autogenous block grafts in implant dentistry. In: Tolstunov L, editor. Horizontal alveolar ridge augmentation in implant dentistry: a surgical manual. Hoboken: John Wiley & Sons; 2016. p. 274–307; with permission.)

One solution for the lack of adequate bone height is short dental implants. Different reports describe short dental implants with varying lengths. Part of the reports show good survival rates,[57] whereas others exhibit lower survival rates.[58] Nevertheless, most do not show long-term results. One should remember crown-to-implant ratio and crown height space may affect

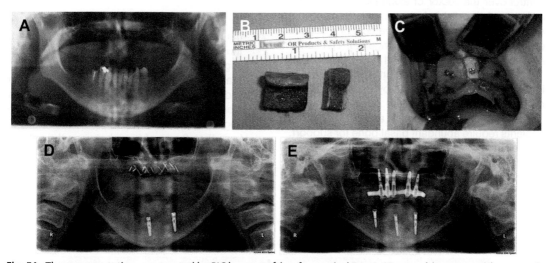

Fig. 54. The representative case treated by PIC bone grafting for vertical RA. A 65-year-old woman with a severely resorbed knife-edge maxillary anterior ridge (*A*) undergoes reconstruction with autogenous PIC block grafting (*B*) and cortical fixation screws (*C, D*). Patient had severe maxillary atrophy due to long-standing edentulism wearing a complete denture since the age of 15. Patient underwent reconstruction with placement of mandibular first and then maxillary implants after vertical and horizontal bone reconstruction (*E*). (*From* Broumand V, Khojateh A, Green III, JM. Vertical alveolar ridge augmentation with autogenous block grafts in implant dentistry. In: Tolstunov L, editor. Horizontal alveolar ridge augmentation in implant dentistry: a surgical manual. Hoboken: John Wiley & Sons; 2016. p. 274–307; with permission.)

implant survival,[59] and it is usually unfavorable in short dental implants.

To overcome this obstacle, there are several augmentation methods available: GBR, bone blocks used as onlay or inlay grafts, ridge splitting, and ADO.

GBR is a vastly used augmentation method.[60] It is commonly used for minor deficiencies, yet it lacks the ability to achieve significant bone height. For medium-sized deficiencies of up to 6 mm, block bone grafts are a good option.[61] Onlay bone graft has a tendency for resorption, and both onlay and inlay bone grafts may result in donor site morbidity.[62] In medium to large alveolar bone deficiency of greater than 6 mm, the authors recommend using the ADO method.

Distraction osteogenesis is a method of generating new bone following an osteotomy with gradual distraction. The method is based on the tension-stress principle described by Dr Ilizarov.[63] DO results in augmentation of both bone and soft tissue. The process of gradual elongation brings about differentiation of stem cells, angiogenesis, and mineralization.[64–66] The method was clinically performed for the first time in 1992 by McCarthy and colleagues[67] on hypoplastic mandibles of syndromic children.

ADO can be divided into unidirectional, bidirectional, and horizontal. Unidirectional ADO results in vertical elongation. In cases of a large mesiodistal deficiency of greater than 3 cm, the use of 2 distraction devices, 1 on each side of the defect, will allow control over the vector of elongation and prevent collapse of the distracted segment. Bidirectional ADO is used for concomitant vertical and sagittal control over the vector of elongation. Horizontal ADO is performed when sagittal deficiencies exist.

ADO devices are divided into extraosseous, intraosseous, and distraction by implants. Extraosseous devices are the most prevalent devices used. Intraosseous distraction and distraction by implants require abundant basal bone for support. In addition, compared with extraosseous devices, they are more prone to negative influences by lateral forces that may affect the vector of elongation and result in bone resorption surrounding the distraction device. Implant distraction devices may be left and used for prosthetic rehabilitation or removed and replaced by osseointegrated dental implants. It is difficult to predict the final location of the implant distraction devices and thus may be difficult to use them for the rehabilitation.[68] Extraosseous distraction devices, on the other hand, require a large subperiosteal lumen, thus affecting the periosteal blood supply and resulting in possible soft tissue dehiscence and exposure. Nonetheless, they are the most abundant distraction devices used.[69]

ADO is composed of several stages. It begins with an osteotomy and placement of the distraction device. Next, there is a latency period of several days in which the callous organizes. Following the latency period, gradual distraction is initiated at a rate of 0.5 mm/d. The final stage is the consolidation period consisting of several months in which maturation and mineralization of the callous are observed (**Fig. 55**).

Indications and Contraindication

Indications

- Severe alveolar bone deficiency of greater than 6 mm
- Lack of soft tissue for closure following bone augmentation
- Patient refuses a second donor site for harvesting the bone graft

Contraindications

- Transported segment height is smaller than 6 mm
- The lingual/palatal periosteal attachment to the transport segment was compromised, thus compromising the blood supply of the segment
- Transport segment does not have enough width (bucco-lingual/bucco-palatal); thus elongation might result in a fracture of the segment
- Less than 2 mm of bone between the osteotomy and the IAN or sinus/nasal floor

Distraction Technique

The first stage of the procedure includes flap elevation. A buccal paracrestal mucoperiosteal

Surgery	Latency period	Rate of bone elongation	Consolidation period	Device removal	Implant placement
	4 d	0.5 mm/d as necessary	3–4 mo		

Fig. 55. Protocol for ADO procedure.

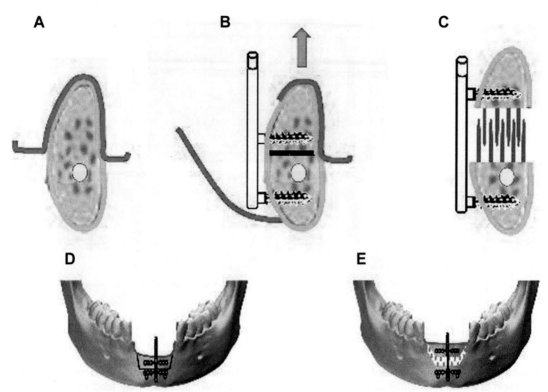

Fig. 56. The alveolar distraction procedure: (*A–C*) illustrate the procedure in the posterior mandible. (*A*) Coronal section of a mandible before distraction osteogenesis. (*B*) Following mucoperiosteal paracrestal buccal flap elevation, osteotomy (black line) and distractor fixation using mini screws. Notice the crestal and lingual mucoperiosteum (red line). Orange line – cortex of the bone. *Arrow* – direction of the transported segment vertically upwards is left intact. (*C*) Following vertical bone elongation (the gray lines represent the newly formed bone trabeculae). (*D, E*) illustrate the procedure in the anterior mandible: (*D*) anterior view following device fixation and (*E*) following bone elongation.

incision is performed maintaining the crestal and lingual/palatal periosteum intact, allowing for proper blood supply to the transport segment (**Fig. 56**). Next, the osteotomies are performed, 2 inclined vertical and 1 horizontal osteotomy, creating a trapezoidal transport segment (see **Fig. 56**D). Following a latency period of several days, bone elongation is commenced, in the case of ADO, at a rate of 0.5 mm/d. The elongation continues according to the required final bone volume and is restricted by the length of the distractor. Next, a consolidation period of 3 to 4 months is required. The final step is device

removal after which endosseous dental implants may be placed followed by prosthetic rehabilitation.

Two-stage reconstruction
In cases of severe bone deficiency, mostly due to trauma or ablative surgery, 2-stage reconstruction can be performed: bone block placement followed by ADO.[70]

Span of the defect
In large-span defects (mesiodistal), there is a difficulty to maintain a proper vector of elongation and

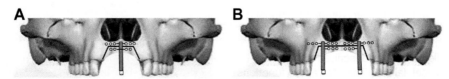

Fig. 57. Number of devices used depends on the span. (*A*) In up to 3 to 4 teeth, 1 device is used. (*B*) In deficiencies of 4 teeth or more, 2 devices are used. (*From* Rachmiel A, Shilo D, Aizenbud D, et al. Three-dimensional reconstruction of post-traumatic deficient anterior maxilla. J Oral Maxillofac Surg 2017;75:2691; with permission.)

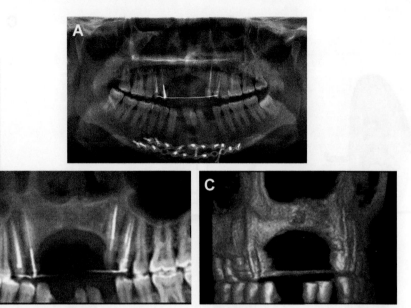

Fig. 58. A 30-year-old woman suffering from a mandibular fracture and avulsion of the premaxilla with loss of the incisors and the supporting bone. (*A–C*) Panoramic radiograph and CBCT show the deficient anterior maxilla.

stability of the transport segment. In these cases, utilization of 2 distractor devices at the lateral aspects of the defect, instead of 1 device in the middle of the defect, will increase stability. The authors recommend using 1 device in cases of 3 to 4 missing teeth, and 2 devices if the span of the deficiency is 4 teeth or larger. When using 2 devices at the lateral edges, the lateral plates of the distractor in the transport segment are removed (**Fig. 57**).[71]

A case of maxillary alveolar distraction can be observed in **Figs. 58–61.**

Complications and Management

- Inferior alveolar and mental nerve injury. This can be avoided by a carefully performed flap elevation and osteotomy.
- Damage to adjacent teeth.
- Compromised vector of elongation. This is one of the main difficulties in the procedure. The transport segment is prone to palatal/lingual inclinations due to periosteal tractions. One can use elastics on teeth, temporary anchorage devices, or personalized tooth-born devices to maintain the proper vector of elongation. The vector of longer mesiodistal transport segment span can be better controlled by using 2 distractors, as described above.
- Mechanical failure. The distractor functions under constant masticatory forces and may fracture or malfunction. This requires another surgical intervention for device replacement.

- Exposure of the device. This is a known complication and may lead to infection, device removal, and improper bony ossification.
- Transport segment or basal bone fracture. Follow the minimal bone segments sizes and distances. Use proper and maintained equipment and accurate osteotomies. In the case of basal bone fracture, immediate surgical repositioning and osteosynthesis are required.

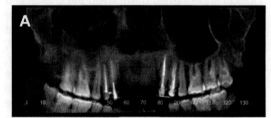

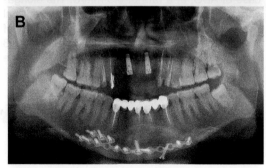

Fig. 59. Same patient as in **Fig. 58** following augmentation. (*A*) CBCT following ADO. (*B*) Panoramic radiograph following placement of two dental implants.

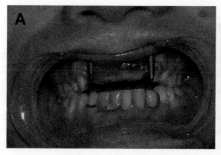
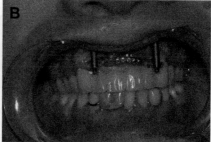

Fig. 60. The patient described before during the consolidation period of the distraction procedure. (*A, B*) Without the temporary prosthetic reconstruction and with the reconstruction.

- Improper vector of elongation or rod position may lead to occlusal interferences. It is important to plan and correctly place the distraction device.
- Improper blood supply leading to transport segment resorption. This may be due to compromise of the crestal and lingual/palatal mucoperiosteal attachment or physical pressure applied on the segment.
- Infection, improper rate of elongation, or exposure of the distraction chamber may lead to improper ossification of the newly created bone.
- Masticatory forces, improper ossification, or short consolidation period may cause relapse.

The most frequent complication is undesirable bone movement followed by mechanical failure.[72]

Advantages and Disadvantages

Advantages of ADO include greater bone gain compared with other methods of augmentation.[73–75] One of the advantages allowing for this increased augmentation is the simultaneous distraction of both bone and soft tissue. Soft tissue coverage without tension is one of the main disadvantages of other methods due to bone graft exposure that leads to complications. Another advantage is that cortical bone and attached

mucosa at the crest are left as the coronal aspect of the ridge at the end of the process, thus allowing for the placement of dental implants in the original attached mucosa and in cortical bone for increased stability. In addition, the method results in increased stability without donor site morbidity and lower infection rates.

Disadvantages of the method include mainly the need for a second operation for device removal (although some advocate the simultaneous dental implants insertion during removal) and pain during the elongation process, which can be managed by the rate and extent of elongation and by pain medication.

Summary

Fig. 62 describes the authors' algorithm for alveolar bone augmentation. ADO results in a more stable outcome than GBR and block grafts,[76] yet 3% to 20% relapse is observed. Thus, overcorrection of a few millimeters should be considered.[77,78] This overcorrection may be reduced easily at the time of device removal and implant placement.

Important Points

1. Proper case selection: medium to severe cases of alveolar deficiency.
2. Correct planning of the osteotomy (transport segment size and anatomic landmarks);

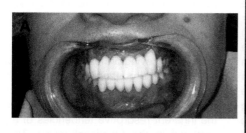
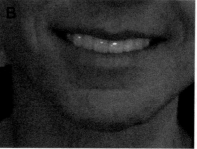

Fig. 61. Same patient as in **Fig. 60** following the permanent prosthetic reconstruction. (*A*) Complete dentoalveolar reconstruction with proper occlusion relations. (*B*) Smile exhibiting proper upper arch exposure with good relations to the soft tissue.

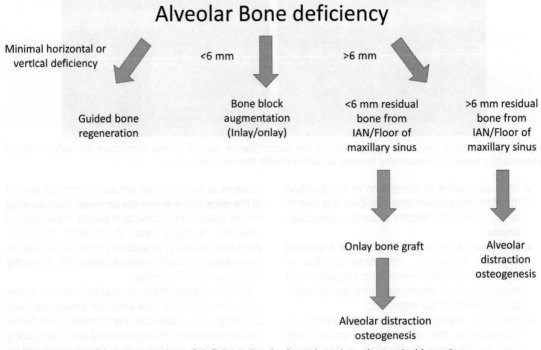

Alveolar Bone deficiency

Minimal horizontal or vertical deficiency

<6 mm

>6 mm

Guided bone regeneration

Bone block augmentation (Inlay/onlay)

<6 mm residual bone from IAN/Floor of maxillary sinus

>6 mm residual bone from IAN/Floor of maxillary sinus

Onlay bone graft

Alveolar distraction osteogenesis

Alveolar distraction osteogenesis

Fig. 62. Algorithm for reconstruction of deficient alveolar bone based on the vertical bone loss.

respect the integrity of the blood supply of the transport segment at the crest and lingual/palatal aspects (see **Fig. 56**).

3. Proper vector of elongation. Remember the vector can change during the active lengthening; thus close monitoring of the patient is mandatory. Use elastics when required.
4. Appropriate rate and rhythm of elongation are crucial.
5. Adequate consolidation period for proper ossification and minimal relapse.
6. Avoid occlusal forces on the transported segment during the distraction and consolidation periods.

SUMMARY

The ultimate decision concerning which bone augmentation procedure to use in each particular case rests in the hands of the operator. When considering the option for reconstruction of the partially or completely edentulous patient with inadequate bone, the surgeon must establish a plan to take the patient from their current state to a fully functional and esthetically pleasing prosthesis. Understanding all stages of this driven process is critical to obtaining an ideal outcome.

The authors demonstrated indications, alternatives, benefits, and risks of the most common alveolar bone augmentation techniques for horizontal and vertical ridge deficiency. A knowledgeable and skilled surgeon should base his or her decision on the most effective and efficient surgical technique that would provide the patient with a long-lasting bony foundation for implant prosthetics. The patient's medical state and competency of an immune system are paramount in making a choice in surgical technique. TE principles may be a part of a decision-making process, including utilization of rhBMP-2, platelet-rich plasma, PRF, mesenchymal stem cells, and other biomimetics, when needed.

In general, the latest trend in bone augmentation fluctuates toward GBR particulate onlay and inlay grafting techniques for mild to moderate alveolar ridge deficiency cases. In larger composite bone defects (related to trauma or pathology cases), autogenous block bone grafts or ADO with TE products, or a combination of techniques in a consecutive manner, accomplish the desired goals of achieving orthoalveolar form. Overcorrection during the grafting procedure has become a common approach[79] because of postsurgical adaptive physiologic resorption. This relates to the inherent resorptive tendencies of a particular graft within the functional milieu. The surgeon should also pay attention to the biologic rationale in selecting a particular bone augmentation technique.

ACKNOWLEDGMENTS

The "Alveolar Ridge-Split Expansion Technique" section was written by Len Tolstunov. The "Guided Bone Regeneration with Particulate Bone Graft" section was written by Eric Hamrick. The "Autogenous Onlay Block Bone Grafting" section was written by Vishtasb Broumand. The "Alveolar Distraction Osteogenesis" section was written by Adi Rachmiel and Dekel Shilo. The authors express sincere appreciation to Evans "Whit" Whitaker, MD, MLIS, a research librarian from UCSF Health Sciences Library in San Francisco, for technical expertise in citations and references when formatting this complex multiauthor article.

REFERENCES

1. Buser D, Chappuis V, Belser UC, et al. Implant placement post extraction in esthetic single tooth sites: when immediate, when early, when late? Periodontol 2000 2016;73(1):84–102.
2. Buser D, Halbritter S, Hart C, et al. Early implant placement with simultaneous guided bone regeneration following single-tooth extraction in the esthetic zone: 12-month results of a prospective study with 20 consecutive patients. J Periodontol 2009;80(1):152–62.
3. Raes S, Eghbali A, Chappuis V, et al. A long-term prospective cohort study on immediately restored single tooth implants inserted in extraction sockets and healed ridges: CBCT analyses, soft tissue alterations, aesthetic ratings, and patient-reported outcomes. Clin Implant Dent Relat Res 2018;20(4):522–30.
4. Aghaloo TL, Moy PK. Which hard tissue augmentation techniques are the most successful in furnishing bony support for implant placement? Int J Oral Maxillofac Implants 2007;22(Suppl):49–70.
5. Jensen OT, Bell W, Cottam J. Osteoperiosteal flaps and local osteotomies for alveolar reconstruction. Oral Maxillofac Surg Clin North Am 2010;22(3):331–46.
6. Bell WH. Revascularization and bone healing after anterior maxillary osteotomy: a study using adult rhesus monkeys. J Oral Surg 1969;27(4):249–55.
7. Bell WH. Biologic basis for maxillary osteotomies. Am J Phys Anthropol 1973;38(2):279–89.
8. Bell WH, Levy BM. Revascularization and bone healing after anterior mandibular osteotomy. J Oral Surg 1970;28(3):196–203.
9. Pikos MA. Block autografts for localized ridge augmentation. Implant Dent 2000;9(1):67–75.
10. Scipioni A, Bruschi GB, Calesini G. The edentulous ridge expansion technique: a five-year study. Implant Dent 1995;4(3):205.
11. Simion M, Baldoni M, Zaffe D. Jawbone enlargement using immediate implant placement associated with a split-crest technique and guided tissue regeneration. Int J Periodontics Restorative Dent 1992;12(6):462–73.
12. Bravi F, Bruschi GB, Ferrini F. A 10-year multicenter retrospective clinical study of 1715 implants placed with the edentulous ridge expansion technique. Int J Periodontics Restorative Dent 2007;27(6):557–65.
13. Bruschi GB, Scipioni A, Calesini G, et al. Localized management of sinus floor with simultaneous implant placement: a clinical report. Int J Oral Maxillofac Implants 1998;13(2):219–26.
14. Duncan JM, Westwood RM. Ridge widening for the thin maxilla: a clinical report. Int J Oral Maxillofac Implants 1997;12(2):224–7.
15. Engelke WG, Diederichs CG, Jacobs HG, et al. Alveolar reconstruction with splitting osteotomy and microfixation of implants. Int J Oral Maxillofac Implants 1997;12(3):310–8.
16. Smiler DG. Advances in endosseous implants: the 'sandwich' split cortical graft for dental implant placement. Dent Implantol Update 2000;11(7):49–53.
17. Casap N, Brand M, Mogyros R, et al. Island osteoperiosteal flaps with interpositional bone grafting in rabbit tibia: preliminary study for development of new bone augmentation technique. J Oral Maxillofac Surg 2011;69(12):3045–51.
18. Jensen OT, Ellis E. The book flap: a technical note. J Oral Maxillofac Surg 2008;66(5):1010–4.
19. Jensen OT, Mogyros R, Owen Z, et al. Island osteoperiosteal flap for alveolar bone reconstruction. J Oral Maxillofac Surg 2010;68(3):539–46.
20. Le B, Rohrer MD, Prassad HS. Screw "Tent-Pole" grafting technique for reconstruction of large vertical alveolar ridge defects using human mineralized allograft for implant site preparation. J Oral Maxillofac Surg 2010;68(2):428–35.
21. Lekovic V, Camargo PM, Klokkevold PR, et al. Preservation of alveolar bone in extraction sockets using bioabsorbable membranes. J Periodontol 1998;69(9):1044–9.
22. Geurs NC, Korostoff JM, Vassilopoulos PJ, et al. Clinical and histologic assessment of lateral alveolar ridge augmentation using a synthetic long-term bioabsorbable membrane and an allograft. J Periodontol 2008;79(7):1133–40.
23. von Arx T, Buser D. Horizontal ridge augmentation using autogenous block grafts and the guided bone regeneration technique with collagen membranes: a clinical study with 42 patients. Clin Oral Implants Res 2006;17(4):359–66.
24. Urban IA, Jovanovic SA, Lozada JL. Vertical ridge augmentation using guided bone regeneration (GBR) in three clinical scenarios prior to implant

placement: a retrospective study of 35 patients 12 to 72 months after loading. Int J Oral Maxillofac Implants 2009;24(3):502–10.

25. Wang HL, Boyapati L. "PASS" principles for predictable bone regeneration. Implant Dent 2006;15(1):8–17.

26. Greenstein G, Greenstein B, Cavallaro J, et al. The role of bone decortication in enhancing the results of guided bone regeneration: a literature review. J Periodontol 2009;80(2):175–89.

27. Fontana F, Santoro F, Maiorana C, et al. Clinical and histologic evaluation of allogeneic bone matrix versus autogenous bone chips associated with titanium-reinforced e-PTFE membrane for vertical ridge augmentation: a prospective pilot study. Int J Oral Maxillofac Implants 2008;23(6):1003–12.

28. Nevins M, Mellonig JT. Enhancement of the damaged edentulous ridge to receive dental implants: a combination of allograft and the GORE-TEX membrane. Int J Periodontics Restorative Dent 1992;12(2):96–111.

29. Fonseca RJ. Reconstruction of the maxillofacial cancer patient. In: Fonseca RJ, editor. Oral and maxillofacial surgery, vol. 7, 1st edition. Philadelphia: Saunders; 2000. p. 361.

30. Yates DM, Brockhoff HC, Finn R, et al. Comparison of intraoral harvest sites for corticocancellous bone grafts. J Oral Maxillofac Surg 2013;71(3):497–504.

31. Jensen OT, Block M. Alveolar modification by distraction osteogenesis. Atlas Oral Maxillofac Surg Clin 2008;16(2):185–214.

32. Schwartz-Arad D, Levin L, Sigal L. Surgical success of intraoral autogenous block onlay bone grafting for alveolar ridge augmentation. Implant Dent 2005;14(2):131–8.

33. Xu R, Ebraheim NA, Yeasting RA, et al. Anatomic considerations for posterior iliac bone harvesting. Spine 1996;21(9):1017–20.

34. Colterjohn NR, Bednar DA. Procurement of bone graft from the iliac crest. an operative approach with decreased morbidity. J Bone Joint Surg Am 1997;79(5):756–9.

35. Kolomvos N, Iatrou I, Theologie-Lygidakis N, et al. Iliac crest morbidity following maxillofacial bone grafting in children: a clinical and radiographic prospective study. J Craniomaxillofac Surg 2010;38(4):293–302.

36. Ahlmann E, Patzakis M, Roidis N, et al. Comparison of anterior and posterior iliac crest bone grafts in terms of harvest-site morbidity and functional outcomes. J Bone Joint Surg Am 2002;84(5):716–20.

37. Bruno BJ, Gustafson PA. Cranial bone harvest, grafting. AORN J 1994;59(1):242–51.

38. Iizuka T, Smolka W, Hallermann W, et al. Extensive augmentation of the alveolar ridge using autogenous calvarial split bone grafts for dental

rehabilitation. Clin Oral Implants Res 2004;15(5):607–15.

39. Gutta R, Waite PD. Cranial bone grafting and simultaneous implants: a submental technique to reconstruct the atrophic mandible. Br J Oral Maxillofac Surg 2008;46(6):477–9.

40. Burchardt H, Enneking WF. Transplantation of bone. Surg Clin North Am 1978;58(2):403–27.

41. Ozkan Y, Ozcan M, Varol A, et al. Resonance frequency analysis assessment of implant stability in labial onlay grafted posterior mandibles: a pilot clinical study. Int J Oral Maxillofac Implants 2007;22(2):235–42.

42. Scheerlinck LME, Muradin MSM, van der Bilt A, et al. Donor site complications in bone grafting: comparison of iliac crest, calvarial, and mandibular ramus bone. Int J Oral Maxillofac Implants 2013;28(1):222–7.

43. Araújo PPT, Oliveira KP, Montenegro SCL, et al. Block allograft for reconstruction of alveolar bone ridge in implantology. Implant Dent 2013;22(3):304–8.

44. Simion M, Rocchietta I, Dellavia C. Three-dimensional ridge augmentation with xenograft and recombinant human platelet-derived growth factor-BB in humans: report of two cases. Int J Periodontics Restorative Dent 2007;27(2):109–15.

45. Waasdorp J, Reynolds MA. Allogeneic bone onlay grafts for alveolar ridge augmentation: a systematic review. Int J Oral Maxillofac Implants 2010;25(3):525–31.

46. Baker RD, Terry BC, Davis WH, et al. Long-term results of alveolar ridge augmentation. J Oral Surg 1979;37(7):486–9.

47. Sbordone C, Toti P, Guidetti F, et al. Volume changes of iliac crest autogenous bone grafts after vertical and horizontal alveolar ridge augmentation of atrophic maxillas and mandibles: a 6-year computerized tomographic follow-up. J Oral Maxillofac Surg 2012;70(11):2559–65.

48. Proussaefs P, Lozada J. The use of intraorally harvested autogenous block grafts for vertical alveolar ridge augmentation: a human study. Int J Periodontics Restorative Dent 2005;25(4):351–63.

49. Khojasteh A, Soheilifar S, Mohajerani H, et al. The effectiveness of barrier membranes on bone regeneration in localized bony defects: a systematic review. Int J Oral Maxillofac Implants 2013;28(4):1076–89.

50. Khojasteh A, Behnia H, Soleymani Shayesteh Y, et al. Localized bone augmentation with cortical bone blocks tented over different particulate bone substitutes: a retrospective study. Int J Oral Maxillofac Implants 2012;27(6):1481–93.

51. Heller AL, Heller RL, Cook G, et al. Soft tissue management techniques for implant dentistry: a clinical guide. J Oral Implantol 2000;26(2):91–103.

52. Davies JE, Ajami E, Moineddin R, et al. The roles of different scale ranges of surface implant topography on the stability of the bone/implant interface. Biomaterials 2013;34(14):3535–46.

53. Pogrel MA, Podlesh S, Anthony JP, et al. A comparison of vascularized and nonvascularized bone grafts for reconstruction of mandibular continuity defects. J Oral Maxillofac Surg 1997;55(11): 1200–6.

54. Rowan M, Lee D, Pi-Anfruns J, et al. Mechanical versus biological stability of immediate and delayed implant placement using resonance frequency analysis. J Oral Maxillofac Surg 2015;73(2):253–7.

55. Liu Y, Enggist L, Kuffer AF, et al. Erratum to "The influence of BMP-2 and its mode of delivery on the osteoconductivity of implant surfaces during the early phase of osseointegration" [Biomaterials 28 (2007) 2677–2686]. Biomaterials 2007;28(35):5399.

56. Albrektsson T, Dahl E, Enbom L, et al. Osseointegrated oral implants. J Periodontol 1988;59(5):287–96.

57. Tawil G, Aboujaoude N, Younan R. Influence of prosthetic parameters on the survival and complication rates of short implants. Int J Oral Maxillofac Implants 2006;21(2):275–82.

58. Lemos CAA, Ferro-Alves ML, Okamoto R, et al. Short dental implants versus standard dental implants placed in the posterior jaws: a systematic review and meta-analysis. J Dent 2016;47:8–17.

59. Anitua E, Alkhraist M, Piñas L, et al. Implant survival and crestal bone loss around extra-short implants supporting a fixed denture: the effect of crown height space, crown-to-implant ratio, and offset placement of the prosthesis. Int J Oral Maxillofac Implants 2014;29(3):682–9.

60. Jensen OT, Greer RO, Johnson L, et al. Vertical guided bonegraft augmentation in a new canine mandibular model. Implant Dent 1996;5(1):59.

61. Jensen OT. Alveolar segmental "sandwich" osteotomies for posterior edentulous mandibular sites for dental implants. J Oral Maxillofac Surg 2006;64(3): 471–5.

62. Laurie SWS, Kaban LB, Mulliken JB, et al. Donor-site morbidity after harvesting rib and iliac bone. Plast Reconstr Surg 1984;73(6):933–8.

63. Ilizarov GA. The tension-stress effect on the genesis and growth of tissues. Clin Orthop Relat Res 1989;(238):249–81.

64. Rachmiel A, Laufer D, Jackson IT, et al. Midface membranous bone lengthening: a one-year histological and morphological follow-up of distraction osteogenesis. Calcif Tissue Int 1998;62(4):370–6.

65. Rachmiel A, Leiser Y. The molecular and cellular events that take place during craniofacial distraction osteogenesis. Plast Reconstr Surg Glob Open 2014; 2(1):e98.

66. Rachmiel A, Rozen N, Peled M, et al. Characterization of midface maxillary membranous bone formation during distraction osteogenesis. Plast Reconstr Surg 2002;109(5):1611–20.

67. McCarthy JG, Schreiber J, Karp N, et al. Lengthening the human mandible by gradual distraction. Plast Reconstr Surg 1992;89(1):1–8.

68. McAllister BS. Histologic and radiographic evidence of vertical ridge augmentation utilizing distraction osteogenesis: 10 consecutively placed distractors. J Periodontol 2001;72(12):1767–79.

69. McAllister BS, Gaffaney TE. Distraction osteogenesis for vertical bone augmentation prior to oral implant reconstruction. Periodontol 2000 2003;33(1):54–66.

70. Rachmiel A, Emodi O, Aizenbud D, et al. Two-stage reconstruction of the severely deficient alveolar ridge: bone graft followed by alveolar distraction osteogenesis. Int J Oral Maxillofac Surg 2018;47(1): 117–24.

71. Rachmiel A, Shilo D, Aizenbud D, et al. Three-dimensional reconstruction of post-traumatic deficient anterior maxilla. J Oral Maxillofac Surg 2017; 75(12):2689–700.

72. Ugurlu F, Sener BC, Dergin G, et al. Potential complications and precautions in vertical alveolar distraction osteogenesis: a retrospective study of 40 patients. J Craniomaxillofac Surg 2013;41(7): 569–73.

73. Rachmiel A, Srouji S, Peled M. Alveolar ridge augmentation by distraction osteogenesis. Int J Oral Maxillofac Surg 2001;30(6):510–7.

74. Jensen OT, Cockrell R, Kuhike L, et al. Anterior maxillary alveolar distraction osteogenesis: a prospective 5-year clinical study. Int J Oral Maxillofac Implants 2002;17(1):52–68.

75. Jensen OT, Ueda M, Laster Z, et al. Alveolar distraction osteogenesis. Quintessence; 2002.

76. Keestra JAJ, Barry O, Jong LD, et al. Long-term effects of vertical bone augmentation: a systematic review. J Appl Oral Sci 2016;24(1): 3–17.

77. Kim J-W, Cho M-H, Kim S-J, et al. Alveolar distraction osteogenesis versus autogenous onlay bone graft for vertical augmentation of severely atrophied alveolar ridges after 12 years of long-term follow-up. Oral Surg Oral Med Oral Pathol Oral Radiol 2013; 116(5):540–9.

78. Saulacic N, Zix J, Iizuka T. Complication rates and associated factors in alveolar distraction osteogenesis: a comprehensive review. Int J Oral Maxillofac Surg 2009;38(3):210–7.

79. Elnayef B, Porta C, del Amo F, et al. The fate of lateral ridge augmentation: a systematic review and meta-analysis. Int J Oral Maxillofac Implants 2018;33(3):622–35.

Biomimetic Enhancement of Bone Graft Reconstruction

Tara L. Aghaloo, DDS, MD, PhD[a],*, Ethan Tencati, BTech, ME[b],
Danny Hadaya, DDS[b]

KEYWORDS

- Bone grafting • Biomimetic enhancement • Scaffolds • Growth factors • Bone augmentation

KEY POINTS

- Bone augmentation procedures are commonly used by practicing clinicians to facilitate oral rehabilitation with dental implant.
- A variety of biomaterials are available for clinical use, each with a specific set of properties that help define their use.
- Here, we describe the clinical application and use of these biomaterials, while focusing on the properties of platelet-rich fibrin (PRF), growth factors, and other scaffolds.

INTRODUCTION

Dental implants are commonly used for the oral rehabilitation of individuals with missing teeth. With an aging population with compromised teeth due to caries and periodontal disease, the use of dental implants becomes an alternative for those seeking tooth replacement.[1] Similarly, treating the partially or fully edentulous aging patient presents unique challenges that are being overcome with various technological advances. Given the aging population, there has been a dramatic increase in the demand for dental implants, with prevalence potentially reaching 23% by 2026.[2] Unfortunately, placing implants in aging patients can be challenging because of bone atrophy, particularly in the posterior maxilla, and diminished healing capacity owing to natural aging and more medically compromised patients.[3] As a result, these patients often require various augmentation procedures before implant placement; despite augmentation procedures, implant failures can still occur.[4] Whereas failure rates may seem insignificant, their incidence following augmentation procedures is likely underreported in the literature. The above factors have led many clinicians to search for ways to ensure greater success of the implants they place, particularly following grafting procedures.

Although autogenous bone-grafting material is considered the gold standard, a substitute that mimics the material's osteoconductive, osteogenic, and osteoinductive properties without the increased morbidity due to a second surgical site is highly sought after.[5] Accordingly, some researchers have shifted their focus toward designing graft materials and protocols that mimic the body's natural structure and elicit natural responses. This type of shift has been a recent trend within much of science and medicine, and is broadly termed biomimetics, which is the understanding of principles of underlying mechanisms through the study of natural phenomena, using nature to obtain new ideas.[6] Although biomimetic

Disclosure Statement: This work was supported, in part, by a Peter Geistlich Research Award from the Osteo Science Foundation.

[a] Section of Oral and Maxillofacial Surgery, Division of Diagnostic and Surgical Sciences, UCLA School of Dentistry, 10833 Le Conte Avenue, CHS Room 53-009, Los Angeles, CA 90095, USA; [b] UCLA School of Dentistry, 10833 Le Conte Avenue, CHS Room 53-076, Los Angeles, CA 90095-1668, USA
* Corresponding author.
E-mail address: taghaloo@dentistry.ucla.edu

Oral Maxillofacial Surg Clin N Am 31 (2019) 193–205
https://doi.org/10.1016/j.coms.2018.12.001
1042-3699/19/© 2018 Elsevier Inc. All rights reserved.

solutions to enhance bone grafts are often relatively safe and less invasive, many clinicians are quickly adopting them into practice without extensive literature support.[7] Here, we discuss these biomimetic solutions and highlight how a true consensus is yet to exist in the literature, as well as present some novel biomimetic concepts that could be incorporated into clinical practice in the future.

PLATELET-RICH FIBRINS
Early Platelet Concentrates

For decades, platelet concentrates have attracted much attention in many surgical fields with the promise of decreased bleeding and swelling at the surgical site, in conjunction with decreased wound healing times.[5,8] Multiple growth factors (GFs) in platelet concentrates, which promote angiogenesis, increased vascularity, enhanced fibroblast proliferation, subsequent collagen synthesis, extracellular matrix production, and endothelial cell proliferation, are released when degranulation of platelet α-granules occurs. As such, incorporating these platelet concentrates into surgical practice for improved biomimetic tissue regeneration is highly desirable.[5,8,9] Although use of platelet concentrates initially began in the 1990s with the introduction of platelet-rich plasma (PRP), these required non-autogenous components to induce platelet degranulation, such as thrombin and calcium chloride, and could take several hours to prepare. These factors limited the appeal of PRP and its incorporation into daily practice. Of note, although early studies showed promising results, later studies involving PRP have shown that it has little effect on bone

formation.[8,10] These conflicting results bring the clinical use of PRP into question. More recently, however, platelet-rich fibrin (PRF) has been gaining popularity as it overcomes these issues.[11]

Platelet-Rich Fibrin Protocols

Although the formation of the clot used in PRF is relatively simple and requires only whole blood and a centrifuge, various centrifuges and centrifugation methods exist.[12] The standard PRF centrifugation protocol, first described by Choukroun and termed leukocyte-rich PRF (L-PRF), requires centrifugation at 2700 rpm (750 g) for 12 minutes[12–15] (**Fig. 1**). Recently, however, there has been a shift toward using protocols that require a lower rpm because this method is believed to cause less damage to the platelets and cellular component of the PRF, and more leukocytes, especially neutrophilic granulocytes, are retained in the fibrin matrix of the clot.[15] The addition of the neutrophilic granulocytes influences bone and soft tissue regeneration because they can contribute to the increased differentiation of monocytes to macrophages.[15] The most popular and well-studied of these protocols is termed advanced PRF (A-PRF) and requires centrifugation at 1300 rpm (200 g) for 14 minutes.[15,16] In addition to reducing the rpm, reducing the centrifugation duration has also shown promising results. A recent study that used 1300 rpm for only 8 minutes, called advanced PRF and time (A-PRF+), demonstrated even greater release of GFs than both L-PRF and A-PRF.[16] Even more recently, an injectable form of PRF (i-PRF) has been developed that requires centrifugation at 700 rpm (60 g) for 3 minutes (**Fig. 2**). Although i-PRF shows promise

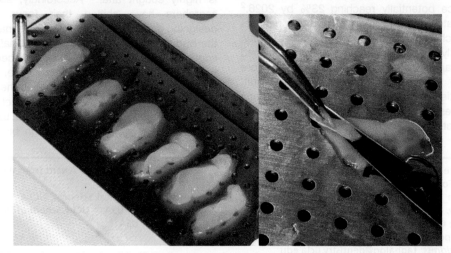

Fig. 1. PRF membrane. Platelet-rich fibrin is commonly used as a membrane to potentially enhance wound healing.

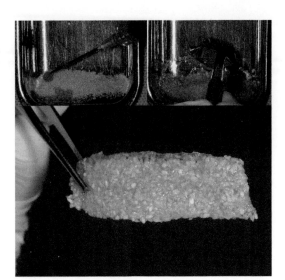

Fig. 2. "Sticky Bone." PRF is also combined with particulate bone to make a more solidified bone graft construct that can be used for many hard tissue augmentation techniques.

for treating temporomandibular joint disorders, almost no clinical research has been carried out on the topic. These PRF protocols are summarized in **Table 1**.

In addition, there is some evidence to suggest that increased levels of undesirable centrifuge vibration can cause diminished levels of GF activity of the PRF clot owing to the destruction of cell populations. A recent study of 4 different centrifuge systems (Intra-spin, A-PRF 12, Salvin 1301, and LW-UPD8) concluded that the Intra-spin centrifuge system produced 4.5 to 6 times less vibration and remained under the resonance threshold, unlike the other 3 machines.[17]

Clinical Applications and Evidence

Clinically, PRF has a variety of applications centered on attempts to improve bone and soft

tissue healing and formation; however, idence to support these notions exists rich fibrin, although not an occlusive m has been used by some to cover def retain graft material (**Fig. 3**); similarly, it has been used as a scaffold for other biologics, as well as a direct application in sites of augmentation or to the surface of an endosseous implant[11,18–23] (**Fig. 4**). Studies have supported its use for a wide range of potential clinical applications including: prevention of infection at the surgical site[24]; reduction of post-extraction socket healing time and complications[25,26]; post-extraction hemostasis[27]; reduction of post-operative hematoma[28]; reconstruction following cyst enucleation and tumor excision; and as an adjunct to palatal wound treatment or alveolar cleft treatment.[29,30] However, evidence remains scant and clinical trials are required to investigate whether these applications are clinically relevant. Platelet-rich fibrin can also be used in the following ways: as an easy-to-suture membrane to cover, protect, and promote re-epithelialization[31]; during sinus augmentation procedures,[32] including as the sole filling material; as a resorbable membrane over an occlusive membrane for soft tissue healing[22,33,34]; in the treatment of peri-implant defects[35–37]; and to improve wound healing in diabetic and immunocompromised patients.[38] In addition, it has been noted that, although no known contraindications for the use of PRF exist,[38] patients receiving anti-coagulation medications can experience significant challenges in formation of the PRF clot.

Whereas PRF shows promise in a variety of applications, and seems to be safe, it has yet to be shown as efficacious in many human clinical studies. Of the evidence that does exist, there is a distinct lack of studies conducted with large numbers of participants and longer follow-up

Table 1
PRF protocols

Protocol	Speed (rpm)	Force (g)	Time (min)	Advantages
L-PRF	2700	750	12	High release of GFs
A-PRF	1300	200	14	Higher release of GFs
A-PRF+	1300	200	8	Highest release of GFs
i-PRF	700	60	3	Injectable

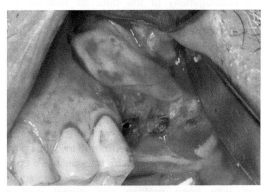

Fig. 3. PRF membrane can be used to cover a bone graft, but is not an occlusive membrane. It can be used over an occlusive collagen membrane to enhance soft tissue wound healing.

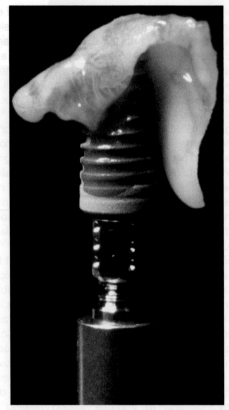

Fig. 4. PRF over the surface of an implant. New applications for PRF membranes are occurring regularly. In this example, it is being placed over an implant for placement in a prepared osteotomy site.

times. Although a recent systematic review did show significantly improved treatment outcomes for use of PRF in sinus elevation, alveolar ridge preservation, and implant therapy, where improved implant stability and less marginal bone loss over time were observed,[22,35,36] meta-analysis could not be performed due in part to the heterogeneity of the data as well as the extremely small sample size from few studies.[32] There are, however, some isolated studies that show modest results. For example, 1 study of 20 patients used resonance frequency measurements to determine implant stability 1 month after implant placement with L-PRF. Mean implant stabilities were 77.1 ± 7.1 for the L-PRF group and 70.5 ± 7.7 for the control.[12] Thus, although the results show promise, the extremely small study size and the fact that this was performed in isolation by no means allows clinicians to draw definitive conclusions on the efficacy of PRF for use in conjunction with bone grafting and dental implant placement.

Although the clinical efficacy of PRF may be poorly characterized, its ability to induce osteogenesis in animal models and in vitro has been the focus of more research. The PRF clot is not uniform in its distribution, with higher concentration of platelets, cytokines, and leukocytes existing toward the red blood cell end of the clot.[39] This likely explains why others have found that low-speed protocols are better at increasing the levels of leukocytes present in the clot.[15,16] Even without the presence of leukocytes, GFs released by the platelets themselves is believed to be one of their primary mechanisms of action. Growth factors commonly found in PRF include: transforming growth factor beta; platelet-derived growth factor; basis fibroblast growth factor; epidermal growth factor; vascular endothelial growth factor; and connective tissue growth factor.[40,41] These GFs, present in the clot, have been shown to induce the migration, differentiation, and proliferation of many different cell types implicated in bone and soft tissue regeneration, including; mesenchymal stem cells and human umbilical vein endothelial cells, osteoblasts, keratinocytes, fibroblasts, and macrophages.[15,42–45]

Likewise, animal studies have shown promise in increasing osseointegration, particularly during the early stages of healing.[22] In particular, PRF used in the treatment of peri-implant defects and during implant placement surgery have shown increased rates of new bone formation as well as an increase in the mean bone-to-implant contact.[22,37] One study performed with a rabbit model showed significant increases in new bone formation and bone-to-implant contact (31.7% versus 12.1% and 52.6% versus 36.0%, respectively) after 1 week when compared with a nil-treatment control. However, by the fourth week, this difference diminished and the differences in new bone formation and bone-to-implant contact were less impressive (39.9% versus 26.4% and 54.6% versus 39.0%, respectively).[22] Similar findings have been reported by other studies.[37] Although PRF has not yet been shown to have a significant effect on bone regeneration,[22,37] its ability to improve soft tissue regeneration leading to rapid wound closures in clinical settings has been well documented.[34]

GROWTH FACTORS
Current Use of Growth Factors

Although researchers are aware of many different GFs, few are currently used, or are proposed to be used, for bone grafting, especially in the oral environment.[46] Within the field of implant dentistry, the most popular and well-studied GFs are recombinant human bone morphogenetic protein-2 (rhBMP-2) and recombinant human platelet-derived growth factor-BB (rhPDGF-BB).[47,48] Other GFs currently under investigation include recombinant human growth/differentiation-5 and rhBMP-7.[47,49,50] All of these GFs function, in one capacity or another, as osteoinductive agents, causing the growth, recruitment, differentiation, and maturation of primitive stem cells or immature bone cells to form healthy bone tissue.[51] Interestingly, although perhaps the most osteoinductive GF, rhBMPs are not mitogenic for many cells and cell types.[46] Nevertheless, the osteoinductive capability of rhBMPs, especially rhBMP-2, is well documented[52–54] (**Fig. 5**).

The use of rhBMP-2 shows much potential for use in many applications within implant dentistry, particularly within alveolar ridge augmentation and preservation, maxillary sinus augmentation, and peri-implant defect repair, and this subject has been the focus of a large amount of research, both clinically and pre-clinically.[55] Notwithstanding this research, however, as is the case with all GFs, effectively delivering rhBMP-2 to the desired location for the required time proves challenging and causes the efficacy of its use to vary considerably. As such, carriers are frequently studied in depth, and the ideal carrier has not been developed for each specific indication.

Growth Factor Carrier Scaffolds

The use of an absorbable collagen sponge (ACS) has been the primary method of delivering rhBMP-2 since it was first approved by the US Food and Drug Administration for spinal fusion in 2002, and then in 2004 for open tibia fracture repair.[56] In 2007, rhBMP-2/ACS was then approved for use in bone augmentation, both in conjugation with tooth extraction sockets and the maxillary sinus, to permit the placement of an osseointegrated dental implant for the rehabilitation of edentulous or partially edentulous patients.[55] Since then, many other scaffolds have been developed and they are used in various dental applications. These include: allogeneic bone grafts; inorganic matrices (hydroxyapatite, β-tricalcium-phosphate, and bioglasses) and polymeric materials (collagen, polytetrafluoroethylene-expanded, polylactic acid, polyglycolic acid, polylactic-polyglycolic acid, polyethylene glycol, polycaprolactone, and composite scaffolds).[57] Although many of these scaffolds show promise for the delivery of GFs, few of these materials have been studied due to the infancy of the use of GFs in implant dentistry. As a result of the limited clinical trials using these novel scaffolds, there is no established safety record and their clinical use is minimal. Aside from the ACS, the only other well-studied carrier scaffold for GFs used in implant dentistry is polylactic-polyglycolic acid (PLGA) (**Fig. 6**), which can be precisely manipulated through 3D printing.[58–61] Of note, polyethylene glycol and polycaprolactone, which are currently used as carriers of polypeptides and mesenchymal stem cells, could also likely be

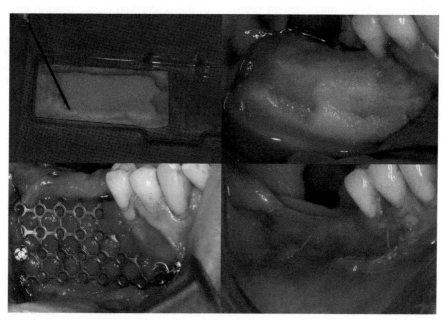

Fig. 5. rhBMP-2 for localized alveolar ridge augmentation. rhBMP-2 on an absorbable collagen sponge (ACS) can be used to increase alveolar bone height and width, but often needs structural support such as a titanium mesh.

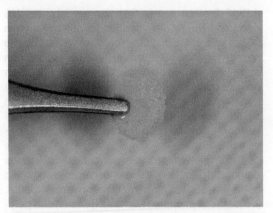

Fig. 6. PLGA scaffold. This PLGA scaffold is fabricated to fit perfectly into an in vivo experimental calvarial defect.

used as carriers of GFs but they are not well-studied and have very long resorption times.[30,61,62]

One novel scaffold carrier of rhBMP-2 that shows a great deal of promise is the use of a biomimetic heparin hydrogel[63] (**Fig. 7**). Although rhBMP-2 has demonstrated excellent potential for bone formation and repair, the rapid release of rhBMP-2 from an ACS carrier has been shown to possibly lead to many undesirable and unpredictable outcomes, such as osteoclastic bone resorption, soft tissue swelling, inappropriate adipogenesis, and ectopic bone formation.[64–71] Despite these undesirable and unpredictable outcomes, however, biomimetic heparin hydrogels, which are still in their infancy, may solve the problem of premature rhBMP-2 release by creating a hydrogel surface that mimics heparin using heparin-mimicking sulfonated molecules, which stabilizes rhBMP-2. These biomimetic heparin hydrogels also have the added benefit of being photo-crosslinkable allowing for precise control of placement by the clinician.[63] Since GFs are still relatively new to clinical and especially oral and maxillofacial applications, much work still needs

to be done to identify the ideal carrier for optimized bone healing and regeneration. Significant research is ongoing and will be necessary before widespread clinical use will occur.

Clinical Applications and Evidence

Unlike PRF, several systematic reviews exist, including human clinical trials, demonstrating that rhBMP-2 is an extremely powerful osteoinductive agent in vitro and in vivo.[47,53,72,73] However, a systematic review of 63 articles of animal studies concluded that there is great variation in carriers for delivery, experimental sites, and evaluation methods.[47] In another systematic review and meta-analysis on GF treatments for implant-based bone grafts, the authors concluded that, although there was initially an increase in new bone formation, after 3 years no statistically significant difference existed for implant survival between the GF treatment and control groups, leaving the indications for such bioactive compounds in question.[73] In a further systematic review and meta-analysis that included 8 articles, the use of rhBMP-2 for maxillary sinus and alveolar ridge augmentation was investigated. Interestingly, although the study concluded in favor of the use of rhBMP-2 for localized alveolar ridge augmentation, it found that, when used for maxillary sinus floor augmentation, rhBMP-2 produced inferior results when compared with the control group.[53] The findings of these systematic reviews highlight the need for more research with larger studies and better characterization of the impact of the scaffolding carrier used in its delivery. To emphasize this, a novel study with rhBMP-2 compared the use of hydroxyapatite with bovine-derived xenograft as the carrier. Both carriers were effective in augmenting the alveolar ridge, but rhBMP-2 with the hydroxyapatite carrier seemed to be more beneficial for use in complicated alveolar ridge defects[54] (**Fig. 8**).

Limited human clinical studies have also been performed using rhPDGF-BB. One such study of

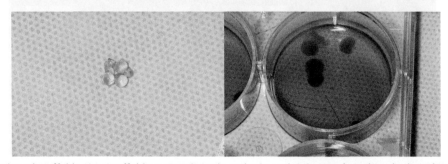

Fig. 7. Hydrogel scaffolds. New scaffolds are consistently under investigation, such as these hydrogels to enhance bone formation in an in vivo experimental defect.

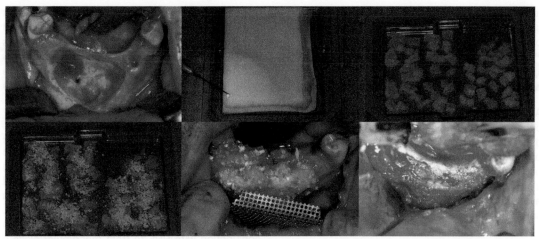

Fig. 8. rhBMP-2 large defect. After removal of a central giant cell granuloma, a combination of rhBMP-2/ACS and mineralized allograft were used to regenerate the mandibular alveolar ridge after 7 months healing.

34 patients found that, after 4 months of recovery, the mean percent remaining of the mineralized allograft was significantly less in the group treated with rhPDGF-BB and had greater bone formation in the test group (41.8% versus 32.5%).[74] Another study of 8 patients found that using rhPDGF-BB along with xenograft material combined with tenting screws to support a resorbable membrane over the graft site led to the formation of vital bone and residual graft particles, which was similar in both treatment and control groups.[75] A novel study was also conducted in dogs to determine the difference between a commercially available rhPDGF-BB formulation coating and a prototype viscous rhPDGF-BB coating that was applied to dental implants before placement. However, after 6 weeks, the commercially available coating was found to have more trabecular bone and higher bone-in-contact to both the prototype viscous coating and the uncoated control.[48] Similar to the case of rhBMP-2, this perhaps demonstrates that the delivery method is an integral part of using GFs to augment bone

grafts and should be an area of focus of future research.[76] Unfortunately, however, the cost of most GFs is high, which has caused its use in clinical practice and research to be limited.

ABSORBABLE COLLAGEN SPONGE

The porous ACS is currently the gold standard scaffold used to support a wide array of biomimetic molecules, such as those discussed above, and is well established in the literature. Collagen has gained popularity as a scaffold because of its biocompatibility, biodegradability, and ability to enhance cellular penetration to form an extracellular matrix material.[77] However, an understanding of the relationship between the scaffold material and the drug to be delivered, as well as the way in which the drug will be delivered, is crucial. Just as drug molecules differ from one another, so too will the way in which they are retained and released by the ACS (**Fig. 9**). Therefore, although the use of the ACS is still prominent, modifications and adjuncts to its use, as well as

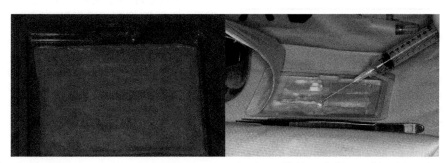

Fig. 9. Absorbable collagen sponge. This ACS is the most simple scaffold available, and has been shown to bind rhBMP-2, with a working time of 15 to 120 minutes.

replacements, are frequently studied because drug delivery is of critical importance when placing biomimetic grafting materials.[76]

NOVEL BIOMIMETIC GRAFTING MATERIALS AND SCAFFOLDS

Autogenous bone-grafting material has long been considered the gold standard because of its osteoconductive, osteogenic, and osteoinductive properties.[5] However, its use is frequently avoided because of its increased morbidity associated with a second surgical site.[78] As a result, xenograft and allograft materials are currently preferred for most surgical procedures. However, these materials only function as osteoconductive scaffolds.[78] Whereas some synthetic graft materials are commercially available, their osteoconductive properties and predictable remodeling and bone formation is not well documented. As such, novel biomimetic scaffold materials are a popular field of research with the goal of developing a material that better mimics the properties of native bone. Some of these newer biomimetic materials are discussed below. Although many of them have yet to reach clinical practice, research continues as clinicians and researchers search for the ideal bone-grafting material.

Marine Sponge

The collagen structure of marine sponges has been proven to be an effective framework to support a wide range of cells and tissues.[79,80] The type IV collagen matrix of the sponge possesses significant vital structural and biochemical cues that allow for the support and maintenance of bone.[81] This has culminated in the development of a biomimetic-engineered tissue matrix using silica, chitin, and collagens from the marine sponge.[82] Although, as of yet, no animal or clinical studies have been completed, as this field matures it could be applied to bone graft regeneration.

Nacre

Nacre, the inner lining of the shell from the giant oyster *Pinctada maxima*, otherwise known as mother of pearl, has shown great promise as a resorbable biomimetic graft material.[83] It has been repeatedly shown to be a natural osteoinductive bone substitute with strong effects on osteoprogenitors, osteoblasts, and osteoclasts during bone tissue formation and morphogenesis.[79,81,84] Nacre has also been shown to possess many other qualities as a potential graft material, including being biocompatible and biodegradable.[84] Its proposed uses include being used to

offer mechanical support in load-bearing defect sites and to fill large bone defects in unloaded bone defects.[84] Although most of the literature is relatively recent, 1 early human clinical study of 8 patients from 1997 showed that powered nacre could be used to successfully reconstruct defects of the maxillary alveolar ridge.[83]

Bioactive Ceramic Composite Granules

Bioactive ceramic composite granules have been proposed for use as a scaffold for bone grafting and tissue engineering, as well as a carrier scaffold for drug delivery.[61,85] As of yet, this concept has gained little traction within implant dentistry. Currently, its use has been demonstrated in conjunction with PRF to treat mandibular class II furcation defects, but it may be applied to other areas of dentistry in the future.[86]

Bioactive Glass

Originally developed in the 1960s, surface reactive glass ceramics composed of calcium sodium phosphosilicates, which naturally occur in various forms in the body, have been attracting more attention in recent years owing to their potential applications in implant dentistry.[87,88] There are many features of bioactive glass, including proven biocompatibility and the capacity to act as a rapid biomimetic mineralizer through osteoconductive and osteostimulatory properties.[89] Although there are still few clinical studies, bioactive glass has shown some satisfactory results as a grafting material for use in maxillary sinus augmentation and alveolar ridge augmentation surgeries.[90]

Calcium Phosphate Granules Coprecipitated with rhBMP-2

Calcium phosphate granules coprecipitated with rhBMP-2, and used in conjunction with deproteinized bovine bone, have been shown to bring osteoinductive properties to the deproteinized bovine bone material.[90] This novel osteoinducer is formed by biomimetically assembling calcium phosphate, layer by layer, and coprecipitating rhBMP-2 into the calcium phosphate granules. Calcium phosphate granules, coprecipitated with rhBMP-2, have been successfully tested as a potent osteoinducer in the repair of critical-sized bone defects in sheep.[91] With further research and maturation of this technology, it may have applications in implant dentistry for bone reconstruction in the future.

Modified Biphasic Graft Materials

In recent years, biphasic calcium phosphate materials have been ever more frequently used in dental applications for use as a scaffolding carrier for drug delivery. In the case of implant dentistry, a biphasic material containing hydroxyapatite and tricalcium phosphate can be used as a bone-grafting material. Augmenting this material with PLGA has been shown to improve the volume of bone formed and prevent bone migration into undesired locations.[92] This novel biphasic material could prove to be the subject of more investigation as the use of rhPDGF-BB coated onto β-tricalcium phosphate for use in periodontal intraosseous defects has also been more thoroughly investigated with promising initial results.[93] It is, therefore, conceivable that the use of a biphasic material with PLGA could prove to be more efficacious than the β-tricalcium phosphate alone.

Biomimetic Synthetic Oligopeptide Surface Modification

Biomimetic surface modification of a scaffold with a synthetic oligopeptide has been proposed in several studies as a means to deliver oligopeptides that correspond to various cell-surface receptors, such as BMP receptor I and BMP receptor II.[94] Earlier studies used a 15-residue peptide from the α-1 chain of type I collagen, which uniquely bound to osteoblasts at BMP receptor I and BMP receptor II.[95] The 15-residue peptide from the α-1 chain of type I collagen proved to be effective at enhancing bone regeneration in both calvarial defects in rabbits, and in L-shaped defects in the edentulous alveolar ridge of beagle dogs.[96,97] Most recently, a unique oligopeptide sequence taken from BMPs that corresponds to the BMP receptor I and BMP receptor II domains, and contains the amino acid sequence DWIVA, was used to enhance bone regeneration in 1-wall intrabony defects in beagles.[94]

SUMMARY

With an aging population and increasing case complexity, bone graft reconstruction before the placement of dental implants is becoming a more prevalent practice that presents a variety of unique challenges. The budding field of biomimetics offers many new ideas and techniques to overcome these challenges. Several of these biomimetic techniques are very alluring, to both patients and clinicians alike, as they can often be performed as simple, relatively safe, cost-effective modifications of existing, well-understood procedures. As many of these procedures and techniques, such as PRF and the use of GFs, continue to become mainstream, more literature to determine their efficacy will no doubt surface. Until that time, however, the modern clinician must exercise caution as

there is relatively little literature available to support many of these procedures as they quickly become incorporated into routine clinical practice. The recent interest in biomimetics has also seen the development of many new and novel bone-grafting materials. Although these bone-grafting materials are still in their infancy, the literature has demonstrated promising initial results and more research is needed. As bone-grafting technology continues to develop, some of these new materials may begin to become incorporated into practice. However, similar to currently used biomimetic techniques, the prudent clinician should be cautious until their use has been better established in the literature.

REFERENCES

1. Rozier RG, White BA, Slade GD. Trends in oral diseases in the U.S. population. J Dent Educ 2017; 81(8):eS97–109.
2. Elani HW, Starr JR, Da Silva JD, et al. Trends in dental implant use in the U.S., 1999–2016, and projections to 2026. J Dent Res 2018;97(13):1424–30.
3. Ting M, Rice JG, Braid SM, et al. Maxillary sinus augmentation for dental implant rehabilitation of the edentulous ridge: a comprehensive overview of systematic reviews. Implant Dent 2017;26(3): 438–64.
4. Starch-Jensen T, Aludden H, Hallman M, et al. A systematic review and meta-analysis of long-term studies (five or more years) assessing maxillary sinus floor augmentation. Int J Oral Maxillofac Surg 2018;47(1):103–16.
5. Aghaloo TL, Hadaya D. Basic principles of bioengineering and regeneration. Oral Maxillofac Surg Clin North Am 2017;29(1):1–7.
6. Hwang J, Jeong Y, Park JM, et al. Biomimetics: forecasting the future of science, engineering, and medicine. Int J Nanomedicine 2015;10:5701–13.
7. Aghaloo TL, Mardirosian M, Delgado B. Controversies in implant surgery. Oral Maxillofac Surg Clin North Am 2017;29(4):525–35.
8. Marx RE, Carlson ER, Eichstaedt RM, et al. Platelet-rich plasma: growth factor enhancement for bone grafts. Oral Surg Oral Med Oral Pathol Oral Radiol Endod 1998;85(6):638–46.
9. Barrientos S, Stojadinovic O, Golinko MS, et al. Growth factors and cytokines in wound healing. Wound Repair Regen 2008;16(5):585–601.
10. Aghaloo TL, Moy PK, Freymiller EG. Investigation of platelet-rich plasma in rabbit cranial defects: a pilot study. J Oral Maxillofac Surg 2002;60(10):1176–81.
11. Simonpieri A, Del Corso M, Vervelle A, et al. Current knowledge and perspectives for the use of platelet-rich plasma (PRP) and platelet-rich fibrin (PRF) in oral and maxillofacial surgery part 2: Bone graft,

implant and reconstructive surgery. Curr Pharm Biotechnol 2012;13(7):1231–56.

12. Oncu E, Alaaddinoglu EE. The effect of platelet-rich fibrin on implant stability. Int J Oral Maxillofac Implants 2015;30(3):578–82.

13. Dohan Ehrenfest DM. How to optimize the preparation of leukocyte- and platelet-rich fibrin (L-PRF, Choukroun's technique) clots and membranes: introducing the PRF Box. Oral Surg Oral Med Oral Pathol Oral Radiol Endod 2010;110(3):275–8 [author reply: 278–80].

14. Dohan Ehrenfest DM, Bielecki T, Mishra A, et al. In search of a consensus terminology in the field of platelet concentrates for surgical use: platelet-rich plasma (PRP), platelet-rich fibrin (PRF), fibrin gel polymerization and leukocytes. Curr Pharm Biotechnol 2012;13(7):1131–7.

15. Ghanaati S, Booms P, Orlowska A, et al. Advanced platelet-rich fibrin: a new concept for cell-based tissue engineering by means of inflammatory cells. J Oral Implantol 2014;40(6):679–89.

16. Fujioka-Kobayashi M, Miron RJ, Hernandez M, et al. Optimized platelet-rich fibrin with the low-speed concept: growth factor release, biocompatibility, and cellular response. J Periodontol 2017;88(1):112–21.

17. Dohan Ehrenfest DM, Pinto NR, Pereda A, et al. The impact of the centrifuge characteristics and centrifugation protocols on the cells, growth factors, and fibrin architecture of a leukocyte- and platelet-rich fibrin (L-PRF) clot and membrane. Platelets 2018; 29(2):171–84.

18. Anitua E, Andia I, Ardanza B, et al. Autologous platelets as a source of proteins for healing and tissue regeneration. Thromb Haemost 2004;91(1):4–15.

19. Anitua E, Orive G, Pla R, et al. The effects of PRGF on bone regeneration and on titanium implant osseointegration in goats: a histologic and histomorphometric study. J Biomed Mater Res A 2009; 91(1):158–65.

20. Anitua EA. Enhancement of osseointegration by generating a dynamic implant surface. J Oral Implantol 2006;32(2):72–6.

21. Lourenco ES, Mourao C, Leite PEC, et al. The in vitro release of cytokines and growth factors from fibrin membranes produced through horizontal centrifugation. J Biomed Mater Res A 2018;106(5):1373–80.

22. Oncu E, Bayram B, Kantarci A, et al. Positive effect of platelet rich fibrin on osseointegration. Med Oral Patol Oral Cir Bucal 2016;21(5):e601–7.

23. Yilmaz D, Dogan N, Ozkan A, et al. Effect of platelet rich fibrin and beta tricalcium phosphate on bone healing. A histological study in pigs. Acta Cir Bras 2014;29(1):59–65.

24. Marenzi G, Riccitiello F, Tia M, et al. Influence of leukocyte- and platelet-rich fibrin (L-PRF) in the healing of simple postextraction sockets: a split-mouth study. Biomed Res Int 2015;2015:369273.

25. Hoaglin DR, Lines GK. Prevention of localized osteitis in mandibular third-molar sites using platelet-rich fibrin. Int J Dent 2013;2013:875380.

26. Yelamali T, Saikrishna D. Role of platelet rich fibrin and platelet rich plasma in wound healing of extracted third molar sockets: a comparative study. J Maxillofac Oral Surg 2015;14(2):410–6.

27. Dohan Ehrenfest DM, Rasmusson L, Albrektsson T. Classification of platelet concentrates: from pure platelet-rich plasma (P-PRP) to leucocyte- and platelet-rich fibrin (L-PRF). Trends Biotechnol 2009; 27(3):158–67.

28. Sammartino G, Dohan Ehrenfest DM, Carile F, et al. Prevention of hemorrhagic complications after dental extractions into open heart surgery patients under anticoagulant therapy: the use of leucocyte- and platelet-rich fibrin. J Oral Implantol 2011;37(6): 681–90.

29. Femminella B, Iaconi MC, Di Tullio M, et al. Clinical comparison of platelet-rich fibrin and a gelatin sponge in the management of palatal wounds after epithelialized free gingival graft harvest: a randomized clinical trial. J Periodontol 2016;87(2):103–13.

30. Jain RA. The manufacturing techniques of various drug loaded biodegradable poly(lactide-co-glycolide) (PLGA) devices. Biomaterials 2000;21(23):2475–90.

31. Eren G, Atilla G. Platelet-rich fibrin in the treatment of localized gingival recessions: a split-mouth randomized clinical trial. Clin Oral Investig 2014;18(8): 1941–8.

32. Castro AB, Meschi N, Temmerman A, et al. Regenerative potential of leucocyte- and platelet-rich fibrin. Part B: sinus floor elevation, alveolar ridge preservation and implant therapy. A systematic review. J Clin Periodontol 2017;44(2):225–34.

33. Choukroun J, Diss A, Simonpieri A, et al. Platelet-rich fibrin (PRF): a second-generation platelet concentrate. Part V: histologic evaluations of PRF effects on bone allograft maturation in sinus lift. Oral Surg Oral Med Oral Pathol Oral Radiol Endod 2006;101(3):299–303.

34. Choukroun J, Diss A, Simonpieri A, et al. Platelet-rich fibrin (PRF): a second-generation platelet concentrate. Part IV: clinical effects on tissue healing. Oral Surg Oral Med Oral Pathol Oral Radiol Endod 2006;101(3):e56–60.

35. Boora P, Rathee M, Bhoria M. Effect of platelet rich fibrin (PRF) on peri-implant soft tissue and crestal bone in one-stage implant placement: a randomized controlled trial. J Clin Diagn Res 2015;9(4):ZC18–21.

36. Hamzacebi B, Oduncuoglu B, Alaaddinoglu EE. Treatment of peri-implant bone defects with platelet-rich fibrin. Int J Periodontics Restorative Dent 2015;35(3):415–22.

37. Lee JW, Kim SG, Kim JY, et al. Restoration of a peri-implant defect by platelet-rich fibrin. Oral Surg Oral Med Oral Pathol Oral Radiol 2012;113(4):459–63.

38. Del Corso M, Vervelle A, Simonpieri A, et al. Current knowledge and perspectives for the use of platelet-rich plasma (PRP) and platelet-rich fibrin (PRF) in oral and maxillofacial surgery part 1: periodontal and dentoalveolar surgery. Curr Pharm Biotechnol 2012;13(7):1207–30.

39. Bai MY, Wang CW, Wang JY, et al. Three-dimensional structure and cytokine distribution of platelet-rich fibrin. Clinics (Sao Paulo) 2017;72(2): 116–24.

40. De Pascale MR, Sommese L, Casamassimi A, et al. Platelet derivatives in regenerative medicine: an update. Transfus Med Rev 2015;29(1):52–61.

41. Speth C, Rambach G, Wurzner R, et al. Complement and platelets: mutual interference in the immune network. Mol Immunol 2015;67(1):108–18.

42. Schar MO, Diaz-Romero J, Kohl S, et al. Platelet-rich concentrates differentially release growth factors and induce cell migration in vitro. Clin Orthop Relat Res 2015;473(5):1635–43.

43. Clipet F, Tricot S, Alno N, et al. In vitro effects of Choukroun's platelet-rich fibrin conditioned medium on 3 different cell lines implicated in dental implantology. Implant Dent 2012;21(1):51–6.

44. He L, Lin Y, Hu X, et al. A comparative study of platelet-rich fibrin (PRF) and platelet-rich plasma (PRP) on the effect of proliferation and differentiation of rat osteoblasts in vitro. Oral Surg Oral Med Oral Pathol Oral Radiol Endod 2009;108(5): 707–13.

45. Marcazzan S, Weinstein RL, Del Fabbro M. Efficacy of platelets in bone healing: a systematic review on animal studies. Platelets 2018;29(4):326–37.

46. Salata LA, Franke-Stenport V, Rasmusson L. Recent outcomes and perspectives of the application of bone morphogenetic proteins in implant dentistry. Clin Implant Dent Relat Res 2002;4(1):27–32.

47. Khojasteh A, Behnia H, Naghdi N, et al. Effects of different growth factors and carriers on bone regeneration: a systematic review. Oral Surg Oral Med Oral Pathol Oral Radiol 2013;116(6):e405–23.

48. Al-Hezaimi K, Nevins M, Kim SW, et al. Efficacy of growth factor in promoting early osseointegration. J Oral Implantol 2014;40(5):543–8.

49. Ayoub A, Roshan CP, Gillgrass T, et al. The clinical application of rhBMP-7 for the reconstruction of alveolar cleft. J Plast Reconstr Aesthet Surg 2016; 69(1):101–7.

50. Roldan JC, Jepsen S, Schmidt C, et al. Sinus floor augmentation with simultaneous placement of dental implants in the presence of platelet-rich plasma or recombinant human bone morphogenetic protein-7. Clin Oral Implants Res 2004;15(6): 716–23.

51. Bowler D, Dym H. Bone morphogenic protein: application in implant dentistry. Dent Clin North Am 2015; 59(2):493–503.

52. Freitas RM, Spin-Neto R, Marcantonio Junior E, et al. Alveolar ridge and maxillary sinus augmentation using rhBMP-2: a systematic review. Clin Implant Dent Relat Res 2015;17(Suppl 1):e192–201.

53. Kelly MP, Vaughn OL, Anderson PA. Systematic review and meta-analysis of recombinant human bone morphogenetic protein-2 in localized alveolar ridge and maxillary sinus augmentation. J Oral Maxillofac Surg 2016;74(5):928–39.

54. Nam JW, Khureltogtokh S, Choi HM, et al. Randomised controlled clinical trial of augmentation of the alveolar ridge using recombinant human bone morphogenetic protein 2 with hydroxyapatite and bovine-derived xenografts: comparison of changes in volume. Br J Oral Maxillofac Surg 2017;55(8):822–9.

55. Spagnoli DB, Marx RE. Dental implants and the use of rhBMP-2. Oral Maxillofac Surg Clin North Am 2011;23(2):347–61, vii.

56. McKay WF, Peckham SM, Badura JM. A comprehensive clinical review of recombinant human bone morphogenetic protein-2 (INFUSE Bone Graft). Int Orthop 2007;31(6):729–34.

57. Ceccarelli G, Presta R, Benedetti L, et al. Emerging perspectives in scaffold for tissue engineering in oral surgery. Stem Cells Int 2017;2017:4585401.

58. DeConde AS, Sidell D, Lee M, et al. Bone morphogenetic protein-2-impregnated biomimetic scaffolds successfully induce bone healing in a marginal mandibular defect. Laryngoscope 2013;123(5): 1149–55.

59. Gentile P, Chiono V, Carmagnola I, et al. An overview of poly(lactic-co-glycolic) acid (PLGA)-based biomaterials for bone tissue engineering. Int J Mol Sci 2014;15(3):3640–59.

60. Lee M, Dunn JC, Wu BM. Scaffold fabrication by indirect three-dimensional printing. Biomaterials 2005; 26(20):4281–9.

61. Rezwan K, Chen QZ, Blaker JJ, et al. Biodegradable and bioactive porous polymer/inorganic composite scaffolds for bone tissue engineering. Biomaterials 2006;27(18):3413–31.

62. Tanataweethum N, Liu WC, Goebel WS, et al. Fabrication of poly-L-lactic acid/dicalcium phosphate dihydrate composite scaffolds with high mechanical strength-implications for bone tissue engineering. J Funct Biomater 2015;6(4):1036–53.

63. Kim S, Cui ZK, Kim PJ, et al. Design of hydrogels to stabilize and enhance bone morphogenetic protein activity by heparin mimetics. Acta Biomater 2018; 72:45–54.

64. Fan J, Pi-Anfruns J, Guo M, et al. Small molecule-mediated tribbles homolog 3 promotes bone formation induced by bone morphogenetic protein-2. Sci Rep 2017;7(1):7518.

65. Govender S, Csimma C, Genant HK, et al. Recombinant human bone morphogenetic protein-2 for treatment of open tibial fractures: a prospective,

controlled, randomized study of four hundred and fifty patients. J Bone Joint Surg Am 2002;84-A(12):2123–34.

66. Irie K, Alpaslan C, Takahashi K, et al. Osteoclast differentiation in ectopic bone formation induced by recombinant human bone morphogenetic protein 2 (rhBMP-2). J Bone Miner Metab 2003;21(6):363–9.

67. James AW, LaChaud G, Shen J, et al. A review of the clinical side effects of bone morphogenetic protein-2. Tissue Eng Part B Rev 2016;22(4):284–97.

68. Kang Q, Sun MH, Cheng H, et al. Characterization of the distinct orthotopic bone-forming activity of 14 BMPs using recombinant adenovirus-mediated gene delivery. Gene Ther 2004;11(17):1312–20.

69. Poynton AR, Lane JM. Safety profile for the clinical use of bone morphogenetic proteins in the spine. Spine (Phila Pa 1976) 2002;27(16 Suppl 1):S40–8.

70. Tang TT, Xu XL, Dai KR, et al. Ectopic bone formation of human bone morphogenetic protein-2 gene transfected goat bone marrow-derived mesenchymal stem cells in nude mice. Chin J Traumatol 2005;8(1):3–7.

71. Wong DA, Kumar A, Jatana S, et al. Neurologic impairment from ectopic bone in the lumbar canal: a potential complication of off-label PLIF/TLIF use of bone morphogenetic protein-2 (BMP-2). Spine J 2008;8(6):1011–8.

72. Avila-Ortiz G, Bartold PM, Giannobile W, et al. Biologics and cell therapy tissue engineering approaches for the management of the edentulous maxilla: a systematic review. Int J Oral Maxillofac Implants 2016;31(Suppl):s121–64.

73. da Rosa WLO, da Silva TM, da Silva AF, et al. Bioactive treatments in bone grafts for implant-based rehabilitation: systematic review and meta-analysis. Clin Implant Dent Relat Res 2018;20(2):251–60.

74. Wallace SC, Snyder MB, Prasad H. Postextraction ridge preservation and augmentation with mineralized allograft with or without recombinant human platelet-derived growth factor BB (rhPDGF-BB): a consecutive case series. Int J Periodontics Restorative Dent 2013;33(5):599–609.

75. Nevins ML, Reynolds MA, Camelo M, et al. Recombinant human platelet-derived growth factor BB for reconstruction of human large extraction site defects. Int J Periodontics Restorative Dent 2014;34(2):157–63.

76. Thoma DS, Nanni N, Benic GI, et al. Effect of platelet-derived growth factor-BB on tissue integration of cross-linked and non-cross-linked collagen matrices in a rat ectopic model. Clin Oral Implants Res 2015;26(3):263–70.

77. Hubbell JA. Biomaterials in tissue engineering. Biotechnology (N Y) 1995;13(6):565–76.

78. Sheikh Z, Hamdan N, Ikeda Y, et al. Natural graft tissues and synthetic biomaterials for periodontal and alveolar bone reconstructive applications: a review. Biomater Res 2017;21:9.

79. Green DW, Kwon HJ, Jung HS. Osteogenic potency of nacre on human mesenchymal stem cells. Mol Cells 2015;38(3):267–72.

80. Lin Z, Solomon KL, Zhang X, et al. In vitro evaluation of natural marine sponge collagen as a scaffold for bone tissue engineering. Int J Biol Sci 2011;7(7):968–77.

81. Green DW, Lai WF, Jung HS. Evolving marine biomimetics for regenerative dentistry. Mar Drugs 2014;12(5):2877–912.

82. Ehrlich H, Ilan M, Maldonado M, et al. Three-dimensional chitin-based scaffolds from Verongida sponges (Demospongiae: Porifera). Part I. Isolation and identification of chitin. Int J Biol Macromol 2010;47(2):132–40.

83. Atlan G, Balmain N, Berland S, et al. Reconstruction of human maxillary defects with nacre powder: histological evidence for bone regeneration. C R Acad Sci III 1997;320(3):253–8.

84. Zhang G, Brion A, Willemin AS, et al. Nacre, a natural, multi-use, and timely biomaterial for bone graft substitution. J Biomed Mater Res A 2017;105(2):662–71.

85. Habraken WJ, Wolke JG, Jansen JA. Ceramic composites as matrices and scaffolds for drug delivery in tissue engineering. Adv Drug Deliv Rev 2007;59(4–5):234–48.

86. Lohi HS, Nayak DG, Uppoor AS. Comparative evaluation of the efficacy of bioactive ceramic composite granules alone and in combination with platelet rich fibrin in the treatment of mandibular class II furcation defects: a clinical and radiographic study. J Clin Diagn Res 2017;11(7):ZC76–80.

87. Sohrabi K, Saraiya V, Laage TA, et al. An evaluation of bioactive glass in the treatment of periodontal defects: a meta-analysis of randomized controlled clinical trials. J Periodontol 2012;83(4):453–64.

88. Wennerberg A, Bougas K, Jimbo R, et al. Implant coatings: new modalities for increased osseointegration. Am J Dent 2013;26(2):105–12.

89. Hench LL. The story of bioglass. J Mater Sci Mater Med 2006;17(11):967–78.

90. Profeta AC, Prucher GM. Bioactive-glass in periodontal surgery and implant dentistry. Dent Mater J 2015;34(5):559–71.

91. Liu T, Zheng Y, Wu G, et al. BMP2-coprecipitated calcium phosphate granules enhance osteoinductivity of deproteinized bovine bone, and bone formation during critical-sized bone defect healing. Sci Rep 2017;7:41800.

92. Khan R, Witek L, Breit M, et al. Bone regenerative potential of modified biphasic graft materials. Implant Dent 2015;24(2):149–54.

93. Calin C, Patrascu I. Growth factors and beta-tricalcium phosphate in the treatment of periodontal intraosseous defects: a systematic review and meta-analysis of randomised controlled trials. Arch Oral Biol 2016;66:44–54.

94. Lee CK, Koo KT, Park YJ, et al. Biomimetic surface modification using synthetic oligopeptides for enhanced guided bone regeneration in beagles. J Periodontol 2012;83(1):101–10.

95. Amso Z, Cornish J, Brimble MA. Short anabolic peptides for bone growth. Med Res Rev 2016;36(4):579–640.

96. Park JB, Lee JY, Park YJ, et al. Enhanced bone regeneration in beagle dogs with bovine bone mineral coated with a synthetic oligopeptide. J Periodontol 2007;78(11):2150–5.

97. Park JB, Lee JY, Park HN, et al. Osteopromotion with synthetic oligopeptide-coated bovine bone mineral in vivo. J Periodontol 2007;78(1):157–63.

Implant Therapy in Alveolar Cleft Sites

R. John Tannyhill III, DDS, MD*, Maria J. Troulis, DDS, MSc

KEYWORDS

- Cleft lip and palate • Alveolar cleft • Dental implant • Root form implant • Bone grafting
- Reconstruction

KEY POINTS

- Thorough knowledge and understanding of the differences in the cleft patient versus the non-cleft patient allow for more predictable and successful outcomes. Each step of surgical planning must be thoughtfully and carefully considered.
- The complexity of the challenges in the cleft patient are minimized with a meticulous clinical and radiographic workup. Treatment planning is much more accurate with the use of advanced imaging, and modern hard and soft tissue grafting techniques provide excellent options for the treating surgeon.
- Communication between the surgeon and the restorative team is critically important to achieve excellent long-term results.

INTRODUCTION

Cleft lip with and without cleft palate is one of the most common birth defects in the United States, with an estimated national prevalence of 10.63 per 10,000 live births in 2004 to 2006, while the estimated prevalence of cleft palate alone was 6.35 per 10,000 live births.[1] Treatment occurs from neonate to young adult and may consist of primary lip/palate repair, nasal repair, orthodontics, secondary bone grafting, orthognathic surgery, and multiple revisions. Prosthetic dental rehabilitation of the cleft palate patient has long been viewed as the capstone event for the patient who has undergone several operations and interventions to correct their cleft deformity. The placement and maintenance of the dental prosthesis is the final step in attempting to gain form and function. With the advent of different bone-grafting techniques and dental implant therapy, more options are now available to the reconstructive team to give the best possible functional and esthetic outcome.

Most patients with access to tertiary care facilities will have access to a cleft lip and palate team consisting of pediatricians, pediatric dentists, orthodontists, plastic surgeons, otolaryngologists, oral and maxillofacial surgeons, and speech and audiology specialists. However, Samama and Tulasne[2] note that, in Europe, there is currently no consensus on the primary and secondary treatment for cleft lip and palate patients. The 2010 Euro Cleft survey identified 194 different protocols for 201 teams. The situation in the United States is similar, with different teams having slightly dissimilar protocols. The lack of consensus leads to widely differing clinical situations facing the restorative dentist and surgeon as they attempt to treat the esthetic sequelae and restore the dentition for function and appearance. It is important to note that by the time many cleft patients seek dental

Disclosure Statement: Supported by the Massachusetts General Hospital, Department of Oral and Maxillofacial Surgery Education and Research Fund and the Francine and Roger Jean Foundation Education and Research Fund in Oral and Maxillofacial Surgery.
Department of Oral and Maxillofacial Surgery, Massachusetts General Hospital, 55 Fruit Street, Boston, MA 02114, USA
* Corresponding author.
E-mail address: rjtannyhill@mgh.harvard.edu

rehabilitation they are no longer associated with their original cleft team. The treatment team subsequently comprises the oral surgeon and the general dentist or prosthodontist. Therefore, it is important that the oral surgeon has an adequate understanding of the challenges that will be faced by the restorative dentist and have the foresight to mitigate those challenges.

This Review will attempt to outline a timeline for treatment, common challenges, and strategic considerations to facilitate optimal outcomes for patients with cleft lip and palate.

HISTORY

The first long-term follow-up of implant placement for dental rehabilitation in the non-cleft patient was published by Brånemark and colleagues[3] in 1977. Since that time, implant therapy has become a common and highly successful means of restoring missing teeth. In a systematic review of survival and success rates of dental implants reported in longitudinal studies with a follow-up period of at least 10 years, Moraschini and colleagues[4] reported a cumulative mean dental implant survival rate of 94.6% (SD 5.97%). These success rates are favorable in comparison with fixed and removable restorations.[5]

Historically, attempts to fully realize optimal form and function for the cleft patient have taken various forms. Agenesis of the lateral incisor tooth on the affected side is reported to be present in 50% to 97.1% of unilateral cleft patients, and 27.2% to 52.8% of the time on the unaffected side.[6,7] The reported figure in the non-cleft population is less than 2%. Removable and fixed prosthetics (conventional or Maryland bridges) have a long history as treatment methods in this demographic. Treatment options expanded once orthodontists began closing cleft spaces through orthodontic tooth movement and sometimes recontouring transposed teeth. The development of endosseous, root-form dental implants and predictable bone-grafting techniques in the 1970s eventually added another treatment option for these patients.

The first report of implant placement into the cleft alveolus was published in 1991 by Verdi and colleagues.[8] In contrast to published data on non-cleft patients, there are very few data on long-term outcomes of dental implant placement in the cleft patient. In a systematic review of clinical outcomes in alveolar cleft patients undergoing dental implant therapy, Wang and colleagues[9] reported a somewhat reduced long-term survival rate of 91.5% ± 4.77% indicating that dental implant therapy is a reliable treatment option for alveolar patients, at least in the short term

(<5 years). Kearns and colleagues[10] reported an implant survival rate of 90% when a two-stage implant procedure was used. The small number of studies is due to many factors and, as a result, there is currently no consensus on best practices.

WHAT MAKES THE CLEFT PATIENT DIFFERENT FROM THE NON-CLEFT PATIENT?

Treatment options for the cleft and non-cleft patient have historically included no treatment, and fixed prostheses and removable prostheses. With the advent of implant therapy, site development in the cleft patient became the greatest challenge to successful outcomes—functional success in the cleft patient may not equate with esthetic success. The ability to optimize a potential implant site with significant hard and soft tissue defects can dramatically alter outcomes. Experience gained in the non-cleft population undergoing implant therapy translates into strategies that can be used in the cleft population. Landes[11] hypothesized that bone-grafted cleft defects would have similar implant outcomes compared with patients who had experienced traumatic anterior maxillary defects. Both groups possessed bony defects and scarred periosteum and soft tissue. He found similar success rates between the groups.

When considering the challenges presented by the cleft patient, the problems of the unilateral and the bilateral cleft patient are similar. Anatomic defects, delays in the formation and eruption of teeth, problems with orthodontic movement, and the presence of prostheses contribute to reductions in bone levels in the areas next to the cleft. Maxillary arch segment irregularities, orthodontic appliances, and persisting soft tissue folds before palatoplasty, as well as the presence of scar tissue after cleft closure, make oral hygiene control difficult[12] (Fig. 1), complicating the number of considerations that must be addressed.

Soft Tissue Challenges

Soft tissue ultimately determines the long-term periodontal health of a tooth or dental implant. Thick, healthy keratinized and non-mobile tissue around teeth and implants is often not the case in the cleft patient. The irregularity of the cleft soft tissues (Fig. 2), the lack of deciduous teeth, and current surgical techniques often result in a preponderance of unattached gingiva rather than attached gingiva. For instance, using an advancement flap to create tension-free closure over an alveolar bone graft takes precedence over having ideal placement of the primordial keratinized band.

If the prosthetic plan does not include a dental implant this concern is lessened. Adjacent teeth

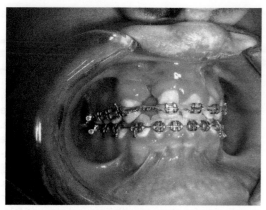

Fig. 1. Right unilateral cleft lip and palate patient with missing tooth no. 7, bony irregularity of alveolus, poor oral hygiene, and minimal attached gingiva.

often have reduced and irregular bone levels on the surfaces facing the cleft. Use of an initial or follow-up bone graft is not only to create continuity of the arch, but also to provide bony (and soft tissue) support to the adjacent teeth. If bony continuity is achieved with a bone graft, and a fixed or removable prosthetic option is chosen, keratinized tissue over the entire crest where the tooth is missing is ideal, but not necessary. Long-term esthetics will be enhanced by keratinized tissue, but periodontal health of the adjacent teeth only requires a keratinized tissue band on the surfaces facing the cleft.

If implant reconstruction is planned, keratinized tissue is desired across the entire crest. This will allow for keratinized tissue not only on the cleft-facing surfaces of the adjacent teeth, but also for the peri-implant tissues. It is difficult, if not impossible, to consistently achieve this at the time of the alveolar cleft advancement flaps. The periodontal and peri-implant soft tissue often need to be

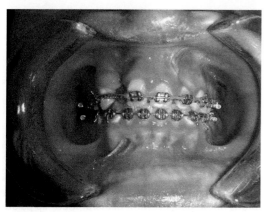

Fig. 2. Discontinuity of the cleft alveolus with irregular bone and soft tissue bilaterally, not only on cleft side.

addressed as part of implant site development. But favorable transformation of soft tissue during the intervening years between the time of the bone graft and placement of the dental implant remains unpredictable. Techniques of soft tissue augmentation involving full-thickness palatal grafts, split thickness connective tissue grafts, rotational flaps, and acellular dermal matrix have all been reported.[13] Successful achievement of keratinized tissue in the periodontal and peri-implant areas of the cleft are critical to good long-term implant-supported outcomes.

Hard Tissue Challenges

After orthodontic expansion of the maxilla, the aim of reconstruction of the alveolar cleft is to provide continuity of the maxillary arch, close the oronasal fistula, permit tooth eruption, provide support of the alar base, and to improve nasal symmetry.[14] Several methods have been reported. These include rib grafts, calvarial grafts, tibial grafts, iliac crest bone grafts, allograft utilization, in vivo tissue engineering,[15] and, more recently, tissue engineering with recombinant human bone morphogenetic protein-2 (rhBMP-2).[16] An excellent systematic review and best evidence synthesis of grafting materials was recently reported by Wu and colleagues.[17] End-stage morphology of the graft, although important, is often not the most important consideration at the time of alveolar grafting, because closure of the oronasal fistula and obtaining bony continuity of the dental arch are preeminent considerations. Once continuity is achieved, there may be a scarcity or sometimes an overabundance of bone. Whether this bone, routinely placed between the ages of 8 and 11 years, will allow for placement of a dental implant several years later depends on many factors including maxillary alveolar growth and development.[11]

If a removable or fixed prosthesis option is chosen, bone and soft tissue morphology is largely esthetic rather than functional. However, if dental implant rehabilitation is planned, alveolar cleft site morphology becomes critical. An alveolar cleft often results in both vertical and horizontal deficiencies. The lack of functional load contributes to this problem.[18] If these deficiencies are not significant (<3 mm), the patient can usually be treated with routine "tertiary" grafting techniques before, or at the time of, implant placement. However, if the graft requirement is significant (>3 mm), further implant site development is warranted. Currently, this decision is usually made using a combination of clinical examination and volumetric 3D cone beam computed tomography (CT) technology. If arch continuity is present but the defect is large enough to prevent implant placement with minor techniques, repeat grafts from sites such as the iliac crest or tibia may be necessary. If the defect is smaller (<3 mm), any combination of routine minor bone-grafting techniques can be used. Once the site is grafted, Dempf and colleagues[19] reported that functional loading of the graft after implant placement seems to preserve the grafted bone in the alveolar cleft.

Practical Concerns

Secondary alveolar bone grafts are commonly carried out done in patients between the ages of 8 and 11 years. Once dental arch continuity is achieved, many years may pass until the site is addressed for prosthetic rehabilitation. As in any dental site not under constant functional stress and stimulation, atrophy of the bone graft may occur. Reports by Takahashi and colleagues[20] and Ronchi and colleagues[21] report that bone resorption may occur as early as 4 to 6 months after cleft osteoplasty. Oesterle and colleagues[22] and Chiapasco[23] have suggested that implant placement after growth completion in late puberty and early adulthood may afford the best chance for successful long-term outcomes. Others recommend implant placement once adjacent permanent teeth have erupted.[24] Delays due to orthodontia may not be avoidable. In addition, grafted bone may result in an implant site that is largely dense and cortical in nature. The adjacent teeth may also have vertical periodontal defects, which predispose a dental implant to peri-implant problems such as subsequent crestal bone loss and peri-implantitis. Performance of a tertiary bone graft is made more difficult because of previous surgical scarring of the periosteum and soft tissue envelope, and a dense cortical bony recipient bed. This is an instance when alveolar distraction may be useful because histogenesis of bone and soft tissue occurs concurrently. However, a baseline amount is required for alveolar distraction to be successful. Even after every attempt has been made to develop the implant site, implant placement is often only possible in a more apical and palatal position. This results in less-favorable crown-to-implant ratios, difficult hygiene problems, and poor long-term esthetic and reduced survival outcomes.

WHAT ARE TREATMENT OPTIONS IN THE CLEFT PATIENT?

Once bony continuity of the dental arch is achieved via secondary alveolar cleft bone grafting, the quality of the bone and soft tissue will largely determine restorative options.

Unilateral Clefts

Fixed or removable prosthetics

Before the advent of dental implant therapy, removable and fixed restorative options were the standard of care for the cleft patient (**Figs. 3–8**). Wegscheider and colleagues[25] described the following prosthetic options: (1) fixed prosthodontics (crowns, bridges, and Maryland bridges); (2) removable prostheses (conventional cast partials, overdentures, and full dentures); and (3) precision prostheses (appliances with bars, splints, and telescopic retainers). Whereby good bony continuity and segment stability have previously been achieved with an alveolar cleft graft, a fixed restorative option may be considered. Adequate tooth spacing and periodontal health of the abutment teeth are considered critical to a good esthetic and functional outcome. Presently, the nature of prosthetic options remains unchanged. If the teeth adjacent to the cleft defect have abnormal morphology, a fixed prosthesis may be considered. A removable prosthesis or Maryland bridge

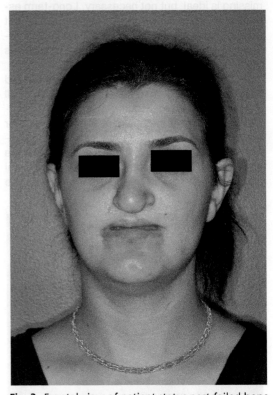

Fig. 3. Frontal view of patient status post failed bone grafts in a patient with bilateral cleft lip/palate. Note deficient midface support. (Photo courtesy of Leonard B. Kaban, DMD, MD, Boston, MA and Maria J. Troulis, DDS, MSc, Boston, MA.)

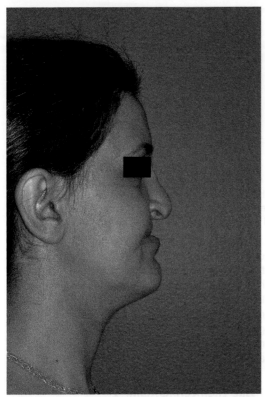

Fig. 4. Lateral view of patient status post failed bone grafts in a patient with bilateral cleft lip/palate. Note deficient midface support and relative mandibular prognathism. (Photo courtesy of Leonard B. Kaban, DMD, MD, Boston, MA and Maria J. Troulis, DDS, MSc, Boston, MA.)

may be considered as an esthetic stop gap while the patient grows to skeletal maturity, or as a long-term option in the appropriate patient. Interestingly, Papi and colleagues[26] reported that patients constructed with implant-supported

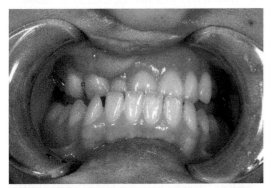

Fig. 5. Poor functional and esthetics of prosthesis due to jaw positioning, status post failed bone grafts, including vascularized free fibula graft, in a patient with bilateral cleft lip/palate. (Photo courtesy of Leonard B. Kaban, DMD, MD, Boston, MA and Maria J. Troulis, DDS, MSc, Boston, MA.)

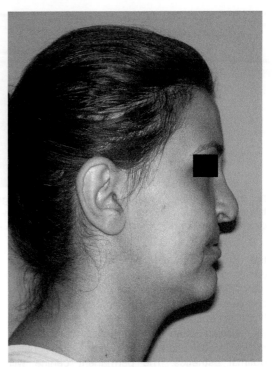

Fig. 6. Lateral view of same patient after status post iliac crest bone graft and bilateral distraction osteogenesis. Note improvement in midface support and relative mandibular prognathism. (Photo courtesy of Leonard B. Kaban, DMD, MD, Boston, MA and Maria J. Troulis, DDS, MSc, Boston, MA.)

dentures are more satisfied than subjects with fixed partial dentures and removable partial dentures.

Orthodontics
Shetye[27] notes that there are 2 options when a lateral incisor is missing. The lateral incisor space can be maintained until skeletal growth is complete, or the space may be closed by transposing

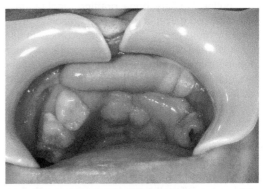

Fig. 7. Intraoral view of same patient status post iliac crest bone graft and distraction osteogenesis. (Photo courtesy of Leonard B. Kaban, DMD, MD, Boston, MA and Maria J. Troulis, DDS, MSc, Boston, MA.)

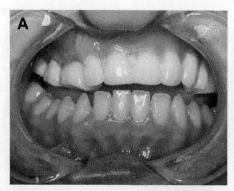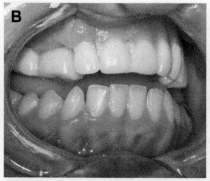

Fig. 8. (*A*) Anterior view and (*B*) lateral view of orthognathic jaw position, status post iliac crest bone graft and bilateral distraction osteogenesis, allowing for a removable partial fixed denture with acceptable results. (Photo courtesy of Leonard B. Kaban, DMD, MD, Boston, MA and Maria J. Troulis, DDS, MSc, Boston, MA.)

the canine tooth medially into the gap, called canine substitution. If the space is maintained, a removable prosthesis can be used until growth is complete and implant reconstruction is complete. If canine substitution is planned for replacement of the missing lateral incisor, then several canine crown modifications are needed to achieve optimal esthetics. The permanent canine will need recontouring on all surfaces. Recontouring is usually done progressively during the orthodontic phase. The first bicuspid would take the canine position and be reshaped to resemble a permanent canine. The second premolar and first and second molars in turn are moved mesially. The patient's orthodontic treatment is finalized as a class II occlusal relationship on the side of the missing lateral incisor. With successful esthetic bonding, excellent results can be achieved with this option.[2]

Traditional bone grafting with dental implant

Volumetric 3D CT analysis after traditional iliac crest bone grafts show the greatest initial bony morphology. This may result in better implant sites after skeletal maturation and, thus, necessitate only routine "tertiary bone grafting" techniques. Rib grafts and calvarial grafts often result in alveolar bony morphology that is largely cortical in nature. It is often difficult to achieve normal alveolar ridge morphology with a scarred, previously operated, soft tissue envelope. Inadequate bone width may lead to implant placement in a non-ideal position, which may impair the final esthetics of the implant-supported denture.[28]

Distraction osteogenesis

The challenges of distraction in the cleft patient are derived from the initial bone structure and morphology. Often, the gap in question is only 7 to 10 mm, making the use of this technique potentially difficult. This option may be considered when agenesis of other teeth exists and the segment is larger,

or when the choice is made to sacrifice an adjacent tooth, such as a central incisor with severe enamel hypoplasia.[7] An excellent update of alveolar distraction techniques for dental implants was recently published by Vega and Bilbao.[29] Distraction osteogenesis for maxillary advancement is often recommended for the cleft patient because of scarring and lack of soft tissue[30] (see **Fig. 4**).

Tissue engineering/rhBMP-2

In a systematic review of growth factor-aided tissue engineering with regard to reconstruction of the alveolar cleft in cleft lip and palate, van Hout and colleagues[16] reported that the main advantage of growth factor-aided tissue engineering is the avoidance of a second surgical site needed for the harvest of autologous bone. This resulted in shortening of the operation time, absence of donor site morbidity, shorter hospital stays, and reduction of overall cost.[16] Favorable results with rhBMP-2 were obtained in terms of quantity of bone formation. They found that the application of rhBMP-2 resulted in shortening of the operation time, absence of donor site morbidity, shorter hospital stays, and reduction of overall cost.[16] In a retrospective review of 40 non-cleft patients to evaluate the clinical effectiveness of alveolar distraction osteogenesis versus rhBMP-2 for vertical ridge augmentation, Reuss and colleagues[31] showed similar values in absolute vertical bone gain. The distraction group showed a better outcome in the vertical regenerative potential, albeit with a more frequent need for re-grafting with implant placement. The BMP cohort showed a lesser need for re-grafting, despite having a higher postoperative complication rate.[31] The benefit of distraction is that histogenesis of bone and soft tissue occurs. It is important to note, however, that both must be present, in some amount initially, to allow for alveolar distraction osteogenesis.

Bilateral Clefts

Fixed or removable prosthetics

Owing to the instability of the premaxilla and the often less than ideal bone height, removable and fixed prostheses are often used for these patients. Large, multiunit, fixed bridges can be esthetically pleasing, and functionally excellent. Primary stability of the premaxilla is required if a fixed prosthesis is to be used. In addition, the rigidity of a fixed bridge may offer support of the premaxilla and bone grafts in the long term.

Orthodontics

Canine teeth may be brought medially into the cleft spaces in the bilateral cleft patient and result in a symmetric change in the occlusion. Advancing both quadrants of teeth medially into a class II occlusion can maintain esthetic and functional symmetry and minimize the need for further surgery. In addition, distraction osteogenesis to advance the maxilla can be used[32,33] (see **Fig. 4**).

Other considerations in the bilateral patient are not dissimilar from the unilateral patient with regard to other options.

Author's Suggested Protocol

Clinical workup

First, a thorough history and clinical examination are performed. It is critical to consider the patient's treatment goals. A systematic examination is undertaken. Height of smile line and gingival show are taken into consideration (**Fig. 9**). Careful consideration is given to the spacing of the adjacent teeth, periodontal health, and degree of hard and soft tissue compromise (**Fig. 10**). Photos and models are routinely taken.

Imaging

Plain film, CT, or cone beam computed tomography images allow for evaluation of the outcome of previous grafting of the cleft site (**Fig. 11**). Careful assessment of the bone levels on the teeth adjacent to the cleft must be undertaken, as tertiary grafting against cementum is rarely successful. The height of the bony crest is evaluated, and the planned crown/implant ratio considered. In patients in whom an unfavorable ratio exists, consideration must be given to a fixed or removable prosthetic option. Techniques such as distraction or interpositional grafting to gain vertical height are possible options, but are very technique sensitive. Elo and colleagues[34] have published high success rates with both options, albeit not in the alveolar cleft population.

Site development

If keratinized tissue is necessary, soft tissue grafting with palatal tissue or acellular dermal matrix is performed. A 3-month period is usually allowed for incorporation and healing. This may also be required after implant placement if the implant is buried in a two-stage protocol.

Although secondary bone grafting is commonly necessary in the cleft patient, de Barros Ferreira[35] reported an overall survival rate of 94.3% in 120 patients receiving secondary grafts with

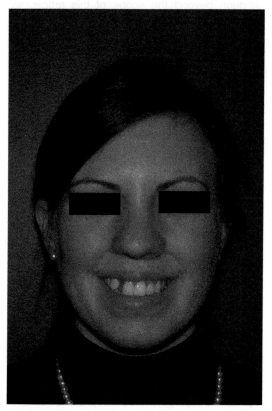

Fig. 9. Smiling view of unilateral partial cleft after iliac crest bone graft, but before implant placement.

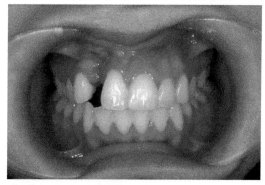

Fig. 10. Intraoral photo of same patient. Note irregularity of periodontal tissues.

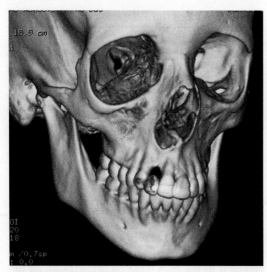

Fig. 11. Computed tomography showing no. 7 site, before secondary grafting, with Maryland bridge prosthesis in place.

subsequent implant placement. If the hard tissue deficit is less than 3 mm, routine techniques of particulate grafting with guided bone regeneration may be used. In these patients with minor bony deficits, implants are commonly inserted at the time of graft placement. Because the amount of baseline bone is usually less in the previously grafted cleft patient, more moderate amounts of bone loss are common. Thus, implant placement is commonly delayed in the cleft population. Generally, 6 months is allowed between secondary bone grafting and implant placement. This is done after further imaging to confirm healing and adequate volumetric outcomes. If the outcome is less successful than planned, re-grafting with or without implant placement may be considered.

If the bony defect is significant, we consider grafting with iliac crest bone from the ipsilateral side of the original harvest. This avoids a new scar for the patient and usually results in more than adequate amounts of cancellous bone. The mandibular ramus and symphysis or maxillary tuberosity are also sites to be considered. This is often mixed with freeze-dried, banked bone. Platelet-rich plasma, and resorbable collagen or platelet-rich fibrin membranes may also be used at this time.[36] Careful attention is paid to the soft tissue envelope, and releasing periosteal or gingival incisions may be made to ensure that the resultant closure is not under tension.

Placement pearls
Careful consideration of angulation and depth of implant placement are important for both esthetic outcome and long-term prognosis.[28] Implants that

are difficult to restore will result in poor esthetic outcomes and increase the likelihood of peri-implantitis and bone loss. Implants that are placed too apically can result in unfavorable implant/crown ratios, poor soft tissue esthetics, difficult hygiene, and decrease long-term survival. Filho and De Almeida[37] reported that, ideally, the implant should be placed at 1 to 3 mm from the cemento-enamel junction of adjacent teeth (**Fig. 12**). The alveolar ridge thickness should also be considered for ideal positioning of the implant. The extent of the edentulous space also influences the final esthetics of the prosthetic crown, because wide spaces lead to wide crowns and reduced spaces lead to narrow crowns.[37]

In the cleft patient, there is a temptation to accept placement that is too deep and too palatal because of the common pattern of healing after the initial grafts. It is critical to develop the implant site, so that placement may be as ideal as possible (**Fig. 13**). If this is not possible, then consideration must be given to fixed or removable options. Forcing placement in a compromised position will not result in a stable, serviceable rehabilitation for the patient.

Restorative pearls
Although beyond the scope of this article, we would add a simple suggestion with regard to the restorative plan. Many restorative dentists are more comfortable with cemented fixed restorations than with screw-retained restorations, but screw-retained options result in a lower incidence of peri-implantitis.[38] Reviews by Renvert and Quirynen[39] and Staubli and colleagues[40] identified excess cement to be a contributing factor to peri-implantitis, especially when the implant is placed deep, which can lead to premature implant

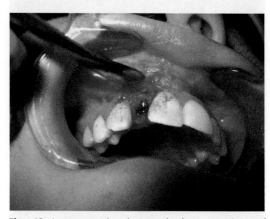

Fig. 12. Intraoperative intraoral photo at time of implant placement. Note adjuvant bone graft on buccal aspect.

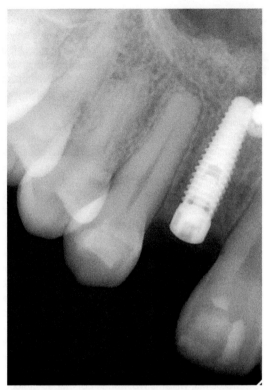

Fig. 13. Postoperative periapical radiograph showing placement of no. 7 implant fixture.

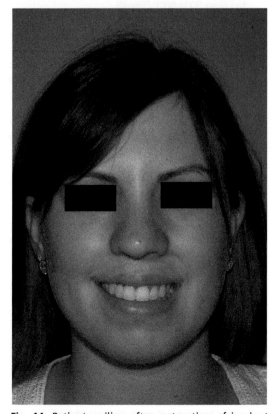

Fig. 14. Patient smiling after restoration of implant with fixed prosthesis.

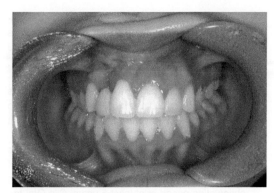

Fig. 15. Intraoral view of final outcome after placement of fixed prosthesis. Note the persistent irregularity of the periodontal tissues.

failure. If the restorative dentist is worried about use of a screw-retained prosthetic treatment plan, referral to a prosthodontic specialist might be considered (**Figs. 14** and **15**). An additional alternative is the use of nitinol retention abutments (Smileloc), which require no cement or screw for crown retention.

Also, occlusal forces must be carefully adjusted to allow for appropriate forces on the implant body and bony support structure. Hyper-occlusion on an implant crown can be catastrophic for the implant and supporting bone, and undo many years of effort by the patient and the surgical team.[41,42]

SUMMARY

Patients born with unilateral or bilateral cleft lip and palate face a long path back to form and function. The final rehabilitation for many of these patients occurs after skeletal maturity. Dental implant rehabilitation restores function, soft and hard tissue support, and confidence. Having a clear understanding of both the challenges and treatment strategies available will allow the oral and maxillofacial surgeon to provide the best of care for these patients. Investigative options abound, as questions of implant outcomes in the cleft patient remain largely unexplored. The difficulty in obtaining these data stem from limited patient volume in any individual practice or center, and difficulty in the long-term tracking of these patients.

REFERENCES

1. Kirby RS. The prevalence of selected major birth defects in the United States. Semin Perinatol 2017;41: 338–44.
2. Samama Y, Tulasne J-F. Dental sequellae of alveolar clefts: utility of endosseous implants. Part I: therapeutic protocols. Int Orthod 2014;12:188–99.

3. Brånemark PI, Hansson BO, Adell R, et al. Osseointegrated implants in the treatment of the edentulous jaw. Experience from a 10-year period. Scand J Plast Reconstr Surg Suppl 1977;16:1–132.

4. Moraschini V, Poubel LA, Ferreira VF, et al. Evaluation of survival and success rates of dental implants reported in longitudinal studies with a follow-up period of at least 10 years: a systematic review. Int J Oral Maxillofac Surg 2015;44(3):377–88.

5. Thoma DS, Sailer I, Ioannidis A, et al. A systematic review of the survival and complication rates of resin-bonded fixed dental prostheses after a mean observation period of at least 5 years. Clin Oral Implants Res 2017;28(11):1421–32.

6. Dewinter G, Quirynen M, Heidbüchel K, et al. Dental abnormalities, bone graft quality, and periodontal conditions in patients with unilateral cleft lip and palate at different phases of orthodontic treatment. Cleft Palate Craniofac J 2003;40(4):343–50.

7. Akcam MO, Evirgen S, Uslu O, et al. Dental anomalies in individuals with cleft lip and/or palate. Eur J Orthod 2010;32(2):207–13.

8. Verdi FJ Jr, Slanzi GL, Cohen SR, et al. Use of the Branemark implant in the cleft palate patient. Cleft Palate Craniofac J 1991;28(3):301–3.

9. Wang F, Wu Y, Zou D, et al. Clinical outcomes of dental implant therapy in alveolar cleft patients: a systematic review. Int J Oral Maxillofac Implants 2014;29(5):1098–105.

10. Kearns G, Perrott DH, Sharma A, et al. Placement of endosseous implants in grafted alveolar clefts. Cleft Palate Craniofac J 1997;34(6):520–5.

11. Landes CA. Implant-borne prosthetic rehabilitation of bone-grafted cleft versus traumatic anterior maxillary defects. J Oral Maxillofac Surg 2006;64(2):297–307.

12. Bousdras VA, Ayliffe PR, Barrett M, et al. Esthetic and functional rehabilitation in patients with cleft lip and palate. Ann Maxillofacial Surg 2015;5(1):108–11.

13. Thoma DS, Buranawat B, Hämmerle CHF, et al. Efficacy of soft tissue augmentation around dental implants and in partially edentulous areas: a systematic review. J Clin Periodontol 2014;41(s15):S77–91.

14. Bajaj AK, Wongworawat AA, Punjabi A. Management of alveolar clefts. J Craniofac Surg 2003;14(6):840–6.

15. Konopnicki S, Troulis MJ. Mandibular tissue engineering: past, present, future. J Oral Maxillofac Surg 2015;73(12, Supplement):S136–46.

16. van Hout WMMT, Mink van der Molen AB, Breugem CC, et al. Reconstruction of the alveolar cleft: can growth factor-aided tissue engineering replace autologous bone grafting? A literature review and systematic review of results obtained with bone morphogenetic protein-2. Clin Oral Investig 2011;15(3):297–303.

17. Wu C, Pan W, Feng C, et al. Systematic review: grafting materials for alveolar cleft reconstruction: a systematic review and best-evidence synthesis. Int J Oral Maxillofac Surg 2018;47:345–56.

18. Honma K, Kobayashi T, Nakajima T, et al. Computed tomographic evaluation of bone formation after secondary bone grafting of alveolar clefts. J Oral Maxillofac Surg 1999;57(10):1209–13.

19. Dempf R, Teltzrow T, Kramer F-J, et al. Alveolar bone grafting in patients with complete clefts: a comparative study between secondary and tertiary bone grafting. Cleft Palate Craniofac J 2002;39(1):18–25.

20. Takahashi T, Fukuda M, Yamaguchi T, et al. Use of endosseous implants for dental reconstruction of patients with grafted alveolar clefts. J Oral Maxillofac Surg 1997;55(6):576–83.

21. Ronchi P, Chiapasco M, Frattini D. Endosseous implants for prosthetic rehabilitation in bone grafted alveolar clefts. J Craniomaxillofac Surg 1995;23(6):382–6.

22. Oesterle LJ, Cronin RJ Jr, Ranly DM. Maxillary implants and the growing patient. Int J Oral Maxillofac Implants 1993;8(4):377–87.

23. Chiapasco M. Use of endosseous implants for dental reconstruction of patients with grafted alveolar clefts. J Oral Maxillofac Surg 1997;55(6):584.

24. Troulis MJ, Williams WB, Kaban LB. Staged protocol for resection, skeletal reconstruction, and oral rehabilitation of children with jaw tumors. J Oral Maxillofac Surg 2004;62(3):335–43.

25. Wegscheider W, Bratschko R, Plischka G, et al. The system of prosthetic treatment for CLAP patients. J Craniomaxillofac Surg 1989;17(Suppl 1):49–51.

26. Papi P, Giardino R, Sassano P, et al. Oral health related quality of life in cleft lip and palate patients rehabilitated with conventional prostheses or dental implants. J Int Soc Prev Community Dent 2015;5(6):482–7.

27. Shetye PR. Update on treatment of patients with cleft—timing of orthodontics and surgery. Semin Orthod 2016;22:45–51.

28. Cune MS, Meijer GJ, Koole R. Anterior tooth replacement with implants in grafted alveolar cleft sites: a case series. Clin Oral Implants Res 2004;15(5):616–24.

29. Vega LG, Bilbao A. Alveolar distraction osteogenesis for dental implant preparation: an update. Oral Maxillofac Surg Clin North Am 2010;22:369–85.

30. Wong GB, Ciminello FS, Padwa BL. Distraction osteogenesis of the cleft maxilla. Facial Plast Surg 2008;24(04):467–71.

31. Reuss JM, Pi-Anfruns J, Moy PK. Dental implants: is bone morphogenetic protein-2 as effective as alveolar distraction osteogenesis for vertical bone regeneration? J Oral Maxillofac Surg 2018;76:752–60.

32. Gürsoy S, Hukki J, Hurmerinta K. Five-year follow-up of maxillary distraction osteogenesis on the dentofacial structures of children with cleft lip and palate. J Oral Maxillofac Surg 2010;68(4):744–50.

33. Ngan P, Moon W. Evolution of class III treatment in orthodontics. Am J Orthod Dentofacial Orthop 2015;148(1):22–36.

34. Elo JA, Herford AS, Boyne PJ. Implant success in distracted bone versus autogenous bone-grafted sites. J Oral Implantol 2009;35(4):181–4.

35. de Barros Ferreira S Jr, Esper LA, Sbrana MC, et al. Survival of dental implants in the cleft area–a retrospective study. Cleft Palate Craniofac J 2010;47(6): 586–90.

36. Alain S, Marco Del C, Alain V, et al. Current knowledge and perspectives for the use of platelet-rich plasma (PRP) and platelet-rich fibrin (PRF) in oral and maxillofacial surgery part 2: bone graft, implant and reconstructive surgery. Curr Pharm Biotechnol 2012;13(7):1231–56.

37. Filho JFF, De Almeida ALPF. Aesthetic analysis of an implant-supported denture at the cleft area. Cleft Palate Craniofac J 2013;50(5):597–602.

38. Weber HP, Kim DM, Ng MW, et al. Peri-implant soft-tissue health surrounding cement- and screw-retained implant restorations: a multi-center, 3-year prospective study. Clin Oral Implants Res 2006; 17(4):375–9.

39. Renvert S, Quirynen M. Risk indicators for peri-implantitis. A narrative review. Clin Oral Implants Res 2015;26:15.

40. Staubli N, Walter C, Schmidt JC, et al. Excess cement and the risk of peri-implant disease–a systematic review. Clin Oral Implants Res 2017;28(10): 1278–90.

41. Goodacre CJ, Kan JYK, Rungcharassaeng K. Clinical complications of osseointegrated implants. J Prosthet Dent 1999;81(5):537–52.

42. Kim Y, Oh T-J, Misch CE, et al. Occlusal considerations in implant therapy: clinical guidelines with biomechanical rationale. Clin Oral Implants Res 2005;16(1):26–35.

Complex Dental Implant Cases
Algorithms, Subjectivity, and Patient Cases Along the Complexity Continuum

Mark Durham, DMD[a],*, Marco Brindis, DDS[b],
Nicholas Egbert, DDS, MSD[a],
Leslie R. Halpern, DDS, MD, PhD, MPH[c]

KEYWORDS

- Algorithms • Complex implant restorations • Interdisciplinary collaboration
- Maxillary and mandibular ridge classification • Provider subjectivity

KEY POINTS

- Complex dental implant cases involve a multiplicity of presurgical and postsurgical considerations that are agreed upon by both patient and practitioner.
- Implant-supported reconstruction in the complex dental implant patient is predicated upon a surgical foundation that promotes both long-term function and esthetics.
- Prosthodontic algorithms are elucidated through a list of the generic operations for providing patients with basic dental implant prosthetics.
- Provider subjectivity is an essential component of complex cases, and specific complex cases are provided to convey the strong subjective component in such cases.

INTRODUCTION

Advances in the discipline of dental implant placement have created choices to enhance the expectations of the dental practitioner and his or her patients with respect to oral rehabilitation. There are more realistic options for restoration of function and esthetics regardless of age, and in most cases, medical disabilities. The latter can improve both better oral health and health-related quality of life in patients who were once considered hopeless "dental cripples." In addition, the bioactivity of implant surface design as well as use of hard and soft tissue augmentation provides a greater enhancement of surgical sites in both the edentulous and the partially edentulous jaw. This millennium has especially provided an increased demand by patients for dental implants, which has cascaded into economic competition by companies that market full mouth rehabilitation whereby the patient regains their teeth regardless of how they lost them. The implant placement, however, although well reported in the literature, can still result in implant failures due to poor patient selection, prior history of oral disease, that is, periodontitis, compliance with oral hygiene instructions, and professional maintenance protocols. These morbidities, whether cause or effect, have their basis in poor treatment planning

Disclosure Statement: The authors have nothing to disclose.
[a] Prosthodontist, University of Utah, School of Dentistry, 530 South Wakara Way, Salt Lake City, UT 84108, USA;
[b] Louisiana State University, School of Dentistry, 1100 Florida Avenue, New Orleans, LA 70119, USA; [c] Oral and Maxillofacial Surgery, University of Utah, School of Dentistry, 530 South Wakara Way, Salt Lake City, UT 84108, USA
* Corresponding author.
E-mail address: Mark.durham@hsc.utah.edu

Oral Maxillofacial Surg Clin N Am 31 (2019) 219–249
https://doi.org/10.1016/j.coms.2018.12.003

strategies.[1–4] As such, a systematic approach to patient assessment must be the number one priority for complex dental implant treatment planning in order to avoid a less than optimized outcome.

With respect to the complex implant case, the doctor must determine whether implants are the best option, especially within a framework of a partially or fully edentulous jaw. In many instances, hard and soft tissue foundations are inadequate for implant placement and must, therefore, be augmented before placing implant fixtures. A promise of a fixed prosthesis may be broken if the treatment turns into a removable appliance, especially when implant placement has resulted in improper positioning to handle the biomechanical stressors during function. **Box 1** lists the most common types of complex cases seen in the oral and maxillofacial surgical practice. These complex cases not only will often require a combination of tissue choices but also will require prosthetic and periodontal reformations for total rehabilitation in the partially and fully edentulous maxilla and mandible.[5] An interdisciplinary approach to restore function and esthetics is most often necessary to offer treatment choices that will be agreeable by both the practitioner and their patient population. The disclosure of the case's complexity is a nonnegotiable need in the management of patient-provider relationship.

This article shares subjective claims regarding the restoration of simple to complex cases, because sharing cases is an important activity in the disambiguation of case complexity for providers. Ultimately disclosing the subjective perception of case complexity aids patients in their need for emotional management and helps meet patient expectations. A series of algorithms for approaching complex dental implant restorations in the partially edentulous and fully edentulous patient is presented. A review of the current literature is used to apply a well-tested systematic assessment

followed by criteria in a checklist format that will determine whether a removable or fixed implant prosthesis is the best option for the patient. Several cases have been chosen to illustrate the algorithms the authors use in order to provide an optimized prognosis for surgical/restorative success.

PATIENT WORKUP

An evidence-based approach was applied to determine patient assessment strategies for complex case rehabilitation that were well tested in other studies.[1,6] A literature search was undertaken using Medline within the PubMed Portal to choose articles within the last 15 years. Only articles in English were chosen for inclusion. Each article's bibliography was further evaluated by hand for relevant publications and reviewed by the authors for inclusion. The keywords chosen included "patient assessment," "complex implant cases and patient selection," "complex planning for dental implants," and "complex restoration of the jaw with dental implants." The level of evidence chosen was based on Sackett's hierarchy of evidence and were predominantly level 1A, 2A, 3A, 4, and 5 (**Box 2**).[6] The following sections describe several algorithms used in the workup of the patient beginning with a medical history and physical examination followed by a series of checklists of hard and soft tissue criteria, radiologic imaging, and prosthetic strategies that the surgeon, prosthodontist, and periodontist can apply to complex implant cases in the maxilla and mandible.

Box 1
Common complex cases of dental implant restorations (All cases may need soft and hard tissue augmentation)

Multi-unit fixed restorations in the esthetic zone

Full-arch restorations that are completely implant supported

Single-unit fixed restorations in the esthetic zone

Full-arch restorations that are implant and tissue assisted

Fixed restorations outside the esthetic zone

Box 2
Criteria for inclusion of articles chosen from PubMed literature search according to Sackett's hierarchy

Level of Evidence	Description
1A	Systematic review/randomized trials (RCT)
1B	RCTs with narrow confidence limit
1C	All or none case series
2A	Systematic cohort
2B	Cohort study/low-quality RCT
3A	Systematic review of case controlled
3B	Case-controlled study
4	Case series/poor cohort case controlled
5	Expert opinion

From Sadowsky SJ, Fitzpatrick B, Curtis DA. Evidence-based criteria for different treatment planning of implant restorations for the maxillary edentulous patient. J Prosthodont 2015;433–46; with permission.

Medical History/Physical Examination

Much debate has centered on whether dental implants are a preferred restorative solution in medically compromised patients, who most often are candidates for complex restorative rehabilitation.[3,4,7] The challenges faced include increased risk of peri-implantitis, recurrence of mucosal disease, and/or development of osteonecrosis due to pharmacotherapy, that is, the use of certain drugs for osteoporosis/bone cancers, and patients who have been exposed to radiation therapy. Diz and colleagues[4] have suggested that risk/morbidity of dental implant placement in medically compromised patients should be predicated upon careful patient workup because new evidence supports successful survival in these patients.[7] Kotsakis and colleagues[3] in a systematic review evaluating implant placement in the maxilla of medically compromised patients conclude that implant survival is acceptable based on disease type and appears more predictable in the mandible than maxilla. Vissink and colleagues[7] in a recent review differentiated between absolute and relative contraindications for dental implant therapy. **Table 1** lists these considerations with measures to allow the feasibility of dental implant placement in patients who are medically challenged.[4,7] Immediate and long-term follow-up of all patients are essential regardless of relative or absolute considerations to complex implant case restorations.

Clinical Examination of Extraoral and Intraoral Hard and Soft Tissues

A systematic approach requires an "interbiologic algorithm" comprising both hard and soft tissue extraoral and intraoral evaluation regardless of whether the practitioner is restoring a single tooth, partial edentulous, or fully edentulous jaw. Factors that influence the ideal restoration must begin with a "checklist approach" across the vertical, transverse, and coronal dimensions of the patient's hard and soft tissue profile.[8,9] In addition, patient concerns of phonation problems and gag reflexes often require a consideration of whether a fixed appliance may be indicated. These criteria are crucial to the design of the restoration because it will ultimately determine the "ideal" position for implant placement. **Table 2** describes the authors' general algorithm for patient treatment planning that sets the stage for the specific criteria to follow based on the patient's treatment preferences.

Extraoral and intraoral hard and soft tissue parameters

The facial appearance provides a foundation for how the hard and soft tissues interact to provide

phonation, function, and esthetics. The following provides an in-depth evaluation of these parameters.

Extraoral hard and soft tissue Table 3 characterizes the extraoral examination based on whether the patient is dentate or edentulous.[8] Skeletal profile, facial contours, soft tissue drape, facial symmetry, lip and cheek support, smile line, and relation of the upper and lower lip provide a guide to optimal placement of the final restoration. These criteria are addressed with and without existing prostheses in order to determine the anatomic limitations precluding stability and retention for a complete denture as well as tolerance for palatal coverage in patients who are refractory gaggers. Regardless of design, facial support becomes critical because dentofacial imbalances also need to be addressed to determine a balance between the esthetic plane and functional occlusion. The balance between upper and low lip esthetics is determined by the convexity or concavity of the patient's profile because prosthetic design can compensate for dentofacial deficiencies. A dentate maxilla provides lip support off the alveolar ridge. In the edentulous upper jaw, lip support is lost due to resorption patterns, and anterior teeth must be placed anterior to the ridge in order to provide lip esthetics and phalange design that compensate for lip length and projection. Maxillary lip length will determine the position of the anterior teeth and therefore short versus long lip length will determine exposure of teeth in repose. All measurements must be calibrated to the age and gender of the patient.[8–10]

Intraoral hard and soft tissue Table 4 shows an algorithm for intraoral examination based on either a fixed or a removable implant prosthesis.[8,9] The intraoral examination includes quantity and quality of bony and mucosal draping. The tissue biotype will set the stage for clinical crown emergence profiles and accompanying abutment angulation of the implants. Alveolar ridge geometry can influence patterns of resorption, which influence the location of implant positioning. Three-dimensional Bony foundations are of primary importance in the reconstruction of the edentulous ridge (see later discussion). Crown inclination, bone relationship, and tooth size will supply adequate lip support and phonation during smiling and speech.

Diagnostic Wax-up Modeling for Treatment Planning

Diagnostic wax-ups are paramount in designing a prosthesis regardless of whether a fixed or removable treatment option is offered. Impressions and study casts are mounted on semiadjustable

Table 1
Type of medical condition and survival of dental-implant placements

Condition	(Relative) Contraindication	Implant Survival Rate	Precautions/Recommendations
Alcoholism	No	Similar	Assure that patients will keep adequate oral health maintenance.
Bleeding disorder	No	Similar	Check coagulation status before placement of implants
Bone disease			
Osteoporosis	No	Similar	Be aware of a slightly higher risk on MRONJ in patients on oral antiresorptive drugs; bone augmentation surgery is allowed
Bisphosphonate use	Yes	Similar/ reduced	Antibiotic prophylaxis; risk of MRONJ is high in patients treated for bone metastasis. When implants in latter patients are indicated, do it early after start of antiresorptive therapy. Also, no augmentation surgery in patients on IV administration unless early after start of usage
Other antiresorptive drugs, for example, denosumab	Yes	Similar/ reduced	Antibiotic prophylaxis; risk of MRONJ is high in patients treated for bone metastasis. When implants in latter patients are indicated, do it early after start of antiresorptive therapy. Also, no augmentation surgery in patients on IV administration unless early after start of usage
Cardiac disease	No	Similar	Assure that patient will keep adequate oral health maintenance, also with regard to control of cardiac disease
Diabetes mellitus			
Uncontrolled	No	Similar/ reduced	Antibiotic prophylaxis; assure that patient will keep adequate oral health maintenance, also with regard to control of diabetes
Controlled	No	Similar	Assure that patient will keep adequate oral health maintenance, also with regard to control of diabetes
Drugs			
Anticoagulants	No	Similar	See bleeding disorder
Antiresorptive drugs	No	Similar/ reduced	See bone disease
Biologicals	No	Similar	See Immunocompromised patients
Chemotherapy	No	Similar	See head neck cancer
Immunotherapy	Yes	Unknown	Implant treatment often can be postponed until end of therapy
Xerostomic drugs	No	Similar	See hyposalivation
Head and neck cancer			
Chemotherapy	No	Similar	Assure that patient will keep adequate oral health maintenance during the course of chemotherapy. After completion, the risk of developing peri-implant health problems is comparable to healthy subjects

(continued on next page)

Table 1
(continued)

Condition	(Relative) Contraindication	Implant Survival Rate	Precautions/Recommendations
Radiotherapy	Yes	Reduced	Preferably place dental implants during ablative surgery. When placed after completion of radiotherapy, implant should be placed under antibiotic coverage (eg, amoxicillin 500 mg tid for 2 wk, starting 1 d before placement of the implants). If cumulative radiation dose in the implant area is >40 Gy, it is recommended to apply hyperbaric oxygen therapy preimplant and postimplant placement
Hypersalivation	No	Similar	
Hyposalivation	No	Similar	Higher risk of per-implant health problems, assure that patient will keep adequate oral health maintenance
Immunocompromised patients			
Biologicals	No	Similar	Discuss with physician whether administration of biologicals has to be adjusted or specific precautions are needed
Crohn disease	No	Similar/ reduced	Antibiotic prophylaxis; older studies mention that implant survival is decreased compared with controls; Recent studies indicate that survival is similar
Mixed connective tissue disease	No	Similar	Antibiotic prophylaxis; higher risk of per-implant health problems, antibiotic prophylaxis
Rheumatoid arthritis	No	Similar	Higher risk of peri-implant health problems, assure that patient will keep adequate oral health maintenance
Scleroderma	No	Similar	Antibiotic prophylaxis; higher risk of peri-implant health problems, assure that patient will keep adequate oral health maintenance
Sjögren syndrome	No	Similar	Antibiotic prophylaxis; higher risk of per-implant health problems, assure that patient will keep adequate oral health maintenance
Systemic lupus erythematosus	No	Similar	Antibiotic prophylaxis; higher risk of per-implant health problems, assure that patient will keep adequate oral health maintenance
Mucosal disease			
Epidermolysis bullosa	No	Similar	Antibiotic prophylaxis; careful treatment if oral mucosa. Slightly higher risk of peri-implant health problems. Assure that patient will keep adequate oral health maintenance
Lichen planus	No	Similar	Antibiotic prophylaxis; slightly higher risk of peri-implant health problems. Assure that patient will keep adequate oral health maintenance. Place implants when mucosal disease is in control
Others (Crohn, SLE)	No	Similar	Antibiotic prophylaxis; slightly higher risk of peri-implant health problems. Assure that patient will keep adequate oral health maintenance. Place implants when mucosal disease is in control

(continued on next page)

Table 1
(continued)

Condition	(Relative) Contraindication	Implant Survival Rate	Precautions/Recommendations
Pemphigoid	No	Similar	Antibiotic prophylaxis; slightly higher risk of peri-implant health problems. Assure that patient will keep adequate oral health maintenance. Place implants when mucosal disease is in control
Pemphigus	No	Similar	Antibiotic prophylaxis; slightly higher risk of peri-implant health problems. Assure that patient will keep adequate oral health maintenance. Place implants when mucosal disease is in control
Smoking	Yes	Similar/ reduced	Implant survival is reduced, in particular for the maxilla, in heavy smokers. Increased risk of per-implantitis
Titanium allergy	Yes	Reduced	Use alternative implant material, for example, zirconium

Abbreviation: MRONJ, medicine related osteonecrosis of the jaw.
From Vissink A, Spijkervet FKL, Raghoebar GM. The medically compromised patient: are dental implants a feasible option? Oral Dis 2018;24:257–8; with permission.

Table 2
General algorithm for all implant cases

Stage	Item Number	Mental Checklist	Material Checklist
Evaluation and treatment planning	1	Evaluate chief complaint, history of present illness, past dental and surgical history, medications, allergies, social history, and review of systems	Written records made
Evaluation and treatment planning	2	Extra-oral and intra-oral examination of soft and hard tissues, not limited to radiograph, dental charting, periodontal probing, diagnostic models, esthetic review, current prosthesis review	Radiographs, models, photographs, and charting complete
Evaluation and treatment planning	3	Deliberation of background information and the generation of potential options	Tentative treatment plan(s) written
Evaluation and treatment planning	4	Referral for consultation to surgical specialist	Narrative for specialist with tentative plan(s) mailed
Evaluation and treatment planning	5	Discussion with specialist about background information and the generation of potential options	Team-based treatment plan(s) created
Restorative phase	6	See specific algorithms (**Tables 6, 7, 9 and 10**)	See specific algorithms (**Tables 6, 7, 9 and 10**)
Maintenance phase	7	Well maintained implant and prosthetic(s)	Home care instructions annotated in notes, and 3- to 6-mo recall visit scheduled, and keratinized tissue band always examined for sufficiency

Table 3
Flow chart for implant treatment: extra-oral variables

Structures	Fixed Implant Prostheses	Removable Overdenture
Facial support	Unnecessary	Evaluate with (out) prosthesis
Esthetic plane	Convex profile	Concave profile
Maxillomandibular relationship (angle class)	Class I/II	Class III (needs compensation)
Lip support	Entire lip thickness display	Thin upper lip
Smile line during function	Low	Average/high during speech
Vestibular space	Little	Increased during smile
Horizontal tooth display	6–10 teeth	10–14 teeth
Length upper lip	Long (26–30 mm) 2.2-mm upper central view	Short (16–20 mm) 3.4 upper central view

From Zitzmann NU, Marinello CP. Treatment plan for restoring the edentulous maxilla with implant-supported restorations: removable overdenture versus fixed partial denture design. J Prosthet Dent 1999;82(2):189; with permission.

articulators with face bow transfer and reproducible Centric Relation, occlusion, and maximum intercuspation. These three-dimensional benchmarks will give the practitioner a position of occlusal function, tooth alignment, and the ability to correct occlusal discrepancies if required. The esthetic zone can be mapped out in order for proper implant placement in relation to the hard and soft tissue of the alveolar ridge. An achievement will allow an achievement of facial form and function that the patient can both comment on and critique so that their perception of the prosthesis is considered as well.[1,8] Most significant is the aid of diagnostic casts in determining the vertical distance of the crown to bone based on the severity of ridge resorption. The distance can provide a "template "for the oral surgeon to build on using bone augmentation strategies.[1] Study casts can also provide a template for surgical guides' radiologic imaging utilizing volumetric.[11]

Bone and Soft Tissue Augmentation Strategies

Surgical-prosthetic reconstruction complexity is increased because this procedure is carried out on a wide variety of patients whose unique alveolar bone positions and facial references require patient-specific surgical-prosthetic customization. Customization almost always increases

Table 4
Flow chart for implant treatment: intraoral variables

Structures	Fixed Complete Denture	Removable Overdenture
Mucosal quality	Keratinized; nonmovable	Nonkeratinized/movable/grafting?
Mucosal quantity	Thick	Thin
Bone quantity		
Ridge palpation buccal/crest	Buccal (convex); crest (round/wide)	Buccal (concave) crest; thin/sharp Bone grafting?
Incisal papilla position	Palatal	Crest/buccal
Crown/bone/interarch space		
Clinical crown length: 10.5 mm	Optimal	Too long (large vertical space)
Tooth size/arch discrepancy	No	Yes
Speech disruption: phonetic	No	Yes
Bone quality	Type I Type II	Type III Type IV

From Zitzmann NU, Marinello CP. Treatment plan for restoring the edentulous maxilla with implant-supported restorations: removable overdenture versus fixed partial denture design. J Prosthet Dent 1999;82(2):190; with permission.

complexity. If the patient has an ideal amount and position of bone on the maxilla and the mandible, and if an ideal amount of prosthetic space is available, then the case is relatively simple. However, as more of these variables that fall outside of ideal, more customization is required. When bone is insufficient, customized bone grafting increases the case complexity. If a patient has insufficient bone in the maxilla or mandible in the vertical or horizontal dimension, bone augmentation is needed, and complexity naturally increases. Vertical augmentation procedures range from the very complex, like distraction osteogenesis, block graft, and interpositional bone grafting, to the moderate sinus augmentation, and to the mild use of particulate grafting.[12] Horizontal bone augmentation is generally mild to moderate in complexity.[12]

There is a wealth of material describing various techniques for bone augmentation, which provides a foundation that either "matures" over a period of months or allows for immediate function by biomechanical loading of implants.[12–16] Classification systems such as the schematic of Lekholm and Zarb[13] allows the surgeon an algorithm to craft the volume and density of bone required for a single unit, partially edentulous and edentulous arch restorations when planning the foundation for complex cases. Most patients who present with complex deficiencies request an "immediate surgical approach" to provide esthetics and function without the removal of an appliance. Jensen[14–16] has published numerous evidence-based studies that measured an "ideal"

vertical and horizontal volume required for immediate loading of dental implants in complex cases. Immediate function is ideally the goal for prosthetic rehabilitation and depends on mechanical fixation of the implant and not how much bone is present or required by augmentation to function. Jensen[17] has developed a complete arch site classification for immediate function using an all-on-4 design in the maxilla and mandible. **Tables 5 and 6** describes the classification system based on length, width, and angulation within the cortical bone in the maxilla and mandible. Jensen's data on 100 consecutive all-on-4 treatment cases, 54 in the maxilla and 46 in the mandible, provided greater than 95% success for immediate function.[17] These results suggest that grafting may not be required as long as there is enough cortical bone that provides a foundation for implant fixation and function. The choice of whether to use an immediate or delayed approach must be based on a discussion by the surgeon with the patient regarding risks and benefits of each method.

Radiologic Imaging

Three-dimensional computed tomography (CT) is the standard of choice to provide a "roadmap" of available bone for dental implant placement, and the introduction of cone-beam computed tomography (CBCT) with virtual reconstruction has provided a new "dimension" for precision of treatment planning.[18] The combination of implant software and imaging allows the surgeon to carefully avoid anatomic barriers, that is, pneumatized

Table 5
Complete arch classification for all-on-4 immediate function

Class of Cortex	Maxilla	Mandible
A		Sufficient vertical bone in posterior; anterior implants placed into canine region; 4 vertical implants placed 20 mm apart, interarch span 60 mm; cantilevered prosthesis not necessary
B		Several millimeter vertical bone above canal; angled implant to avoid mental foramen; implants can be placed in second premolar region and cantilevered; 2 anterior implants can be placed perpendicular to ridge; 4 implants are spaced 15 mm apart with interimplant arch between 40 and 345 mm; 5 mm vertical bone above the nerve
C		Little or no vertical above the foramen; angled implant forward in the first premolar region;10-mm cantilever and no first molar; anterior implants spread equally angled 30° to midline and extending apically in a V formation; anterior/posterior spread between 10 and 12 mm; interimplant distance of 4 implants between 30 and 40 mm. Can have an all-on-3 to increase A/P spread
D		<10 mm vertical height; 3 implants with posterior angled toward midline. IAN visible; implant perforate inferior border; 1 single central implant A/P spread 8 and 12 mm with interimplant span 25–35 mm; 3 implants adequate for immediate function

Table 6	
Complete maxillary arch classification for All-On-4 immediate function	
Class of Cortex	**Maxilla**
A	This class has a thick palatal wall of bone. Anterior implants are placed 20 mm or > forward. And angled back to create an M shape at 30°. A; engage at the M for maximum bone mass which is mostly seen in men
B	Class B has moderate bone atrophy with a relatively thin palatal wall. Posterior implants are placed at the 2nd premolar area and angled 30° forward to form an M. Anterior implants are placed in the canine area and angled back towards the M point
C	Class C maxilla alveolar bone is absent, and trans-sinus implant placement is required. Second premolar location is an alternative. The M point is reduced in volume and anterior implants engage the midline bone referred to as the V point. Anterior implants are angled at 30° forward from canine into the nasal crest; vomer implants. All converge toward the Midline; 2 of which were grafted in sinus and 2 at vomer area. A/P spread is 10–15 mm with 45 mm inter-arch span.
D	Has no M point but has V point. Good for zygomatic implant Placement. BMP needed if no sinus grafting Pterygoid implants are a choice. A V-4 approach can be used but 2 anterior implants must have a high torque value but if not available then zygomatic implants are recommended with delayed loading.

Data from Jensen OT. Complete arch site classification for all – on – 4 immediate function. J Prosth Dent. 2014;112:741–51.

sinuses and resorbed nerve canals, and can also aid in fabrication of surgical guides, which reproduce mutual landmarks improving accuracy between virtually planned and "real-life" insertion of implants.[19] A systematic review by Tahmaseb and colleagues[19] characterized greater accuracy with implants, CT, and the final surgical guide for immediate loading of mini-implants. Although

these approaches have significant benefits, caution is indicated. Intraoperative mishaps can occur, such as movement of the guide during placement of implants. Another frequent complication is the fracture of the surgical guide, which must be considered before so that an alternative surgical plan can be implemented in order to avoid early loss of implants due to lack of primary stability.[19] An impaired surgical guide is of great concern in complex cases where a "domino effect" can occur, resulting in both early and late complications with irreparable damage to anatomically vital structures and future rescue restorations. Future studies measuring template stability are being tested, especially in fully edentulous patients who are devoid of reference markings when compared with partially dentate ridges that provide greater accuracy due to surrounding supporting hard tissue. (The reader is referred to the references for further information.)

COMPLEX CASE PRESENTATIONS

Why is the perception of a case's simplicity/complexity necessary, when the steps to completing a case can be rationally arranged and then carried out according to the logical order of operations?

If patients did not require the emotional management of expectations, executing this rationale of arranged steps would be the only activity necessary, and grading the case's complexity would be valueless. Patients with complex restorative issues require a tremendous amount of emotional management of expectations, and the disclosure of the provider's subjective perception, including the case's perceived level of complexity, is imperative.[20,21] The following represents 4 basic categories of implant restoration that can be considered complex: (a) implant-supported single crown; (b) implant-supported fixed-partial denture; (c) implant-supported/attachment-retained removable overdentures; (d) implant-supported fixed dentures (hybrid).

Implant-Supported Single Crowns

Table 7 depicts the algorithm applied to a single-unit fixed implant treatment plan. If the bone and soft tissue are in the ideal place, then the single-unit fixed implant case can be considered simple. Generally speaking, however, a single, anterior, edentulous space rarely has the bone and soft tissue at an ideal position and therefore is not likely to be considered simple. To verify if the case is simple or complex before extraction of an apparently ideal looking site, bone around the mesial, facial, and distal surfaces are measured to see if the patient has less than or equal to 3 mm, 5 mm, and

Table 7
Specific algorithms for the implant-supported fixed single crowns and partial denture cases

Stage	Item Number	Mental Checklist	Material Checklist
Evaluation and treatment planning	1	Smile height for esthetic cases	Photograph of high smile and document prosthetic-tissue interface's position relative to the lips
Evaluation and treatment planning	2	Bone considerations for implant placement	CBCT reviewed
Evaluation and treatment planning	3	Interarch and intra-arch spacing considerations	Measure distances on mounted models and CBCT
Evaluation and treatment planning	4	Evaluation of the surrounding dentition's color and translucency	Evaluate the patient
Evaluation and treatment planning	5	Evaluation of the potential esthetic prognosis	Bone sounding and visual examination of smile
Presurgical work	6	Optimize the surgical experience	Fabricate surgical template and temporary
Surgical phase	7	Idealized implant placement is communicated	Surgical template is used by surgeon
Surgical phase	8	Patient has reasonable temporization	Temporary is delivered to surgeon and surgeon delivers temporary
Surgical phase	9	Patient is healed and approved by surgeon for restoration	Approval letter with implant size(s) and brand(s)
Restorative phase	10	Soft tissue site is idealized with temporary	Photograph or view of site approved by patient
Restorative phase	11	Impression coping(s) seating position is verified by radiograph	Radiograph of seated impression coping(s), opposing model, bite record, shade, photographs
Restorative phase	12	High-quality impression of implant(s) and relevant dental anatomy	Elastomeric impression with impression coping seated with implant replica
Restorative phase	13	High-quality prosthetic(s) fit on laboratory cast	Master models with implant replica and prosthetic(s)
Restorative phase	14	High-quality single-unit prosthetic(s) delivered to patient	Radiograph of prosthetic(s) torqued to manufacturer's recommendation, and any excess cement removed and patient satisfaction are documented
Restorative phase	15	Patient aware of oral hygiene and maintenance needs	Oral hygiene and maintenance instructions documented, including need to keep implant clean
Maintenance phase	16	Well-maintained implant and prosthetic(s)	Home care instructions annotated in notes, and 3- to 6-mo recall visit scheduled

3 mm, respectively, from the mesial to distal of the contact point and free-gingival margin to the bone. If the space does not exceed these distances, and there is adequate width and height of bone, then the case will be relatively simple. Whereas, a case whose bone sounding measures depths beyond those shown in **Fig. 1**, like in **Fig. 2**, will be moderate to very difficult, as the tissue will relapse to positions that are not in accordance with the ideal. The complexity will then be based on the provider's competence in using technology, interpersonal effectiveness within a multidisciplinary team, and knowledge of justified true-beliefs for the development of the insufficient tissues.

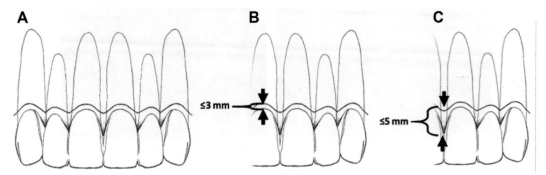

Fig. 1. (*A*) The ideal free-gingival margins and the ideal alveolar bone crests. (*B, C*) The ideal space between the contact point and free-gingival margins and the alveolar bone crests. Note that the distance at the buccal surface on (*B*) is 3 mm from the contact point and free-gingival margin to bone, and on (*C*) it is 5 mm on the mesial and distal surfaces.

Anterior maxillary single teeth

Single-tooth replacement in the anterior maxilla should include gingival position, bone levels at the alveolar crest, dimensional proportions of teeth adjacent to the replacement region, and bone quality; that is, apical levels, canine eminence, and prior periapical disease.[22] Surgical methods for socket preservation and/or bony augmentation of ridges vary, as well as timing of implant placement and loading.[14,23] The latter are predicated upon previous invasive surgery as well as whether an immediate implant is scheduled for placement. Grafting of the extraction site, however, does not guarantee anatomic resolution of the gingival margins. Adjunctive soft tissue grafting and crown lengthening have been used with good success. In a retrospective study by Axiotis and colleagues,[23] the one-piece implant with a smooth concave neck preserved marginal bone levels as well as increased space for soft tissue maturation and the establishment of a biologic width.[24,25]

If the position of the ideal free-gingival margins of the papilla and zenith point is located away from the alveolar bone crest, and the contact point is in the ideal esthetic position, then one can assign the complexity as simple. Ideally, the tissue would look like the illustration in **Fig. 1** and will have adequate bone height and width. If the alveolar bone and attached/free-gingival tissues are not in the ideal positions, like in **Fig. 2**, then the case moves away from the simple side of a complexity continuum. For instance, if before extraction, in a pending implant site, the free-gingival margin extends from the ideal position of the papilla to the interproximal bone in less than 5 mm, then the case is likely simple (see **Fig. 1**). If in the same case, the ideal free-gingival margin extends from the zenith point in a distance greater than 3 to 4 mm, then the case is likely going to be complex. In **Fig. 3**, vertical aspects of the natural tissue were missing at the time of placement of the implant, and this led to the often times overlooked complexity of delivering an ideal-looking outcome, despite the fact that the supporting tissues are not present. When aspects of the natural tissue are not in the ideal position, then competence in using technology, interpersonal effectiveness within a multidisciplinary team, and knowledge of justified

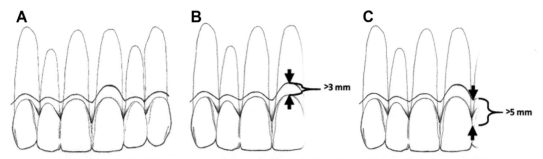

Fig. 2. (*A*) The nonideal gingival margins and the nonideal alveolar bone crests. (*B, C*) The nonideal space between the contact point and free-gingival margins and the alveolar bone crests. Note in (*A*) that the distance at the buccal surface is greater than 3 mm from contact point and free-gingival margin to bone. Note in (*B*) that the space is greater than 5 mm on the mesial and distal surfaces. These illustrations are models of complex cases.

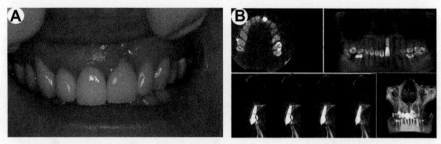

Fig. 3. The definitive effect of an implant placed in a site where the presurgical relationship of the nonideal free-gingival margin and the nonideal alveolar bone crest were greater than the ideal distances. (*A*) Facial photograph showing the nonideal tissue appearance. (*B*) CBCT scan showing the high apical positioning of the implant platform. (*Courtesy of* Nicholas Egbert, DDS, MSD, Salt Lake City, UT.)

true-beliefs, will be challenged as the provider subjectively determines the complexity of a case. **Fig. 4** portrays a case where the mesiodistal bone width was limited, due to congenitally missing lateral incisors. Although the surgeon might have opted to exercise a multidisciplinary team and widen the space with an orthodontist, the use of a smaller-diameter implant technology simplified the case and allowed for the outcome shown in the radiograph. The latter supports how subjectivity of complexity depends on the provider's innovative ability with technology in creating a successful prosthetic foundation.

Following the surgical preparation of this case, the restorative dentist's capacity for using material technology, interpersonal effectiveness with a laboratory team, and knowledge of justified true-beliefs regarding restorative materials are used to resolve the complexity of the case. In the case described, the restorative options pictured in **Fig. 5** could be considered. The breadth of options underlines the potential complexity due to material options in restoring single units. This case is in the esthetic zone so the complexity is inherently greater than one in the nonesthetic zone, but because the implants were one-piece implants and therefore the abutments could not be altered for position or color, the case became more complex. Although it would seem that if by using a one-piece implant and not adding more material

abutments to the situation this would simplify the process, why is it more complex? The complexity comes from the absolute necessity of knowing the justified true-beliefs requisite to mask the silver one-piece implant abutment. The case becomes more complex, when, in addition to masking, the ceramic must also be translucent enough to match the surrounding dentition's translucency. Finally, there is the issue of interpersonal effectiveness of working with a laboratory team that can also add to the complexity. In this case, the implant company no longer made components to impress this case after the patient experienced trauma that compromised the anterior crowns, following years of successful integration. The creative workflow for restoring the one-piece implants is shown in **Fig. 6**, which the laboratory and the restorative dentist underwent to fabricate the proper laboratory materials, and the final restorative image is shown in **Fig. 7** on the day of delivery.

Horizontal biologic issues like the aforementioned case are challenging; however, the vertical biologic issues are usually more difficult. **Fig. 8** shows a case whereby the vertical bone was compromised and the CBCT scan confirmed the vertical buccal bone problems. The management of this issue starts at the diagnostic appointment. If the scan cannot be obtained, then bone sounding can be used to help with the diagnosis and prognosis. The bone

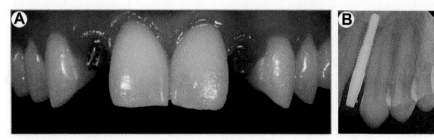

Fig. 4. A patient with minimal space between the central incisors and the canines. (Images were made at least 5 years after the implant placement.) (*A*) Facial photograph showing the final placement of one-piece implants in sites 7 and 10. (*B*) Periapical image of number 10 showing the very narrow space between teeth 9 and 11. (*Courtesy of* [*A*] Juan Olivier, CDT, MDT, FACE, Draper, UT.)

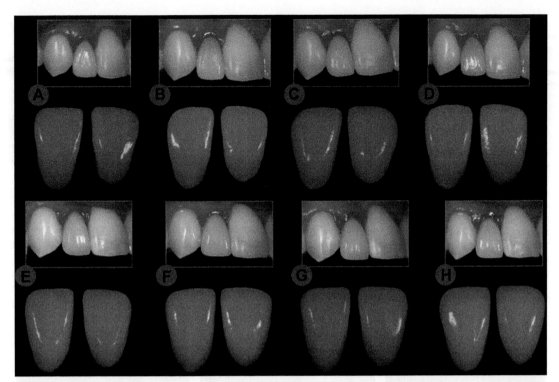

Fig. 5. Clinical images of a small sampling of potential restorative options available to restorative dentists. Notice the translucency differences. (These crowns were fabricated to fit the patient shown previously in **Fig. 4**, but were fabricated and photographed for educational purposes only by Juan Olivier.) (*A*) Multilayered, full-contour (moderate-strength), zirconia crown with glaze/stain. (*B*) Monochromatic, full-contour (high-strength), zirconia crown with glaze/stain. (*C*) Zirconia substructure (high-strength) with porcelain on the entire substructure. (*D*) Full-contour, high-translucency, lithium-disilicate crown with glaze/stain. (*E*) Low-translucency, lithium-disilicate substructure with porcelain stacked/layered on the entire substructure. (*F*) Medium-translucency, lithium-disilicate substructure with porcelain stacked/layered on the entire substructure. (*G*) Medium-opacity, lithium-disilicate substructure with porcelain stacked/layered on the entire substructure. (*H*) High-opacity, lithium disilicate substructure with porcelain stacked/layered on the entire substructure. (Courtesy of Juan Olivier, CDT, MDT, FACE, Draper, UT.)

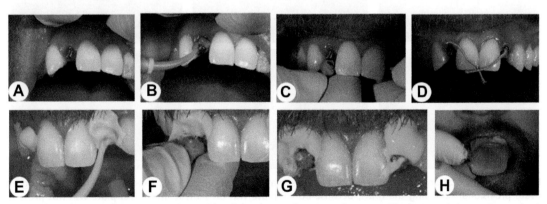

Fig. 6. Clinical image showing a patient with minimal space between the central incisors and the canines, who is going through the steps to restore two single-piece implant body implants. Because the Implant is no longer manufactured, the appropriate parts for impressing are not available. (*A*) Shows the implant site to be impressed. (*B*) Shows the use of bite registration replica to capture the emergence profile. (*C*) Shows the captured emergence profile. (*D*) Shows gingival retraction. (*E*) Shows a light viscosity elastomeric impression. (*F*) Shows the emergence profile replica to be used to ensure a better capture of the emergence profile. (*G*) Shows the use of the bite-registration replica to retract the gingival tissues. (*H*) Shows the elastomeric impression material within a custom tray for the final impression. (Courtesy of Juan Olivier, Draper, UT.)

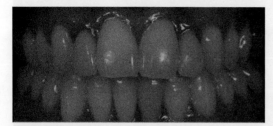

Fig. 7. The final patient case restored on 2 one-piece dental implants. Medium-translucency, lithium-disilicate crowns, with porcelain layered on the entire substructure for teeth 7 and 10. The objective was to copy the adjacent shade and translucencies, while still masking out the silver abutments that were positioned facially, relative to the ideal, due to the natural trajectory of one-piece implants following the natural pitch of the maxilla (see **Fig. 4**). These competing variables make the restoration more complex. Laboratory attribution to/photography from Juan Olivier. (Courtesy of Juan Olivier, CDT, MDT, FACE, Draper, UT.)

sounding will allow the provider to find large vertical discrepancies and determine if additional considerations might be needed. For instance, if a provider bone sounded an ideal looking free-gingival margin to discover bone loss like that pictured in **Fig. 9**, then additional esoteric understanding of biologic nuances would be needed to reconstitute an ideal-looking periodontal architecture. **Fig. 8** shows how the provider managed the vertical defect using a host of carefully executed biologic processes to obtain an ideal outcome.

Posterior maxillary/mandibular single tooth

The placement of a posterior implant and subsequent loading has been debated due to forces on the site restored. It is advantageous to graft in the hopes of restoring ideal width and height to withstand the biting forces. Careful designing of flaps to avoid vascular compromise as well as watertight closure for graft maturation is the primary goal in implant surgery of the posterior jaw.[12,17,22,24]

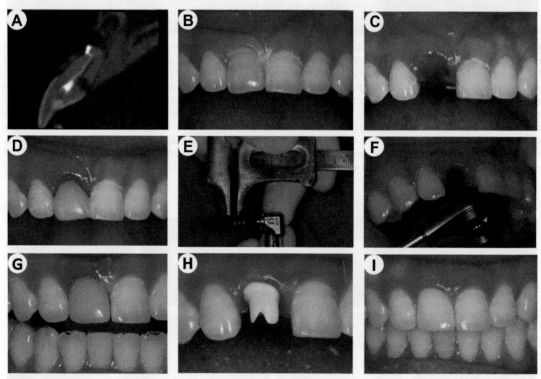

Fig. 8. These clinical photographs show socket preservation with a temporary, fixed-partial denture, using an ovate provisional occluding the graft, because buccal plate was present. If the buccal plate was not present, more aggressive GBR with a membrane would be necessary. After 4 months of healing, an immediate fixed "tissue-molding" screw-retained provisional, out of occlusion, was delivered and properly managed. Case attribution to/photographs from Dr Nicholas Egbert. (*A*) Diagnostic CBCT imaging of tooth number 8. (*B*) Presurgical photograph. (*C*) The extraction site and socket preservation. (*D*) Temporary, fixed-partial denture, with an ovate pontic occluding the grafted site. (*E*) Measuring to obtain a 3-mm distance to the ideal contact point and free-gingival facial margin. (*F*) The implant placement. (*G*) The implant-supported provisional to immediately temporize the implant. (*H*) High-strength zirconia abutment to optimize the crown and gingival colors. (*I*) The final restoration with ideal free-gingival margins. (Courtesy of Nicholas Egbert, DDS, MSD, Salt Lake City, UT.)

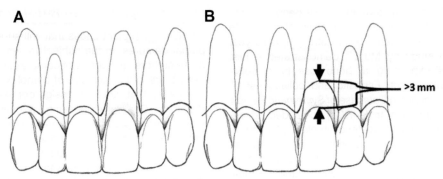

Fig. 9. (*A*) The nonideal gingival margins and the nonideal alveolar bone crests. (*B*) The nonideal space between the free-gingival margins and the alveolar bone crests. Note that the distance at the buccal surface is greater than 3 mm from free-gingival margin to bone. This is a complex case.

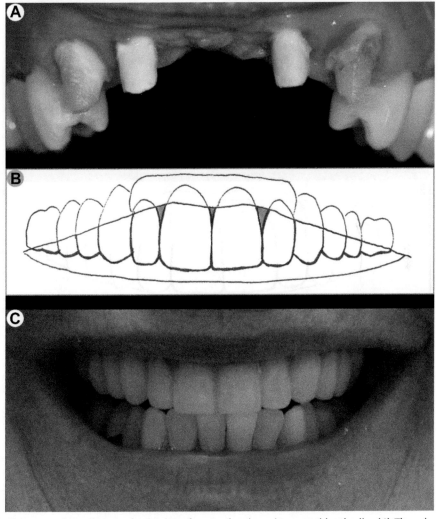

Fig. 10. (*A–C*) A case where the prosthetic's interface to the tissue is covered by the lip. (*A*) The edentulous site when the lip is fully retracted. (*B*) Why the lip is so useful in simplifying these cases. (*C*) A restorative image of the case showing the benefit of hiding the prosthetic-tissue interface.

Successful outcomes of 95% have been reported with regard to long-term predictability of immediate function in the posterior jaw. A retrospective 5-year follow-up study by Mura[24] demonstrated a less than 0.56-mm marginal bone loss in posterior implant placement. Esposito and colleagues[25,26] using the *Cochrane Database of Systematic Review* randomized clinical trials (RCT) concluded advantages in immediate posterior implant placement/functioning by patient esthetics and satisfaction. Although these results are encouraging, care must be taken in interpreting their generalizability. Practitioner protocols exist with respect to preservation of alveolar bone, overall oral health of the patient, type of bone substitutes, and timing of follow-up of patients postoperatively. (The reader is referred to the list of references.)

Implant-Supported Fixed-Partial Denture

All multiunit implant cases that will support fixed-partial dentures, in the subjective assessment of these authors, are worthy of complex status. However, there is a continuum of complexity in multiunit cases that can help assign complexity more distinctly. Generally speaking, a multiunit case whose tissue-prosthetic interface (**Fig. 10**) hides behind the lip is considered relatively simple on a multiunit complexity continuum. A multiunit case whose tissue-prosthetic interface is visible below the maxillary lip is notably more complex on a multiunit complexity continuum (**Fig. 11**). The case shown in **Fig. 10** only required adequate bone and connective tissue to support the dental implants; then prosthetic replica tissues were simulated to manage the existing defects below

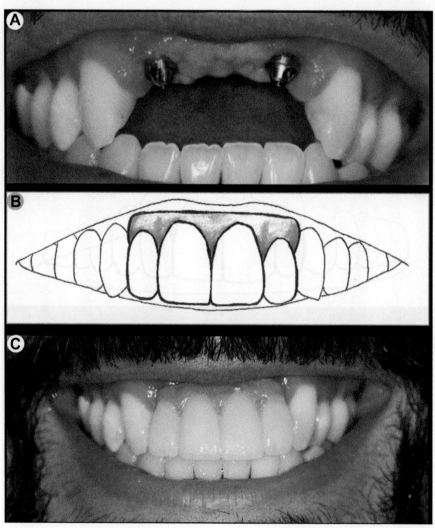

Fig. 11. A case where the prosthetic's interface to the tissue is visible. (*A*) The edentulous site. (*B*) Why the harsh borders of the prosthesis are so hard to disguise when visibly placed below the lip. (*C*) A restorative image of the case showing the entire tissue-prosthetic interface.

the lip. Although this case is admittedly complex, these cases are far simpler than when the interface is visible. So the case in **Fig. 11** is more challenging than the one pictured in **Fig. 10**, because it requires the margin of the replica gingival tissue

that sits against the periodontium to be both hygienic and esthetic. Because it is the case that ideal hygiene can exist only when esthetics are deprioritized, the margin interface usually has a very artificial appearance, because this interface,

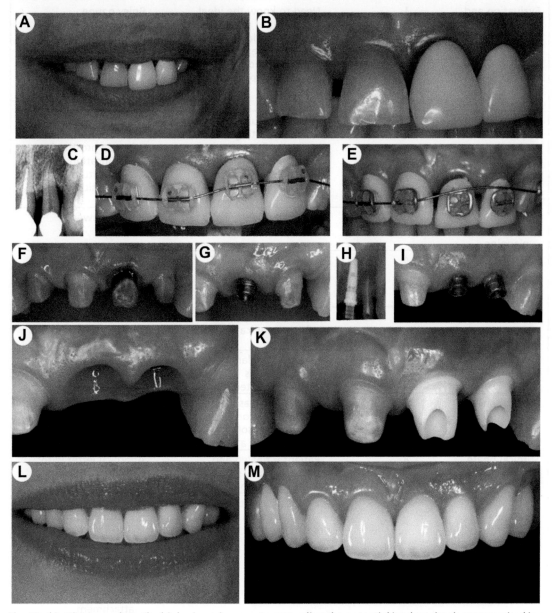

Fig. 12. (*A–M*) A case where the biologic environment surrounding the potential implant sites is compromised in a multitooth space. (*A*) Preoperative smile photograph. (*B*) Preoperative intraoral photograph. (*C*) Preorthodontic periapical film showing extent of bone loss. (*D*) Photograph of preorthodontic starting position with patient in provisionals. (*E*) Outcome of the extrusion of teeth 9 and 10 to improve biologic architecture. (*F*) Postorthodontic photograph. (*G*) One tooth extracted with immediate implant placement, followed by healing; then, the next tooth was extracted with immediate implant placement, for interimplant papilla preservation. (*H*) Radiographic view of bone levels during interimplant papilla preservation. (*I*) Preparing for site-sculpting using temporary abutments that will hold acrylic temporaries. (*J*) After site-sculpting from acrylic temporaries, with optimized emergence profile and well-matured ideal biologic architecture. (*K*) Zirconia abutments in sites 9 and 10. (*L*) Postoperative smile photograph. (*M*) Final intraoral photograph of the idealized multiunit implant sites. (*Courtesy of* Marco Brindis, DDS, New Orleans, LA.)

Table 8
Specific algorithms for the implant/attachment-supported removable dentures for edentulous cases

Stage	Item Number	Mental Checklist	Material Checklist
Evaluation and treatment planning	1	Need to know the ideal amount of prosthetic space needed and how much bone needs to be removed to obtain the ideal space	Boley gauge measurement of prosthetic space of current denture entered into the notes, and the amount of bone reduction needed
Evaluation and treatment planning	2	Define the current status of the existing prosthesis or determine if a new prosthesis is warranted	Document whether the current denture will have a prosthesis modification or a new overdenture prosthetic will be made
Evaluation and treatment planning	3	Bone considerations for implant placement	CBCT reviewed
Presurgical work	4	Optimize the surgical experience	Fabricate surgical template, bone reduction guide, and temporary
Surgical phase	5	Idealized bone position is communicated	Surgical bone reduction template is used by surgeon
Surgical phase	6	Idealized implant placement is communicated	Surgical implant placement template is used by surgeon
Surgical phase	7	Patient has reasonable temporization (most temporary solutions will require a reline)	Temporary is delivered to surgeon and surgeon delivers temporary
Surgical phase	8	Patient is healed and approved by surgeon for restoration	Approval letter with implant size(s) and brand(s)
Restorative phase	9	Definitive prosthetic fabrication is arranged	Patient is scheduled for attachment pick up if the old prosthetic will be modified, or, if a new prosthetic is to be made, the patient is scheduled for the fabrication of an attachment overdenture
Restorative phase	10	Patient is satisfied with attachment overdenture	Abutments torqued to manufacturer's recommendation, resilient liners placed with documented instructions, and patient satisfaction is documented

(continued on next page)

Table 8
(continued)

Stage	Item Number	Mental Checklist	Material Checklist
Restorative phase	11	Patient is aware of oral hygiene and maintenance needs	Oral hygiene and maintenance instructions documented, including need to keep implants clean
Maintenance phase	12	Well-maintained implant and prosthetic(s)	Home care instructions annotated in notes, and 3- to 6-mo recall visit scheduled

unlike natural tissue, must be separated from the tissue for access of hygienic instrumentation.

Both of the cases in **Figs. 10** and **11** are simpler than cases whereby the tissue-prosthetic interface shows, and biologic tissue must be used to replace missing natural tissue. Prosthetic gingiva is more predictably manipulated to the ideal positions than the biologic tissues. If a practitioner desires to bring deficient tissues down to the ideal positions using biologic materials and not use prosthetic gingiva, despite a low lip line, the case would be more complex than if prosthetic gingiva was used. Prosthetic gingiva under a low lip line allows for a less complex scenario.

Some of the more challenging cases occur when multiple adjacent teeth have to be removed, because extraction of adjacent teeth leads to a cascade of massive periodontal tissue loss. Even though much of the periodontal tissue loss has occurred before the implant placement, the removal of the teeth with the implant placement really can exasperate the appearance of this tissue loss. Diagnosing and treating these situations is extremely complex and regularly requires the use

of a multispecialty team. **Fig. 12** shows an example of a ridge with periodontal disease that has caused severe bone loss in the esthetic zone, and the culmination of this loss manifests itself with 2 adjacent teeth, whose dual extraction would lead to even greater periodontal tissue loss.[27] However, the provider manages a multiplicity of biologic variables with a multidisciplinary team to deliver ideal outcomes. **Table 7** provides the algorithms for implant-supported fixed single crowns and fixed partial dentures.

Implant-Supported/Attachment-Retained Removable Overdentures

Maxillary and mandibular attachment-retained, implant-supported, removable "overdentures" for edentulous arches are relatively simple, as long as the necessary prosthetic space is accounted for and the implant health is maintained. **Table 8** shows the specific algorithms for executing the treatment involved in providing implant-supported removable dentures to patients. Complete dentures that do not need to incorporate

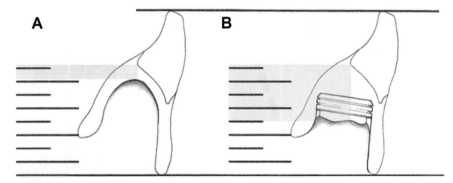

Fig. 13. (*A, B*) Sagittal section illustrations of prosthetics for an edentulous mandible. (*A*) A complete denture. Note the thin space from ridge crest to denture tooth. (*B*) An implant/abutment-supported removable denture for the edentulous arch (implant overdenture). Note the displacement of the ridge away from the denture tooth to provide space for the acrylic denture and the attachments.

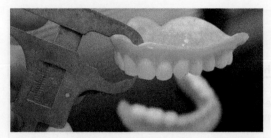

Fig. 14. A denture is measured from the incisal/occlusal surface to the intaglio surface opposite that tooth. This is the entire distance energy will be absorbed by the materials before reaching the attachment. If the amount of material within the distance measured is less than ideal, the denture will break. **Table 8** shares minimum distances from incisal/occlusal surfaces to the residual ridge to help provide sufficient material bulk to avoid prosthetic breakage.

attachments for implants can be far thinner than overdentures, because they do not need space for retaining the attachment or additional energy absorbing acrylic. Energy absorption is not necessary in conventional complete dentures because complete dentures do not have weak points caused by the cavitation into the acrylic that houses the attachment (**Fig. 13**), and because forces on complete dentures are far less than forces on implant-supported removable dentures. Because overdentures must incorporate attachments and be thick enough to withstand the weak points surrounding the attachment cavity, additional prosthetic space is necessary. **Figs. 14** and **15** depict how to determine the minimal amount of prosthetic space between the occlusal/incisal surface

to the opposite intaglio surface, to avoid the common breakages accompanying overdentures with insufficient space. **Table 9** provides the minimal amount of space necessary for edentulous prosthetic solutions.

The use of implants as a restorative alternative in patients with severely resorbed ridges is commonly chosen in cases of limited prosthetic space. Complications due to deficiencies of soft tissue foundation, that is, keratinized gingiva, soft tissue hypertrophy, shallow vestibular depth, and elevated floor of the mouth, gingival hyperplasia, and mucosal irritation, will impede long-term success of implant structure and function. When bone has to be removed to accommodate for the lack of prosthetic space, or when attached tissue has to be added around mucosal-surrounded implants, cases become somewhat more complex. Traditional preprosthetic surgery, originally conceived as the only therapeutic option for complete dentures, provides a stable foundation for implant overdentures. **Fig. 16** depicts a combined "lip switch" and free palatal gingival graft surgical treatment that both increased the vestibular depth and width of keratinized gingiva that "embraces" the transmucosal components of the implant without increasing tension on the mentalis muscle. As a result, the prosthesis becomes periodontally stable for long-term function. The timing of surgery has been debated with respect to simultaneous preprosthetic surgery and implant placement versus implant placement 2 to 3 months after preprosthetic augmentation before loading.[28,29]

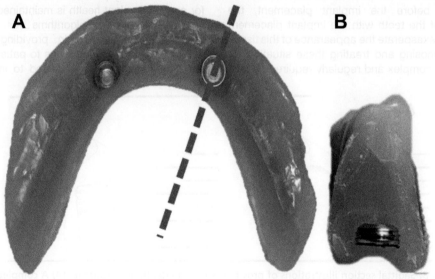

Fig. 15. (*A*) The most probable location for attachment overdenture breakages. (*B*) The overdenture from the sagittal section allows the viewer to make a visual inference as to why the breakage regularly occurs at this specific location.

Table 9
Prosthetic space considerations

Vertical	Maxillary Anterior	Maxillary Posterior	Mandibular Anterior	Mandibular Posterior	Horizontal
Attachment overdenture					
S Person	10	8	11	8	Mx. 12 mm, Md. 10 mm
M Person	12	9	13	9	
L Person	14	10	14	10	
Bar/attachment-overdenture					
S Person	12.5	10.5	13.5	10.5	Mx. 13 mm, Md. 11 mm
M Person	15	12	16	12	
L Person	17.5	13.5	17.5	13.5	
Acrylic hybrid					
S Person	11.5	9.5	12.5	9.5	Mx. 13 mm, Md. 11 mm
M Person	14.5	11.5	15.5	11.5	
L Person	17	13	17	13	
Hybrid with porcelain stacked to metal bar					
S Person (height of clinical crown)	9	6	8	6	Maxillary anterior 9 mm
M Person (height of clinical crown)	10	7	9	7	Maxillary posterior 10 mm Mandibular anterior 8 mm
L Person (height of clinical crown)	11	8	10	8	Mandibular posterior 10 mm
Hybrid with crowns cemented to metal bar					
S Person	10	10	10	10	Maxillary anterior 10 mm
M Person	10	10	10	10	Maxillary posterior 12 mm
L Person	11	10	10	10	Mandibular anterior 9 mm Mandibular posterior 12 mm

*Note these numbers are all minimum, and clinical judgment is necessary.

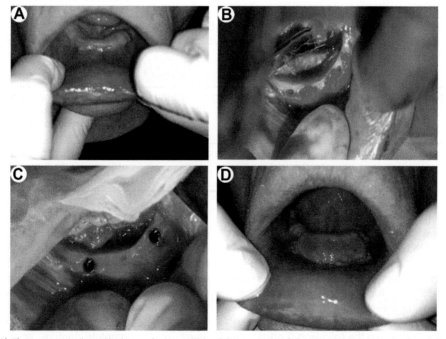

Fig. 16. (*A*) The presurgical vestibule on the mandible. (*B*) Exposure of the site. (*C*) Implants in situ. (*D*) Two-week postoperative deepened vestibule with covered implants for subsequent loading. (Courtesy of David Adams, Salt Lake City, UT.)

Table 10
Specific algorithms for the implant/attachment-supported removable denture for dentate cases

Stage	Item Number	Mental Checklist	Material Checklist
Evaluation and treatment planning	1	Dental labial and overjet:overbite ratio determined	Ideal length of teeth documented, including overbite changes
Evaluation and treatment planning	2	Need to know the ideal amount of prosthetic space needed and how much bone needs to be removed to obtain the ideal space	CBCT reviewed
Evaluation and treatment planning	3	Get ideal position of teeth to plan case	Mounted models of ideal positions of teeth
Presurgical work	4	Optimize the surgical experience	Fabricate surgical template, bone reduction guide, and temporary
Surgical phase	5	Idealized bone position is communicated	Surgical bone reduction template is used by surgeon
Surgical phase	6	Idealized implant placement is communicated	Surgical implant placement template is used by surgeon
Surgical phase	7	Patient has reasonable temporization (most temporary solutions will require a reline and immediates will require additional restorative follow-up)	Temporary is delivered to surgeon and surgeon delivers temporary (appointment(s) with restorative dentist will be needed for the immediate denture)
Surgical phase	8	Patient is healed and approved by surgeon for restoration	Approval letter with implant size(s) and brand(s)
Restorative phase	9	Definitive prosthetic fabrication is arranged	Patient is scheduled for attachment pick up if the immediate will be modified, or, if a new prosthetic is to be made, the patient is scheduled for the fabrication of an attachment overdenture
Restorative phase	10	Patient is satisfied with attachment overdenture and instruction provided	Abutments torqued to manufacturer's recommendation, resilient liners placed with use instructions, and patient satisfaction is documented
Restorative phase	11	Patient aware of oral hygiene and maintenance needs	Oral hygiene and maintenance instructions documented, including need to keep implants clean
Maintenance phase	12	Well-maintained implant and prosthetic(s)	Home care instructions annotated in notes, and 3- to 6-mo recall visit scheduled

Procedures for patients who want to convert their natural teeth to overdentures are more complicated than those for patients who are converting an edentulous ridge with a complete denture to an overdenture. **Table 10** shows the specific algorithms for converting compromised dentitions to implant-supported removable dentures. Patients with natural teeth who will convert to an overdenture have the following 3 additional factors that add complexity to the case. First,

natural overbite and overjet relationships in natural teeth are rarely ideal to transfer to the immediate denture, because the excessive overbite/overjet ratio of natural teeth would be destabilizing in overdenture occlusion (**Fig. 17**). Because of a need to correctly engineer a smaller overjet/overbite ratio for overdentures, additional complexity is added. Second, patients without teeth have never worn a complete denture, an overdenture, or an immediate denture, and the abrupt change

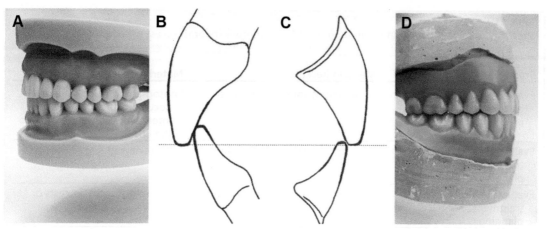

Fig. 17. (*A*) A typodont showing an ideal overbite to overjet ratio of about 3:3 mm. (*B*) The ideal dental overbite. (*C*) The reality of the overjet to overbite ratio with complete denture prosthetics, needed to minimize overbite's destabilizing force made from protrusive movements. (*D*) A complete denture with the classic shallow overbite used to avoid complete denture dislodgement.

from natural teeth to removable teeth can be functionally and psychologically distressing for a couple of months, while they await osseointegration to use the implants to stabilize the overdenture. Third, patients converting from natural teeth may have infections within the bone or other reasons with the extraction sockets that prevent the immediate placement of implants,

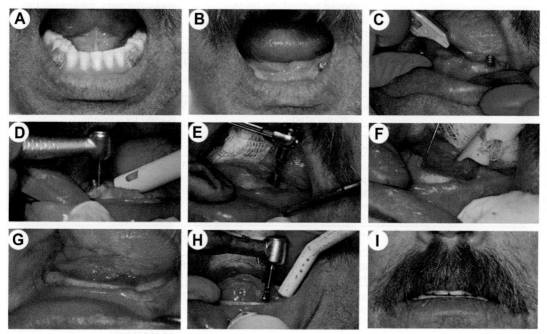

Fig. 18. A patient who likely had a deep bite in his dentition and was likely converted to an immediate without the ideal repositioning of the bone to account for the ideal position of the incisal edge nor the ideal prosthetic space. The patient underwent revision surgery to redo the implant placement and have the implants and bone placed at the ideal positions. Redoing cases can add complexity. (*A*) A significant amount of incisor display, and insufficient acrylic showing through with noticeable pink acrylic on the facial of the premolars. (*B*) Attachments are visible without retraction of the patient's lips. (*C*) Preparing the flap for surgery. (*D*) Trephining out the implants. (*E*) Removing the implants from the jaw. (*F*) Bone reduction to afford a more ideal amount of space between the attachments and the incisal/occlusal surfaces. (*G*) The leveled alveolar bone. (*H*) Placement of the implants at a more apical position. (*I*) The final restoration with a more ideal dentolabial position of the lower incisors.

Table 11
Specific algorithms for the implant-supported fixed denture (hybrid) cases

Stage	Item Number	Mental Checklist	Material Checklist
Evaluation and treatment planning	1	Smile height for esthetic cases	Photograph of high smile and document prosthetic-tissue interface's position relative to the lips
Evaluation and treatment planning	2	Bone considerations for implant placement	CBCT reviewed
Evaluation and treatment planning	3	Inter-arch and intra-arch spacing considerations	Measure distances on casts or CBCT
Evaluation and treatment planning	4	Dental labial and overjet/overbite ratio determined	Ideal length of teeth documented, including overbite changes
Evaluation and treatment planning	5	Get ideal position of teeth to plan case	Mounted models of ideal positions of teeth, and the prosthetic-tissue interface's position relative to the lips
Evaluation and treatment planning	6	Need to know the ideal amount of prosthetic space needed and how much bone needs to be removed behind the lip to obtain the ideal prosthetic space and prosthetic-tissue interface position	CBCT measurement of necessary prosthetic space combined with mounted model measurements, determine the amount of bone reduction needed
Presurgical work	7	Optimize the surgical experience	Fabricate surgical template, bone reduction guide, and temporary
Surgical phase	8	Idealized bone position is communicated	Surgical bone reduction template is used by surgeon
Surgical phase	9	Idealized implant placement is communicated	Surgical implant placement template is used by surgeon
Surgical phase	10	Patient has reasonable temporization (interim temporary solutions will require additional restorative follow-up)	Temporary is delivered to surgeon and surgeon delivers temporary (appointment(s) with restorative dentist will be needed for the interim hybrid)
Surgical phase	11	Patient is healed and approved by surgeon for restoration	Approval letter with implant size(s) and brand(s)
Restorative phase	12	Improvement of the interim hybrid	Reline, repair, and polish the interim
Restorative phase	13	Impression coping(s) seating position is verified by radiograph	Radiograph of seated impression coping(s), opposing model, bite record, shade, photographs
Restorative phase	14	High-quality impression of implant(s) and relevant dental anatomy	Elastomeric impression with impression coping seated with implant replica
Restorative phase	15	Cast's implant positions and mouth's implant positions are precisely the same positions	Verification jig is able to fit precisely on the implants on the cast and in the mouth, and

(continued on next page)

Table 11
(continued)

Stage	Item Number	Mental Checklist	Material Checklist
			radiographs are made and documented
Restorative phase	16	Wax try in on fixed appliance is approved	Photograph and/or documentation of patient's acceptance of the appearance obtained
Restorative phase	17	Coordination with laboratory for the substructure completed	Computer-aided design files approved for fabrication of milled bar
Restorative phase	18	High-quality prosthetic(s) fit on laboratory cast	Master models with implant replica and prosthetic(s)
Restorative phase	19	High-quality single-unit prosthetic(s) delivered to patient and patient is satisfied	Radiograph of prosthetic(s) torqued to manufacturer's recommendation and photographs and documentation of patient's satisfaction obtained
Restorative phase	20	Patient aware of oral hygiene and maintenance needs	Oral hygiene and maintenance instructions documented and include cleaning in-between prosthesis and the tissue for optimal implant and tissue health, and the need to report any problems immediately
Maintenance phase	21	Well-maintained implant and prosthetic(s)	Home care instructions annotated in notes, and 3-mo recall visit scheduled

thereby adding additional wait time for socket healing before initiating the subsequent osseointegration of the implants. Delaying the utility of the overdenture adds more psychological distress to the patient, which has to be managed by the provider.

Fig. 18 depicts a case whereby the complexity of a patient converting to an overdenture from natural teeth was misperceived, and the case had to be redone. This case did not account for the ideal placement of the prosthetic teeth nor did it account for prosthetic space needs with accompanying bone reduction, before the delivery of the overdenture. Redoing any case requires careful management of trust with the patient, and conservative preservation of the effected tissues during the reparative transformation.

Mandibular overdentures are far simpler than maxillary overdentures. Maxillary overdentures are built in bone that has a historically higher failure rate for implants, and more uncertainty surrounds the maxillary overdenture because it has far less research available to inform providers about its essentials. Once the overdentures are in use, as long as the implant health is maintained, both the maxillary and the mandibular maintenance are about the same. However, if an implant's health becomes problematic from an ailing or failing implant in either of these arches, both these arches become complex; because the maxillary arch uses more implants and has poorer-quality bone, the maxillary overdenture is more at risk for higher complexity. Both arches are usually designed with just enough implant support, and not extra implant support in terms of the number of implants. Therefore, when one implant ails or fails, the entire overdenture system is weakened and uncertainty arises regarding the prognosis of the remaining implants that now have to carry more load than originally designed, which adds complexity to the case.

Implant-Supported Fixed Dentures (Hybrid)

Among the available implant options patients consider, the implant- and bar-supported fixed denture (a hybrid) is generally the most complex. **Table 11** shares the specific algorithms for the workflow necessary to provide patients with

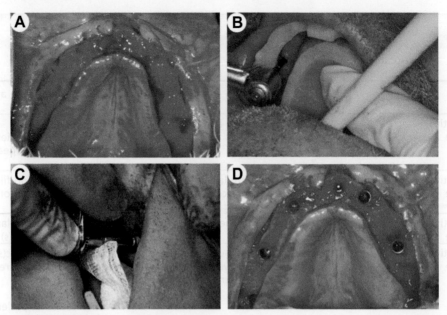

Fig. 19. The hybrid generally is supported by 4 or more maxillary implants. These photographs give a very simplified generic outline of the process of the surgical work leading up to the hybrid prosthetic protocols. (*A*) Incision and flap. (*B*) Osteotomies. (*C*) Implant delivery. (*D*) Implants placed.

implant-supported fixed dentures (hybrids). Only the multiunit fixed partial dentures on patients with visible transition lines that are managed with biologic site development rival these complex cases. These cases often present the most complexity because the technology is extremely esoteric; interpersonal effectiveness within a multidisciplinary team is paramount, and knowledge of justified true-beliefs is very specialized. **Figs. 19** and **20** provide a brief overview of the surgical steps to deliver implants to support hybrids and the prosthetic protocols to immediately load

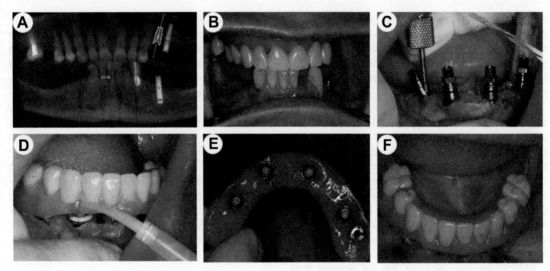

Fig. 20. The conversion process undertaken to replace mandibular dentition with an immediately loaded implant-supported fixed denture. Case attribution to/photography from Dr Nicholas Egbert. (*A*) Presurgical CBCT for planning the placement of implant bodies. (*B*) Preoperative photograph of mandibular dentition. (*C*) Placement of implants into the mandible. (*D*) Preparing for the bonding stage wherein the prosthesis is connected to the implants abutments. (*E*) The intaglio surface showing the cured acrylic or resin surface integrating with the attachments or abutments. (*F*) The completed immediate prosthesis. (Courtesy of Nicholas Egbert, DDS, MSD, Salt Lake City, UT.)

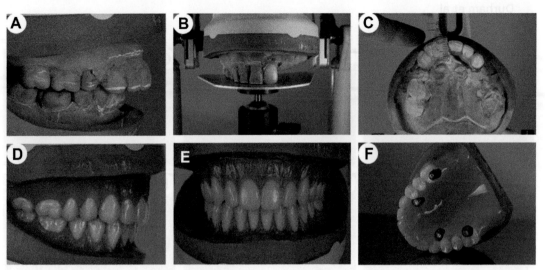

Fig. 21. The workflow to prepare an immediate denture to be used for the transition to an immediate implant-supported hybrid prosthesis. Laboratory attribution to/photography from Eugene Royzengurt. (*A*) White lines on the dental casts signify the references the dentist gave to the laboratory technician to idealize the prescriptive positions of the teeth. (*B, C*) The laboratory technician placing the acrylic teeth in the ideal positions. (*D*) Relative to (*A*), the laboratory technician has optimized the positions of the teeth. (*E*). An immediate denture processed in acrylic from the laboratory technician's wax-up seen in (*F*) This immediate denture will be converted into a temporary hybrid at the day of surgery and used during the healing of the implants. (Courtesy of Eugene Royzengurt, laboratory technician, Sandy, UT.)

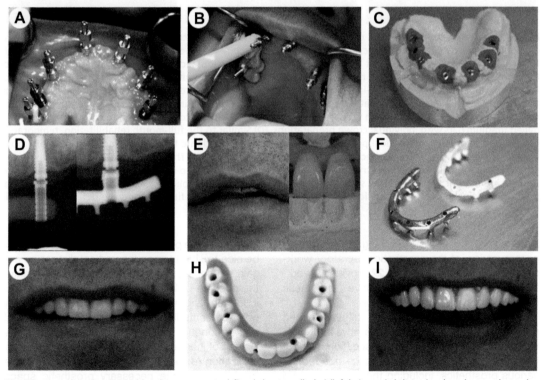

Fig. 22. A patient having an implant-supported fixed denture (hybrid) fabricated. (*A*) An implant impression using open tray impression copings is prepared. (*B*) An elastomeric impression material captures the positions of the copings. (*C*) A dental model is made using implant replicas in the same relative positions as the implants, so indirect dentistry can be performed in the laboratory. (*D*) In the left radiograph, a verification jig is used and shows that it is not seating; therefore, the image on the right containing the final titanium bar will also not seat. The verification jig needs to sit passively in order to fabricate a bar that also sits passively. (*E*) Conventional steps in the fabrication of dentures are carried out, like wax rim and wax try-in prescriptions. (*F*) The replica bar is copied or a computer aided design bar is milled to produce a titanium substructure. (*G*) The final try-in with the titanium bar and acrylic teeth set in wax. (*H*) The definitive prosthesis is processed indirectly in the laboratory. (*I*) The final restoration is delivered.

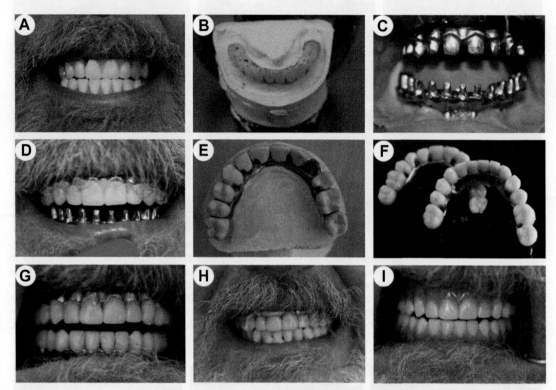

Fig. 23. An implant-supported fixed denture (hybrid) made with ceramic teeth on individual preparations to increase the longevity of the prosthetic. This level of complexity combines the difficulty of hybrid construction with full-mouth crown rehabilitation, but it requires far less bone reduction because the materials are far more effective at managing masticatory forces than acrylic. (*A*) The process begins with the approval from the patient/doctor of the wax try-in. (*B*) The wax try-in is either digitized or acrylized for either digital or mechanical preparing of the denture teeth, similar to how natural teeth are prepared. In the picture shown here, the denture was acrylized, and each acrylic tooth was then prepared for a crown and then sent to a technician to copy and mill. (*C*) The milled titanium bars with individual crown preparations. (*D*) Similar to the full-mouth rehabilitation, temporaries can be used to determine the ideal positions of the teeth and to elucidate the vertical and horizontal bite position. (*E*) The crowns are milled to specification and heated in a furnace. (*F*) The completed prosthetics without the gingival veneering. (*G*) The ceramic try-in and bite verification. (*H*) An up-to-date record of the tissue is desired to provide intimate fit with the ridge, so an impression will be made to replicate these tissue/prosthetic relationships. (*I*) The final porcelain or acrylic pink veneer (acrylic shown here) is finalized and the definitive prosthetic is delivered.

hybrids on the day of surgery. **Fig. 21** provides a case overview of the prosthetic laboratory workflow for the interim hybrid. **Fig. 22** provides a workflow overview of the definitive prosthetic considerations.

Like the overdentures, these full-arch hybrid prosthetics require enough restorative materials to withstand the forces of mastication without breaking. **Table 9** shows the space needed for various prosthetics, including the full-arch hybrid varieties. Again, the space between the lingo-incisal/occlusal surfaces and the gingival tissue made up by restorative materials can be referred to as the prosthetic space and is measured with a Boley gauge (see **Fig. 14**). Because of the uniqueness of every patient, many times patients present with bone that obstructs the volume

needed for the prosthetic space. Although it would be nice to simply open the vertical dimension and gain the necessary prosthetic space by changing the position of the teeth from the ideal length to a longer length, unfortunately, this lengthening often presents its own set of esthetic, functional, and phonetic issues. Therefore, oftentimes, instead of increasing vertical dimension, case customization requires the reduction of bone in order to provide for the necessary prosthetic space. Reducing bone adds complexity to the case because this procedure requires the coordination and execution from the surgical and restorative team of the precise amount of bone that must be removed.

Table 9 shows that the hybrid made of cemented individual crowns on a metal bar, and

Complexity Ranking	Surgical Prosthetic Procedure	Provider Complexity Range
	Table 12 **Subjectivity continuum**	
1	Redoing or implant failure with items ranked 2–7 below	Extremely difficult
2	Crowns on metal preparation hybrids (see **Fig. 23**) with zygomatic implants	Extremely difficult
3	Stacked ceramo-metal hybrid with zygomatic implants	Extremely difficult
4	Crowns on metal preparation hybrids (see **Fig. 23**) with sinus grafting	Extremely difficult
5	Stacked ceramo-metal hybrid with grafting	Extremely difficult
6	Acrylic/titanium hybrid with zygomatic implants	Extremely difficult
7	Acrylic/titanium hybrid with grafting	Extremely difficult
8	Redoing or implant failure with 9	Extremely difficult
9	Implant-supported fixed multiunit crowns, vertical biologic issues, visible interface (see **Figs. 11** and **12**)	Extremely difficult
10	Redoing or implant failure with items ranked 11–13 below	Extremely difficult
11	Crowns on metal preparation hybrids (see **Fig. 23**) with ideal bone	Difficult
12	Stacked ceramo-metal hybrid with ideal bone	Difficult
13	Acrylic/titanium hybrid with ideal bone	Difficult
14	Redoing or implant failure with item ranked 15	Difficult
15	Implant-supported fixed partial dentures, vertical biologic issues, hidden interface (see **Fig. 10**)	Difficult
16	Redoing or implant failure with item ranked 17	Difficult
17	Implant-supported single crown with visible interface and vertical biologic issues (see **Fig. 8**)	Difficult
18	Redoing or implant failure with items ranked 19–20	Difficult
19	Maxillary implant/attachment-supported removable overdenture with grafting	Difficult
20	Mandibular implant/attachment-supported removable overdenture with grafting	Difficult
21	Redoing or implant failure with items ranked 22–23	Moderate
22	Maxillary implant/attachment-supported removable overdenture with ideal bone	Moderate
23	Mandibular implant/attachment-supported removable overdenture with ideal bone	Moderate
24	Redoing or implant failure with items ranked 25–26	Moderate
25	Implant-supported single crown with visible interface and ideal periodontium	Moderate
26	Implant-supported single crown with hidden interface and ideal periodontium	Moderate

the hybrid where porcelain is stacked on the metal bar, do not need very much prosthetic space, and therefore, would not be as complex. However, although the surgical work is less complex if bone reduction is not necessary, these prosthetics are highly technical and surpass the acrylic hybrid in restorative complexity. **Fig. 23** shows some of the unique steps in fabricating one of these more complex prosthetics. Both the porcelain stacked to the metal bar and the

crowns cemented to the metal bar combine elements of full-mouth dental reconstruction with the elements required to provide standard hybrids. If one of the implants ails or fails under the interim or definitive full-arch hybrid, the case can become very complicated if the failing implant is essential for the support of the prosthesis. Because many hybrid prostheses are made with the bare minimum amount of implants to support a hybrid, the failure of one implant can mean short- and long-term reconsiderations. Many of these patients selected the hybrid because it is fixated to the jaw, and these patients are unwilling to have any removable prosthetic. When a definitive prosthetic, fixed to the patient's jaw, has a supporting implant that is failing, in a patient who will not tolerate short-term removable prosthetics, the case becomes very complex. These patients will need to revert to their interim hybrid, and have another implant placed and heal, before a new definitive prosthetic can be delivered. Although these are again somewhat complex operations, as well as expensive and time-consuming reconstructions, much of the additional complexity comes from managing a potentially tense patient-provider relationship.

SUBJECTIVELY HELPING PATIENTS

Although evidence-based dentistry has done much to improve dental procedures by radically augmenting providers' subjective limitations with objectively demonstrated science, the patient-provider relationship will likely always be enormously grounded in sharing subjective beliefs.[29,30] Patient expectations often are misaligned with reality because he or she does not have the experience to form a strong understanding of the impact complex implant procedures might have on their lives. The more complex the procedure, the more likely the expectations of patients may not be managed well enough to avoid a loss of trust in the patient-provider relationship. To aid expectation management in complex implant cases, **Table 12** provides a subjective ranking of case complexity for providers.[29,30] (The reader is referred to the references for further interest.)

SUMMARY

This article has provided a series of algorithms and checklists in the treatment planning of the complex dental implant patient from both the surgeon and the restorative dentist's perspectives. Cooperation among interdisciplinary fields is paramount in order to both reestablish a functional occlusion and provide a long-term esthetic benefit to the patient. Although more of an art than a science, most experienced oral-health care physician know that effectively relating to patients on a subjective level may prove at times to be just as important to the patient as the providers' knowledge of clinical science. The key to success will always be an honest recommendation based on her or his specialization and experience. Cost, advantages,

disadvantages, and treatment alternatives must be predicated upon the hard and soft tissue foundations and how well they can be crafted to create a prosthesis that the surgeon, restorative dentist and patient are satisfied with. Both an algorithmic and a subjective description of complex implant cases have been provided so as to provide the restorative dentists' perceptions and realities involved therein. This form of communication allows dental implant teams to provide higher standards for baseline performance and success in the complex implant patient.

REFERENCES

1. Zitzmann NU, Margolin MD, Filippi A, et al. Patient assessment and diagnosis in implant treatment. Aust Dent J 2008;53(1Suppl):S3–10.
2. Jivraj S, Corrado P, Chee W. An interdisciplinary approach to treatment planning in implant dentistry. Br Dent J 2007;202:11–8.
3. Kotsakis GA, Ioannou AL, Hinrichs JE, et al. A systematic review of observational studies evaluating implant placement in the maxillary jaws of medically compromised patients. Clin Implant Dent Relat Res 2015;17(3):598–608.
4. Diz P, Scully C, Sanz M. Dental implants in the medically compromised patient. J Dent 2013;41(3):195–206.
5. Tucker MR, Narcisi ER, Ochs MW. Implant treatment: advanced concepts and complex cases. In: Hupp JR, Ellis E, Tucker MR, editors. Contemporary oral and maxillofacial surgery. 6th edition. St Louis (MO): Elsevier Mosby Health Sciences; 2014. p. 264–94.
6. Sadowsky SJ, Fitzpatrick B, Curtis DA. Evidence-based criteria for different treatment planning of implant restorations for the maxillary edentulous patient. J Prosthodont 2015;24:433–46.
7. Vissink A, Spijkervet FKL, Raghoebar GM. The medically compromised patient: are dental implants a feasible option? Oral Dis 2018;24:253–60.
8. Zitzmann NU, Marinello CP. Treatment plan for restoring the edentulous maxilla with implant-supported restorations: Removable overdenture versus fixed partial denture design. J Prosthet Dent 1999;82(2):188–96.
9. Pinho T, Neves M, Alves C. Multidisciplinary management including periodontics, orthodontics, implants, and prosthetics for an adult. Am J Orthod Dentofacial Orthop 2012;142:235–45.
10. Mills EJ, Dunson BC, Koch P. Evaluation, diagnosis, and treatment planning of complex implant cases. J Oral Implantol 1996;22(1):12–6.
11. D'Haese J, Ackhurst J, Wismeijer D, et al. Current state of the art of computer-guided implant surgery. Periodontol 2000 2017;73:121–33.
12. Moy PK, Pozzi A, Palacci P, et al. Hard and soft tissue augmentation [Chapter 8]. In: Moy PK, Pozzi A,

John B III, editors. Fundamentals of implant dentistry, vol. 2. Chicago: Quintessence; 2016. p. 205–58.

13. Lekhom U, Zarb GA. Patient selection and preparation. In: Branemark P-I, Zarb GA, Albreksson T, editors. Tissue –integrated prostheses: osseointegration in clinical dentistry. Chicago: Quintesscence; 1985. p. 199–209.

14. Jensen OT. Site classification for the osseointegrated implant. J Prosthet Dent 1989;61:228–34.

15. Jensen OT, Adams MW, Cottam JR, et al. The all-on-four shelf: Maxilla. J Oral Maxillofac Surg 2010;68: 2520–7.

16. Jensen OT, Adams MW, Cottam JR, et al. The all-on-four shelf mandible. J Oral Maxillofac Surg 2011;69: 175–9.

17. Jensen OT. Complete arch site classification for all-on-4 immediate function. J Prosthet Dent 2014;112:741–51.

18. Handelsman M. Surgical guidelines for dental implant placement. Br Dent J 2006;201(3):139–51.

19. Tahmaseb A, De clerck R, Wismeijer D. Computer-guided implant placement: 3D planning software, fixed intraoral reference points, and CAD/CAM technology: a case report. Int J Oral Maxillofac Implants 2009;24:542–6.

20. Emanuel EJ, Emanuel LL. Four models of the physician –patient –relationship. JAMA 1992;267(16):2221–6.

21. Polanyi M. Personal knowledge. Corr. edition. Chicago: University Of Chicago Press; 1974.

22. Block MS, Jackson WC. Techniques for grafting the extraction site I the preparation for dental implant placement. Atlas Oral Maxillofac Surg Clin N Am 2006;14(1):1–25.

23. Axiotis JP, Nuzzolo P, Barausse C, et al. One-Piece implants with smooth concave neck to enhance soft tissue development and preserve marginal bone levels: a retrospective study with 1-6- year follow-up. Biomed Res Int 2018. https://doi.org/10.1155/2018/2908484.

24. Mura P. Immediate loading of tapered implants placed in post extraction sockets: retrospective analysis of the 5-year clinical outcome. Clin Implant Dent Relat Res 2012;14(4):565–74.

25. Esposito MA, Koukoulopoulou A, Coulthard P, et al. Interventions for replacing missing teeth: dental implants in fresh extraction sockets (immediate, immediate-delayed and delayed implants). Cochrane Database Syst Rev 2006;(4):CD005968.

26. Cillo JE, Finn R. reconstruction of the shallow vestibule edentulous mandible with simultaneous split thickness skin graft vestibuloplasty and mandibular endosseous implants for implant- supported overdentures. J Oral Maxillofac Surg 2009;67:381–6.

27. Kan JYK, Rungcharassaeng K. Interimplant papilla preservation in the esthetic zone: a report of six consecutive cases. Int J Periodontics Restorative Dent 2003;23(3):249–59.

28. Cortell-Ballester I, Figuerido R, Gay-Escoda C. Lowering of the mouth floor and vestibuloplasty to support a mandibular overdenture retained by two implants: a case report. J Clin Exp Dent 2014;6(3):310–2.

29. Carlsson G. Review of some dogmas in clinical prosthodontics. J Prosthodont Res 2009;53:3–10.

30. ADA policy statement on evidence-based dentistry. Available at: http://www.ada.org/en/about-the-ada/ada-positions-policies-and-statements/policy-on-evidence-based-dentistry. Accessed January 27, 2019.

Single-Implant Treatment

Michael S. Block, DMD

KEYWORDS

- Single-tooth implant • Navigation planning • Structural strength

KEY POINTS

- The replacement of one tooth using one implant involves a set of unique criteria for long-term success.
- Successful therapy should be based on long-term function and health of the adjacent tissues.
- Sections of this article examine these critical criteria that when working together can result in successful long-term tooth replacement.

THE IMPLANT
Structural Strength

The implant should not fracture at any part of the treatment, from insertion to long-term cyclic loading. Implants made from commercially pure (CP) titanium must have sufficient thickness to withstand loading forces. When narrow implants are used, less than 3.5 mm in diameter, with internal connections, the walls at the coronal aspect of the implant may be thin and hence more susceptible to fracture. Manufacturers may provide strict instructions to withstand insertion torque on these thinner-walled implants.

There are implants made from titanium alloy, which strengthen the implant. Such implants must be carefully evaluated for surface roughness because the blasting and etching protocols will have to be modified to reach a surface roughness comparable with implants made from the softer CP titanium.[1]

Surface Considerations

The process of surface osteogenesis begins with fibrin adhesion from the initial contact of the implant with blood. Fibrin adhesion increases as the surface roughness increases. Platelet aggregation will be proportioned to the degree of fibrin adhesion. The platelets release factors for cell recruitment and angiogenesis, with eventual bone deposition, which all starts with the implant's surface character.[2–4]

Thread Patterns

Most implants have threads that allow the implant to be placed with accuracy, precision, and primary stability. Threads can have flat surfaces, angled surfaces, rounded edges, and other unique designs. Each manufacturer will market the implant's thread design to the best extent possible, yet there is minimal evidence base of clinical evidence that supports one design over other. When threads are closer together, a full turn of the implant deepens the implant less than when the thread pattern is wider and thought to be more "aggressive." This factor is important to take into consideration when placing the implant with a specific timing of the antirotation component, and an angled platform implant. The deeper threads and wider threads are proposed to result in greater primary stability of the implant.[5–7]

Insertion Method

The common theme is atraumatic implant site preparation, which results in minimal bone damage at the implant bone interface. Some implants are placed at slow speed using a drill. Others are seated by hand ratcheting. Manufacturers often

Disclosure Statement: Dr M.S. Block owns X-Nav, Inc. stock and is a consultant for Implant One.
Private Practice, 110 Veterans Memorial Boulevard, #112, Metairie, LA 70005, USA
E-mail address: drblock@cdrnola.com

Oral Maxillofacial Surg Clin N Am 31 (2019) 251–258
https://doi.org/10.1016/j.coms.2018.12.004

oralmaxsurgery.theclinics.com

recommend drill sizes to compensate for soft or hard bone quality. Some implants are placed after forming thread patterns in the bone for ease of placement. The key is to use a drill set that does not burn bone.

When a cutting drill rotates clockwise, it removes bone. When a drill is rotated counter-clockwise, it will tend to compact bone rather than remove it. When placing an implant in porous bone, or in a molar socket with thin interdental bone, a drill that compacts rather than removes bone may be beneficial.[8,9]

Abutment-Implant Connection

The original Branemark implants had an external hex on the platform. The hex was used to drive the implant into a prepared site that had threads formed within the bone. In the edentulous patient with cross-across-arch stabilized prostheses, the retentive copings did not engage the external hex. When these implants were used for single-tooth restorations, engaging the relatively short external hex, there was screw loosening over time. After using increased torque on the screws, with good yet mixed success, implant manufacturers began using an internal connection. The internal connections had an internal hex pattern for antirotational features, a flat interface where the abutments met the implant internal surface, or conical connections that were mechanically sound after loading the screw.

Attention has been given to the obvious contamination of the space within the internal connection that exists between the bottom of the screw and the bottom of the internal connection. Some investigators consider that leakage of these contaminants may be a cause of bone loss.[10–12] The conical connection has been implied to be optimal for sealing the interface and to prevent bone loss from contaminated parts, yet is difficult to prove in clinical trials.

The diameter of the parts fitting into an implant is an important consideration for single-tooth restorations. If the insertion diameter of the abutment is small, and the crown is perhaps a molar tooth that has lateral forces placed on it, the narrow parts engaging the implant may be prone to fatigue and fracture. Thus an abutment-implant system with a relatively small diameter interface may use solid abutments rather than hollow abutments with screw retention to strengthen these narrow abutments.

When using a conical connection, the final seating of the abutment is achieved by using a torque driver set at a manufacturer-derived force value. This approach seats the abutment an extra distance, which may be small but needs to be taken into consideration by the restoring dentist. If the crown on the abutment is fitted with the abutment not in its final position, the crown may not seat completely because of contact interferences. Careful attention to these details is important when seating a crown on a single-implant restoration, otherwise the interface between the crown and abutment may not be sealed. The design of the interface should take this into consideration.[13]

Depth Placement

In a single-tooth restoration, the implant's vertical position plays an important role in the eventual crestal bone levels and esthetics of the restoration. In the molar sites, the implant is usually placed at the level of the crest. The thickness of the alveolar bone on the crest may be 1 mm thick, so subcrestal implant placement in the molar region may result in lack of crestal cortical bone stability. In the anterior maxilla the implant can be placed subcrestal to allow for ideal implant emergence. Evidence-based evaluations indicate that crestal bone levels are better maintained with subcrestal placement, although this may be related more to the design of the abutment-implant interface rather than pure subcrestal placement.[14,15]

Placement Timing: Delayed or Immediate Extraction

Single implants can be placed at the time of tooth removal or after the site has healed. The criteria for immediate placement include, but are not limited to:

1. Lack of purulent exudate
2. Satisfactory bone availability for primary stability of implant
3. Healthy gingiva without erythema or hyperplasia
4. Ability to place implants and avoid the nerves
5. Ability to place implant in ideal location for final prosthetics

Criteria for delayed placement include, but are not limited to:

1. Need to graft site to provide sufficient bone for implant stability and ideal placement location
2. Lack of bone within extraction socket to stabilize implant
3. Avoidance of excessive occlusal trauma to implants with patients wearing removable provisionals

Implant dimensions are important to consider when placing into an immediate extraction socket. In general, implant diameter of choice is restoration dependent. For a molar, choose a wider diameter implant rather than a narrow one. In the anterior region an implant in the small to mid size (4.3 mm) works well compared with wide-diameter implants, owing to emergence profile issues.

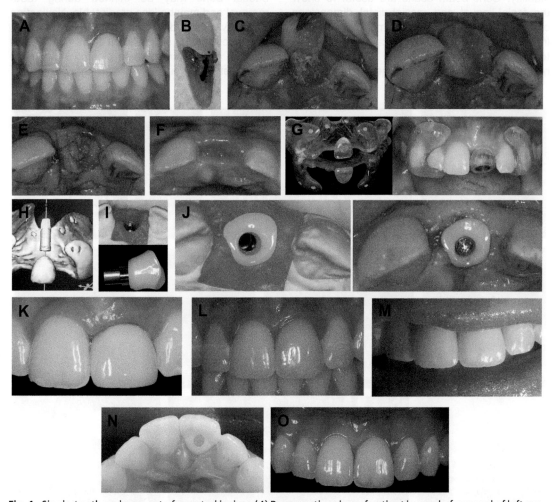

Fig. 1. Single-tooth replacement of a central incisor. (*A*) Preoperative view of patient in need of removal of left central incisor. Note the thin gingiva with darkened appearance from translucent gingiva over a crown. (*B*) Extracted tooth showing external resorption. (*C*) After tooth had been removed, a subperiosteal tunnel was made to allow placement of a subepithelial connective tissue graft from the palate. After placement of the connective tissue graft, the socket was filled with allograft. (*D*) The connective tissue graft was long enough to both augment the labial contour and cover the grafted extraction socket. (*E*) The connective tissue graft sutured to the palatal edge of the grafted socket. (*F*) The edentulous site 4 months following extraction and soft-tissue graft, Note the healthy, stippled thick gingiva. (*G*) Radiographic stent with gutta-percha fiducial markers with a simulated central incisor tooth form. This was used to fabricate a static surgical guide to place the implant in an ideal position. (*H*) Plan from the computed tomography planning software showing the virtual implant placement to provide 3 mm of depth from the planned gingival margin and angulation to allow for screw retention of the final crown. (*I*) An implant analog was placed into the guide stent using a prosthetic guide coping. From the model, a custom healing abutment with ideal subgingival contour was designed and milled for attachment at the time of implant placement to contour the gingiva during the implant integration period. (*J*) Side-by-side photos showing the orientation of the healing abutment on the model and in the patient after implant placement. (*K*) After allowing 4 months for implant integration, a provisional crown was made. There seems to be excess gingival profile. It is advised to leave this tissue in place and allow the natural healing response to crosslink and contract. (*L*) One year after implant placement the final crown has an agreeable esthetic appearance. (*M*) The lip line shows an attractive show of the crown in this 25-year-old woman. (*N*) Eight-year follow-up photo shows maintenance of gingival profile with minimal changes. (*O*) 8 year follow up showing excellent retention of the gingival form and esthetics.

Because the width of the extraction socket in general follows these parameters, a molar-immediate site will use a wider diameter implant greater than 5 mm to engage bone for primary stability. Cone-beam scans are useful to show the facial-lingual and mesial-distal dimensions of the tooth, which aids in implant selection. In addition, the cone-beam scan can be used to identify the location of the inferior alveolar nerve, which allows the surgeon to avoid it when preparing the implant site. The clinician needs to have a reference point to guide implant placement at the time of tooth removal. The height of the lingual bone may be useful. The buccal bone may be thinned during tooth removal and may be less predictable. Navigation definitely aids in depth control in the immediate extraction site. It is important to remember the location of the nerves when placing implants to avoid sensory changes.

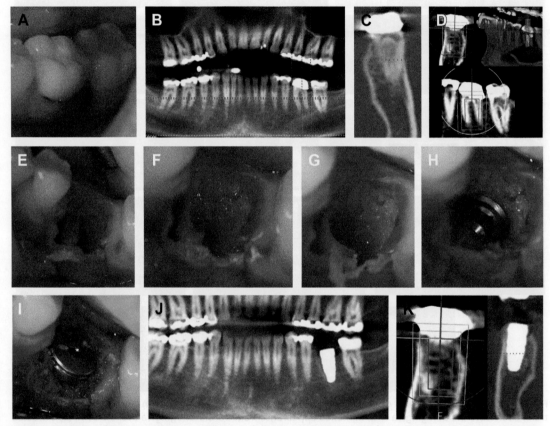

Fig. 2. Immediate molar placement: mandibular left first molar. (*A*) Photo of mandibular left first molar before extraction. (*B*) Panoramic reconstruction from cone-beam scan showing molar position. This tooth had recurrent decay with insufficient feral for restoration. (*C*) Cross section showing position of tooth in ridge. Note that the tooth is toward the buccal with thin buccal bone. (*D*) Three pictures showing the virtual 3-dimensional planning using the dynamic navigation system. Note that the virtual implant is placed in the ideal position for the crown. (*E*) A sulcular incision was used with vertical release to visualize the buccal bone. The tooth was removed with the aid of a piezosurgery periotome tip to separate the tooth from the bone and preserve the thin buccal cortical bone. Note the thin interdental septi. (*F*) A small round bur was used to make a purchase and a pilot drill, under navigation, was used to locate the middle of the implant preparation site. A series of drills was then used using reverse counterclockwise rotation to compact bone and shape it to implant size, rather than remove the bone. Note the bending and reshaping of the interdental bone using the counterclockwise drills (Verseh). (*G*) Reverse-turning drills are used in gradating size until the final size and shape of the preparation site is accomplished. Note the new shape of the preparation site. (*H*) The implant is placed with 50-Ncm insertion torque. (*I*) A healing abutment was placed. Allograft was placed in the root sockets. The gingival margins were approximated similar to as they were before the tooth extraction. (*J*) Panoramic reconstruction form postoperative cone-beam scan showing ideal implant placement in the immediate molar site. (*K*) (*Left*) Virtual plan and (*right*) actual implant placement showing how the navigation system provides guidance for very accurate implant positioning. ([*D*] *Courtesy of* X-Nav, Inc, Lansdale, PA; with permission.)

If a graft is necessary to restore the socket's dimensions for ideal implant placement, the surgeon may wait until the density of the site is similar to that of adjacent bone. In some patients this can occur early and in some it may take in excess of 6 months for the socket to form bone of sufficient density to provide implant stability. In general, the larger the bone defect and presence of inflammation and osteolysis, the longer it will take to achieve bone repair. Cone-beam scans are very useful in making this decision after the graft is allowed to heal.

Restoration Considerations

The single-implant restoration should result in a crown attached to an implant body that looks like a tooth, can be maintained like a tooth, and functions like a tooth. This requires several key criteria for success:

The portion of the restoration that is subgingival should be shaped like a tooth form that is concave to straight emergence in the anterior and can be more convex for posterior restorations. The abutment chosen is critical for success. If a stock abutment is used it must be able to be placed with the crown form developing the profile of the final restoration. A custom machined abutment can be used to develop an anatomically correct form, taking into consideration the form of the final restoration. The form of the final restoration is the sum of the abutment and crown.

The interface between the crown and abutment should be smooth and should not have defects from lack of seating a crown. If the crown is not seated with a crevice present at the interface of the crown to abutment, plaque and eventual bone loss can occur. This situation is iatrogenic and must be corrected.

The restoration should respect the principle of biological width. Placement of the crown close to bone will result in bone loss similarly to that seen when a restoration is placed within 3 mm of the

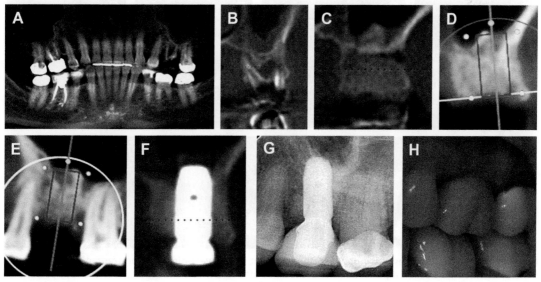

Fig. 3. Maxillary molar single tooth site with immediate sinus elevation. (*A*) Panoramic reconstruction from cone-beam scan showing the location and status of the maxillary left first molar, in need of removal. (*B*) Cross-sectional image of maxillary left first molar. Note the loss of bone with 2 mm of bone in the furcation. (*C*) At the time of tooth removal the tooth was removed. A piezosurgery cutting tip was used to cut between the root sockets to isolate the furcation bone. The mobilized furcation bone was gently intruded superiorly to increase the vertical dimension of the socket. Xenograft was placed in the area of the sinus intrusion and allograft in the remainder of the socket. The incision was closed after periosteal release. This cross section shows the bone height 4 months after the tooth was removed and the graft placed. (*D*) After 4 months a virtual 5.8 × 10.5-mm implant was placed on the planning software. Note that a small additional sinus floor elevation may be needed at the time of implant placement. (*E*) Sagittal view of the planned implant placement. Note that the height of the ridge was very close to the planned implant height selection of 10.5 mm. (*F*) The implant was placed by preparing the implant site to 9 mm depth, using the dynamic navigation system for depth control. Osteotomes were used to bump up the intact bone on the floor. Xenograft was placed and the implant placed. (*G*) Follow-up radiograph at 2 years after restoration showing excellent bone around the implant including the apical portion. (*H*) Clinical photo of the final crown at 2-year follow-up.

crestal bone.[16–18] The abutment should be shaped to avoid adjacent bone, accomplished by using a concave emergence profile of the abutment until it clears the adjacent bone, which then can be formed to follow the anatomic form. It typically emerges 3 mm to the junction of the crown abutment interface.[19–21]

A provisional restoration can be used to shape the gingival tissues to gain similar form of the tooth to be preplaced. These provisionals should be smooth and polished, with an interface that avoids plaque development. If cemented, the cement needs to be removed from the sulcus if present.

If cement is not cleaned from the provisional, inflammation will occur with gingival changes and hard-tissue changes, both of which can result in esthetic problems.

Gingival Considerations

The single implant should follow the same fundamental rules of dentistry. There is a need for a band of attached, keratinized gingiva around a tooth, and similarly around an implant. The resilience of the soft tissue to avoid recession is based on gingival thickness.[22] The clinician must assess

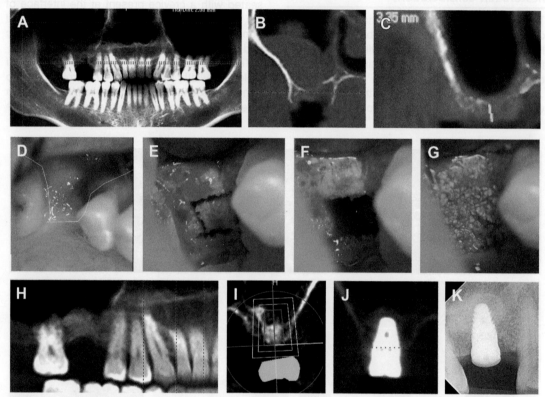

Fig. 4. Maxillary site with crestal window and then implant. (A) 47-year-old man had tooth #3 removed by his general dentist who noticed a perforation into the sinus after a difficult extraction. Note the lack of bone on the floor. (B) Cross section of the extraction site 7 days after extraction. Note the communication between the osseous defect and the sinus with sinus congestion. Conservative therapy was used and healing occurred across the site with no oral-antral fistula. (C) Six weeks after extraction the sinus congestion has resolved. Note the 1- to 2-mm of ridge thickness. (D) At the time of grafting the edentulous area had epithelialized. The incision is drawn on this photo, showing that the incision margins are not directly over the planned crestal window site. (E) The flap is elevated, exposing the thin yet intact maxillary crest. A piezosurgery cutting tip was used to outline a window, leaving the membrane intact. (F) The crestal window island of bone was gently elevated superiorly to 9 mm. (G) Xenograft was placed into the bone defect with the crest now elevated 9 mm into the sinus. (H) Cone-beam scan 4 months after grafting, showing increase in vertical bone height in the edentulous site. (I) There was bone resorption and consolidation resulting in 6 mm of bone height. The virtual implant position shows the intended bump-up of the sinus floor planned at the time of implant placement. (J) The cross section was taken immediately after implant placement. At the time of implant surgery the site was prepared to 5-mm depth. Osteotomes were used to elevate the bone of the floor to 9 mm. Xenograft was placed and the implant placed. (K) Radiograph at 4 months after implant showing adequate bone healing, with bone completely surrounding the implant including the apical region.

the quality and quantity of gingival at the margin of the implant.

In the posterior mandible, the band of keratinized gingiva may be 2 mm, and it should be split and placed around the abutment. If not present it can be recreated by using a graft, usually from the palate. In the maxilla there is usually a much wider band of keratinized attached gingiva, which can be split and moved labially to provide keratinized gingiva around the implant. When using a static guide in the mandible, the clinician may elect to bisect the band of keratinized gingiva and move it to avoid its resection during implant site preparation.

With regard to converting thin to thick gingiva, thin gingiva tends to follow the underlying bone. If the bone around an implant resorbs over time, thin gingiva recedes following bone loss. Thick gingiva tends to stay in position when the underlying bone changes over time, resulting in an attached, deeper pocket, which can usually be maintained. The clinician can examine the patient and if the gingiva is relatively translucent, has minimal stippling, does not have a think band of attached gingiva, and bleeds easily on probing, the gingiva can be termed thin. If the clinician can see the probe through the gingiva, it is thin.[23,24]

Thin gingiva should be converted to thick gingiva at some time during the implant process. Often a subepithelial connective graft, from the palate, is placed under the thin gingiva at the time of tooth removal; this can be done at the time of implant placement. It may be difficult to gain the desired result if the grafting is performed after the abutment connection is made on the implant. The author prefers to perform the soft-tissue procedure at the time of tooth removal.[25]

When removing a single incisor that has thin bone and thin gingiva, the incision is made around the tooth within the sulcus. The gingiva is reflected to the crest. A subperiosteal tunnel is created on the labial bone. The tooth is removed with preservation of the remnants of the thin labial bone. A subepithelial connective tissue graft is harvested from the palate, typically 10 to 15 mm in length and 8 mm in width. A resorbable suture is placed from the vestibule into the tunnel to emerge into the socket. The graft is engaged by the suture, which is then passed from the socket through the tunnel, emerging into the vestibule adjacent to the entry point. The suture is used to pull the graft into position, under the labial gingiva. Allograft is typically used as the graft in the socket, although graft choice is clinician dependent. After the bone graft material is firmly packed into the socket, the remaining edge of the connective tissue graft is sutured to the palatal aspect of the socket. After the socket heals with bone, an implant can be placed.

CASE EXAMPLES

See **Fig. 1** for a single-tooth replacement of a central incisor. See **Fig. 2** for immediate molar placement of a mandibular left first molar. See **Fig. 3** for a maxillary molar single-tooth site with immediate sinus elevation. See **Fig. 4** for maxillary site with crestal window followed by implant.

REFERENCES

1. Ogawa T, Al-Amieh B, Ishimura I, et al. The evolution of modern implant surfaces. Chapter 2. In: Moy PK, Pozzi A, Beumer J III, editors. Fundamentals of implant dentistry, vol. 2. Chicago: Quintessence Publishing; 2016. p. 25–49.
2. Branemark P-I. Introduction to osseointegration. Chapter 1. In: Branemark P-I, Zarb G, Albrektsson T, editors. Tissue- integrated prostheses—osseointegration in clinical dentistry. Chicago: Quintessence; 1985. p. 11–76.
3. Davies JE. In vitro modeling of the bone/implant interface. Anat Rec 1996;245(2):426–45.
4. Davies JE. Mechanisms of endosseous integration. Int J Prosthodont 1998;11(5):391–401.
5. Lee SY, Kim SJ, An HW, et al. The effect of the thread depth on the mechanical properties of the dental implant. J Adv Prosthodont 2015;7(2):115–21.
6. Gehrke SA, Marin GW. Biomechanical evaluation of dental implants with three different designs: removal torque and resonance frequency analysis in rabbits. Ann Anat 2015;199:30–5.
7. Abuhussein H, Pagni G, Rebaudi A, et al. The effect of thread pattern upon implant osseointegration. Clin Oral Implants Res 2010;21(2):129–36.
8. Oliveira PGFP, Bergamo ETP, Neiva R, et al. Osseodensification outperforms conventional implant subtractive instrumentation: a study in sheep. Mater Sci Eng C Mater Biol Appl 2018;90:300–7.
9. Trisi P, Berardini M, Falco A, et al. New osseodensification implant site preparation method to increase bone density in low-density bone: in vivo evaluation in sheep. Implant Dent 2016;25(1):24–31.
10. Ozdiler A, Bakir-Topcuoglu N, Kulekci G, et al. Effects of taper angle and sealant agents on bacterial leakage along the implant-abutment interface: an in vitro study under loaded conditions. Int J Oral Maxillofac Implants 2018. https://doi.org/10.11607/jomi.6257.
11. Tallarico M, Canullo L, Caneva M, et al. Microbial colonization at the implant-abutment interface and its possible influence on periimplantitis: a systematic

review and meta-analysis. J Prosthodont Res 2017; 61(3):233–41.

12. Albrektsson T, Canullo L, Cochran D, et al. "Peri-Implantitis": a complication of a foreign body or a man-made "disease". Facts and fiction. Clin Implant Dent Relat Res 2016;18(4):840–9.

13. Gilbert AB, Yilmaz B, Seidt JD, et al. Three-dimensional displacement of nine different abutments for an implant with an internal hexagon platform. Int J Oral Maxillofac Implants 2015;30(4):781–8.

14. Madani E, Smeets R, Freiwald E, et al. Impact of different placement depths on the crestal bone level of immediate versus delayed placed platform-switched implants. J Craniomaxillofac Surg 2018; 46(7):1139–46.

15. Saleh MHA, Ravidà A, Suárez-López Del Amo F, et al. The effect of implant-abutment junction position on crestal bone loss: a systematic review and meta-analysis. Clin Implant Dent Relat Res 2018. https://doi.org/10.1111/cid.12600.

16. Pozzi A, Tallarico M, Moy PK. The implant biologic pontic designed interface: description of the technique and cone-beam computed tomography evaluation. Clin Implant Dent Relat Res 2015;17(Suppl 2): e711–20.

17. Judgar R, Giro G, Zenobio E, et al. Biological width around one- and two-piece implants retrieved from human jaws. Biomed Res Int 2014;2014:850120.

18. Negri B, López Marí M, Maté Sánchez de Val JE, et al. Biological width formation to immediate implants placed at different level in relation to the crestal bone: an experimental study in dogs. Clin Oral Implants Res 2015;26(7):788–98.

19. Iezzi G, Iaculli F, Calcaterra R, et al. Histological and histomorphometrical analysis on a loaded implant with platform-switching and conical connection: a case report. J Oral Implantol 2017;43(3):180–6.

20. Sánchez-Siles M, Muñoz-Cámara D, Salazar-Sánchez N, et al. Crestal bone loss around submerged and non-submerged implants during the osseointegration phase with different healing abutment designs: a randomized prospective clinical study. Clin Oral Implants Res 2016. https://doi.org/10.1111/clr.12981.

21. Chappuis V, Bornstein MM, Buser D, et al. Influence of implant neck design on facial bone crest dimensions in the esthetic zone analyzed by cone beam CT: a comparative study with a 5-to-9-year follow-up. Clin Oral Implants Res 2016;27(9):1055–64.

22. Kois JC. Predictable single tooth peri-implant esthetics: five diagnostic keys. Compend Contin Educ Dent 2001;22(3):199–206.

23. Kan JY, Rungcharassaeng K, Lozada JL, et al. Facial gingival tissue stability following immediate placement and provisionalization of maxillary anterior single implants: a 2- to 8-year follow-up. Int J Oral Maxillofac Implants 2011;26(1):179–87.

24. Kan JY, Rungcharassaeng K, Morimoto T, et al. Facial gingival tissue stability after connective tissue graft with single immediate tooth replacement in the esthetic zone: consecutive case report. J Oral Maxillofac Surg 2009;67(11 Suppl):40–8.

25. Block MS. Techniques for grafting and implant placement for the extraction site. Chapter 7. In: Block MS, editor. Color atlas of dental implant surgery. St Louis (MO): Elsevier; 2015. p. 295–303.

Maxillofacial Reconstruction Using Vascularized Fibula Free Flaps and Endosseous Implants

Stavan Y. Patel, DDS, MD*, Dongsoo D. Kim, DMD, MD,
Ghali E. Ghali, DDS, MD, FRCS(Ed)

KEYWORDS

- Fibula free flap • Endosseous dental implants • Maxilla • Mandible • Reconstruction • Prosthesis
- Radiation

KEY POINTS

- Use of fibula free flap and endosseous implant-supported prosthesis for reconstruction of maxillofacial subunits greatly improves patients' function, form, and quality of life.
- Flap selection and primary versus secondary implant placement for reconstruction should be individualized based on patients' history, prognosis, comorbidities, needs and wishes.
- Coordination and communication between the reconstructive surgeon and prosthodontist is important in achieving optimal results.
- Special attention should be given to patient selection, surgical planning, implant placement, soft-tissue management and prosthodontic considerations to avoid complication and achieve stable long-term outcomes.
- Patient motivation, meticulous hygiene, and long-term follow-up are important for maintenance and success of the reconstruction.

INTRODUCTION

The maxillomandibular complex is an intricate structure with multiple functions such as mastication, breathing, swallowing, speech, and lip competency, located in a cosmetically demanding region of the head and neck. Head and neck reconstruction has been revolutionized with the use of free tissue transfer and microvascular surgery, which provide adequate reliable bone and soft tissue from distant sites for reconstruction of the defect. Use of endosseous implants has modernized dental, oral, and facial rehabilitation

because it provides a stable, reliable, and long-term option for reconstruction. Prosthetic rehabilitation of maxillofacial subunits using free tissue transfer and endosseous implants has been well described in the literature. The first reports of dental prosthetic rehabilitation of the mandible using free tissue transfer and endosseous implants dates back to 1989.[1] Since then this technique has been further refined, and nowadays dental prosthetic rehabilitation of large maxillofacial defects using free tissue transfer and endosseous implants is considered the standard of care.

Disclosure: The authors have nothing to disclose.
Division of Head and Neck Oncology and Microvascular Reconstructive Surgery, Department of Oral and Maxillofacial Surgery/Head and Neck Surgery, Louisiana State University Health Science Center, 1501 Kings Highway, Shreveport, LA 71103, USA
* Corresponding author.
E-mail address: spate9@lsuhsc.edu

Oral Maxillofacial Surg Clin N Am 31 (2019) 259–284
https://doi.org/10.1016/j.coms.2018.12.005

Types of maxillofacial deficiencies that can be reconstructed using this technique include severely atrophic jaws, post–jaw-resection defects, traumatic defects, or congenital abnormalities. A team approach to reconstruction of these patients is critical.[2–4] Coordination and communication between the reconstructive surgeon and prosthodontist is important in achieving optimal functional and esthetic outcomes and improving the quality of life.

This article reviews the use of endosseous implants in fibula free flap (FFF) for dental, oral, and facial rehabilitation. Under discussion are existing data, the rationale for use of vascularized fibula bone, effects of radiation on endosseous implants, role of virtual surgical planning (VSP), advantages and disadvantages of primary versus secondary implant placement, specifics of FFF and endosseous implant placements, soft-tissue management, prosthodontic considerations, and commonly encountered complications.

REQUIREMENTS FOR RECONSTRUCTION

For any given defect, the goals of reconstruction include maintenance of integrity, maximizing function, reestablishing form, minimizing morbidity, and improving the quality of life (QOL). To achieve these goals in patients requiring free tissue transfer and rehabilitation using an endosseous implant-supported prosthesis, several factors need to be considered. Patient motivation, survival, and long-term prognosis are among the most important. Outlining the individual's goals of reconstruction, managing patient expectations, availability of a reconstructive team, and communication between the patient, reconstructive surgeon, and prosthodontist are equally important. The prosthodontist should be well versed in rehabilitating compromised surgical sites and should be willing to see the patient to the end of the treatment, and thereafter follow the patient periodically for maintenance of prosthesis and hygiene. Anatomic factors, such as favorable anatomy for harvest of distant tissue and microvascular anastomosis, maxillomandibular relationship, volume and location of bone, existing status of remaining dentition, mouth opening, and function of tongue, lips, and pharyngeal wall, are critical when evaluating a patient for reconstruction. Patient-related factors such as comorbidities preventing free tissue transfer or history of head and neck irradiation should also be taken into consideration. Timing of surgeries, steps involved in rehabilitation, need for meticulous oral hygiene, and cost of implant placement

and rehabilitation should be discussed before starting treatment.

TYPE OF BONE FLAP

Several donor sites of vascularized bone free flaps for head and neck reconstruction have been described in the literature, including radius, scapula, rib, ilium, femur, fibula, and metatarsal bone. Of these the fibula, ilium, and scapula are the most common,[5] and are well studied in regard to endosseous implant placement and rehabilitation. They each have advantages and disadvantages based on whether reconstruction of maxilla or mandible is performed, volume and length of bone and soft tissue needed, and location, extent, and type of defect to be reconstructed. Donor sites of these flaps have varying morbidity, and the flaps have differing properties based on quantity, quality, length of bone available, possibility of osteotomy, length of vascular pedicle, availability, and nature soft-tissue skin paddle.

Comparing Fibula with Iliac Crest, Scapula, and Radius Bone Grafts

When comparing the 3 most common vascularized bone flaps (**Fig. 1**)—FFF, iliac crest free flap (ICFF), and scapula free flap (SFF)—the volume of the transplanted FFF bone has the least resorption and is most stable over time, followed by ICFF and SFF.[5] They also have comparable recipient site morbidity.[6–8] When looking at flap survival rates, Brown and colleagues[9] in a systematic review concluded that mandibles reconstructed with ICFF had a statistically significant higher failure rate when compared with FFF, osteocutaneous radial forearm free flap (RFFF), or SFF. These investigators hypothesized that this was likely due to shorter ICFF vascular pedicle and increased technical skill needed for harvest and anastomosis.

Advantages of using a FFF include its ease of harvest, availability of long span of bone, segmental periosteal blood supply, length of vascular pedicle, pliability of skin paddle, reliable vascular anatomy, and ability to use a 2-team approach.[6,10] Disadvantages include bone with insufficient vertical height, inflexible skin paddle, donor site morbidity of poor skin graft take, immobilization of leg, and potential vascular compromise of the foot.[6,10–12] Split-thickness skin graft take on the FFF donor site can be unpredictable, but its poor take has not been a common occurrence noted at the authors' institution.

The biggest criticism of the FFF bone is the lack of vertical height (**Fig. 2**). The average height of the

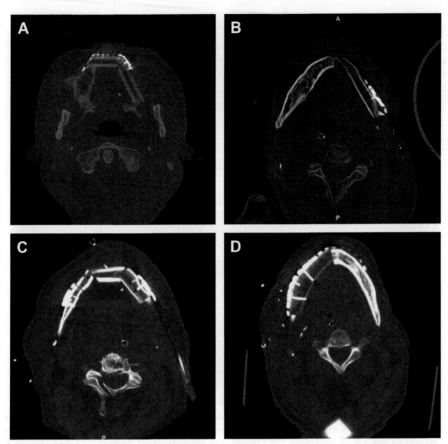

Fig. 1. Maxillofacial reconstruction performed using various common vascularized bone grafts. Radiographs showing varying adaptability, cortical thickness, density, marrow character, volume, and quality of each bone graft. (*A*) Axial view of maxillary reconstruction performed using osteotomized fibula bone. (*B*) Axial view of mandibular reconstruction performed using one-piece scapula bone. (*C*) Axial view of mandibular reconstruction performed using osteotomized scapula bone. (*D*) Axial view of mandibular reconstruction using one-piece iliac crest bone graft.

fibula bone is 13 to 15 mm, which is about half the vertical height of an adult dentate mandible and close to the normal height of an atrophic edentulous mandible.[10] There are several techniques to circumvent the issues of decreased bone height in the fibula. These include vertical distraction osteogenesis, double barreling,[13,14] placing the fibula bone at the height of the alveolus while securing the reconstruction plate at the inferior border to closely represent the ideal mandibular contour[10,15] (**Fig. 3**), and adding nonvascularized corticocancellous autograft to reconstruct the alveolus.[16,17] Vertical distraction of the fibula is unpredictable and can cause lingual tipping of the superior segment, fracture of basal fibula, higher implant failure rate, and increased marginal bone loss.[18] Placing immediate, well-positioned implants in a double-barreled fibula is challenging[19] and generally avoided. At the authors' institution, double-barreled fibulas are routinely

reconstructed with secondary placement of implants. The fibula and reconstruction plate can also be placed 5 to 10 mm *higher*[10,19] than the inferior border of the mandible. This approach would leave a slight cosmetic defect at the inferior border that can be corrected by tucking a deepithelialized vascularized fibula skin paddle over the reconstruction plate to augment higher placement of fibula bone and soft-tissue loss from surgical resection of tumor or from trauma. At the authors' institution a deepithelialized skin paddle lateral to the reconstruction plate is routinely placed in patients who will likely undergo adjuvant irradiation in the postoperative period to prevent the risk of plate exposure during or after radiation therapy. In nonirradiated patients, the fibula and reconstruction plate can be placed at the inferior border of the mandible, and an autologous corticocancellous bone graft or remaining fibula used to graft the alveolus.[16,17]

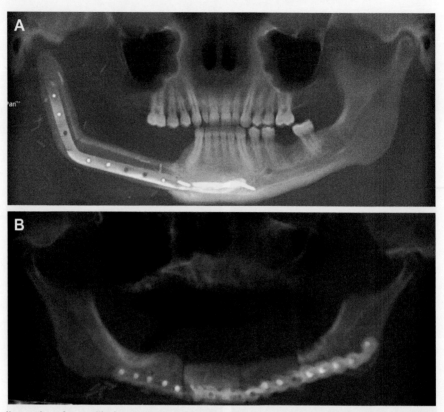

Fig. 2. Radiographs of mandibular reconstruction showing vertical height discrepancy at the alveolus. (*A*) Mandibular reconstruction performed using fibular free flap in a dentate patient. Note that the fibula is half the vertical height of the native mandible. (*B*) Mandibular reconstruction performed using scapula free flap in a recently edentulated patient. The scapula bone offers a closer vertical height match when compared with fibula.

When comparing various vascularized bone flaps, the FFF and ICFF have the most appropriate dimensions for accepting standard-size implants, followed by SFF, and then RFFF.[20] Vascularized bone flaps are superior in comprehensive oral bony reconstruction and improving QOL when compared with reconstruction performed with a combination of reconstruction plate and a soft-tissue flap.[21] There is a gender effect on the implantability of vascularized bone whereby male bone has been reported to be more implantable than female bone.[20,22] The ICFF provides higher mass and volume of bone around the body of the implant but not around its neck.[23] Primary stability of implants placed in fibula bone is higher when compared with iliac crest and scapula, and is ideal for early loading of implants. Furthermore, the rate of peri-implantitis is lowest in vascularized FFF when compared with vascularized ICFF or non-vascularized autologous bone grafts.[24,25] When comparing SFF and ICFF, they have similar bone density and cortical thickness. Cortical thickness in SFF decreases as one moves from cranial

to caudal. SFF cortical bone thickness increases with age, and this flap is ideal for older adults because it has low donor site morbidity and the skin paddle is less bulky in comparison with ICFF.[6,26] One of the major drawbacks of SFF is the inability to use a 2-team approach. Also, a significant number of patients with SFF are unable to undergo reconstruction with implants owing to lack of apical bone width.[26]

Comparing Fibula with Iliac Crest Bone Graft

Overall, FFF and ICFF have comparable donor site morbidity, pain scores, walking ability, wound healing, speech, oral competence, esthetic, and QOL outcomes.[11,27,28] When looking at implant placement, they both have sufficient comparable bone volumes, similar and low (<1 mm) bone resorption around implants, and equal stability at the time of uncovering.[25,29,30] Patients who underwent reconstruction with FFF did have decreased gait and neurosensory changes at the extremity when compared with ICFF, and complications of

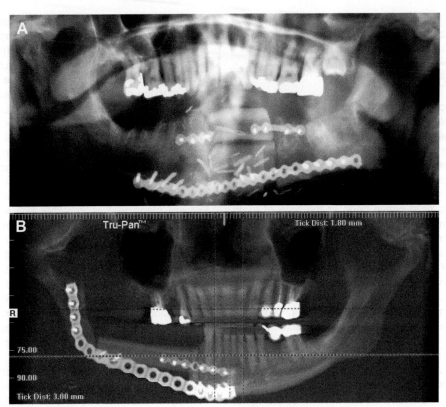

Fig. 3. Radiographs showing techniques to correct vertical height discrepancy when using a fibula free flap. (*A*) Use of a double-barrel fibula graft. (*B*) Placing the anterior fibula segment higher, at the alveolus, while maintaining the reconstruction plate at the inferior border of the mandible.

seroma, hematoma, and herniation were limited to the ICFF donor site.[11,27] Swallowing was significantly better in patients reconstructed with FFF, likely secondary to bulky skin paddle of the ICFF.[28] Another factor to consider is that because of its bulk, the ICFF intraoral skin paddle may require significant debulking for appropriate emergence profile and hygiene of implants.[31] In dentate patients, ICFF is the initial choice for mandibular angle and body defects that are also necessitating bulkier soft-tissue skin paddle. FFF reconstruction is preferred in edentulous patients or dentate patients requiring reconstruction of longer-span defects (subtotal or total mandibulectomy) and those requiring condylar reconstruction.[8,32] Although the deep circumflex iliac artery offers a higher vertical bone dimension, keeping in mind the aforementioned data FFF is a better choice for maxillofacial reconstruction in most patients, with ICFF being a reliable corresponding backup for selected patients.

The Fibula Bone Graft

The efficacy and prognosis of implants placed in FFF has been extensively studied. Size of defect,

pathology, and irradiation were not statistically significant factors affecting implant survival.[33] Success rates of implants placed in nonirradiated fibulas are comparable with those placed in native bone. The overall survival of implants placed in FFF is on an average 93.5%, with a range of 83%–97% at 1–5 years after placement.[33–50] The average 10-year survival of these implants is 80% (range 78%–83%),[38,46,49] and 20-year reported survival is 69%.[49]

Prosthetic (fixed or removable) rehabilitation of implants placed in FFF results in improved function (speech and swallowing), esthetic outcomes, and QOL.[3,15,34,36,51] This approach has led to less dyspnea and fewer patients being dependent on feeding tubes.[36] Maxillofacial subunit reconstructed with implant-supported prosthesis and FFF is resilient over the long term, with high implant survival rate, decreased loss of crestal bone (<1 mm), and low complication rates.[12,19,38,41] Overall implant loss[44] and peri-implant bone loss is higher in implants placed in FFF compared with native bone, particularly in implants placed in maxilla reconstructed with FFF.[48] Implants placed in fibulas attained a statistically significant higher primary stability at the time of implant placement,[25] and the FFF is noted to be suitable bone for implant placement, osseointegration, function, and rehabilitation.

EFFECT OF RADIATION

The effect of radiation therapy on endosseous implant placement in native bone and vascularized free bone graft has been fairly well examined. There are mixed data reported regarding the successful osseointegration of endosseous implants in irradiated vascularized bone. Primary implant placement in FFF is done at the time of FFF harvest and inset, or in native bone at the time of tooth extraction before starting radiation therapy. Secondary implant placement in FFF is done after allowing a usual time of 4 to 6 months for consolidation of the fibula graft. For secondary implant placement after irradiation, there is somewhat of a general consensus on the safe time period for placement of endosseous implants. Although time of implant placement after irradiation is not a factor in overall implant survival,[52,53] most studies recommend waiting at least 6 to 12 months[54–63] after completion of radiation therapy. Shorter waiting periods after irradiation do not guarantee vascularization and suitability of bone for endosseous implant placement.[64]

Implants placed in the irradiated field have a high success rate, with an average overall implant survival of 91.3% over 1 to 5 years[44,50,52,55,57,65–67] and a long-term implant survival rate of 78% to 85% at 15 years.[56,66] Implants placed in irradiated maxilla have a lower survival rate than ones placed in the irradiated mandible,[56] and implants placed in irradiated FFF have lower survival than those placed in native maxilla or mandible.[44] Furthermore, implants placed in previously irradiated FFF or bone that has previously developed osteoradionecrosis (ORN) have significantly higher risk of implant loss.[44,57,65,67] From their data, Ch'ng and colleagues[44] in 2016 concluded that prior therapeutic radiation, 60 to 72 Gy of intensity-modulated radiation therapy, may be a relative contraindication to placement of implants in FFF. Most implant failures in the irradiated and nonirradiated fibulas occur in the first 6 to 12 months after placement.[65,67] Average loss of crestal bone in an irradiated field is twice that of a nonirradiated field, and is highest in the first 12 months after placement of the implants.[55]

In the literature, several factors have been suggested to cause lower implant survival in the irradiated field. These factors include timing of implant placement, type of radiation therapy, dose of radiation therapy (>50 Gy),[35,52,57,67] and female gender.[52] Older data suggested that implant survival was lower when placed in previously irradiated mandibles.[46,68] Newer data suggest that timing of radiation therapy before or after implant placement did not affect implant survival.[35,43] Also, there was no significant difference in implant survival when placed in irradiated versus nonirradiated bone.[67] This finding can possibly be explained by the change in mode of radiation delivery, from conventional conformal radiation therapy to intensity-modulated radiation therapy, which has shown to have statistically higher implant survival.[52] Metallic objects in the radiation field do alter adjacent-tissue radiation doses.[69] Primary placement of implants before radiation therapy can cause backscattering, dose escalation in the bone in front of the implant, and shielding behind the implant.[70,71] Larger implant sizes lead to increased local x-ray or gamma-ray backscatter and would lead to higher local doses of radiation and increased likelihood of ORN. Cobalt-60 radiation can cause 36% increase in radiation, and other high-energy x-rays can cause up to a 20% increase.[71] Owing to backscatter there is a 15% increase in dose at the implant and bone interface, which decreases to negligible within 1 to 2 mm of the interface.[72] Multivectored radiation therapy reduces the effects of backscatter. Given this effect, one should consider placing the smallest available and clinically feasible implants to avoid increased backscatter and higher radiation dose at the bone implant interface, which could possibly be a risk factor for ORN. A systematic review performed by Zen Filho and colleagues[63] in 2016 reported that neither the dose of radiation nor the time of implant placement after radiation therapy are significant factors for implant loss.

Use of hyperbaric oxygen therapy in the peri-implant placement time is controversial, and current data suggest that its use is not a factor in implant survival[19,44,52,53,56,57]; neither does its use improve implant survival, nor does it prevent ORN after implant placement,[73] and it is associated with a statistically significantly higher risk of implant failure.[46]

ROLE OF VIRTUAL SURGICAL PLANNING

VSP, which consists of computer-aided surgical planning and fabrication of surgical guides using computer-aided design and manufacturing (CAD/CAM) technology, plays a huge role in primary and secondary placement of implants. VSP allows for accurate evaluation of anatomy, fabrication of a patient-specific plan for precise placement of FFF and implants into the defect, and execution of this plan with custom-fabricated cutting and implant placement guides (**Figs. 4** and **5**). Use of this

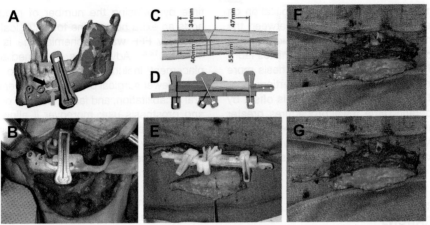

Fig. 4. Role of virtual surgical planning in tumor resection and fibula free flap reconstruction. (*A*) A 3D computer-generated model of the mandible with left mandibular mass. Osteotomy site is virtually planned and a mandibular cutting guide is generated with slots to perform the osteotomy (*green arrow*) and to identify and lateralize the inferior alveolar nerve (*blue arrow*). Black arrow shows the mental foramen. (*B*) Intraoperative use of the mandible cutting guide. (*C*) A 3D computer-generated model of the fibula and tibia bone, with planned osteotomies to reconstruct the mandibular body and ramus/condyle. (*D*) Virtual fibula cutting guide. (*E*) Intraoperative use of the fibula cutting guide. (*F*) Flap after closing osteotomies are made. (*G*) The "V"-shape wedge of osteotomized bone is discarded to allow for appropriate angulation and positioning of the 2 fibula segments.

technology allows for planning of both immediate and delayed endosseous implant placement while avoiding the reconstruction plate and screws. Prefabricated fibula cutting and implant placement guides created using VSP allows for planning of osteotomies in the defect site and for precise cutting and fit of the fibula segments in patient-specific reconstruction plates. Furthermore, it provides for ideal placement of endosseous implants with predetermined angulation and position

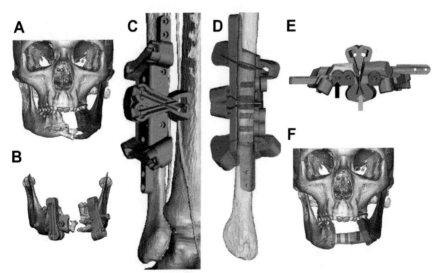

Fig. 5. Role of virtual surgical planning in reconstruction of traumatic injuries with fibula free flap and primary placement of endosseous implants. (*A*) A 3D computer-generated model of the facial skeleton with mandibular defect secondary to ballistic injury and malocclusion. (*B*) Mandibular osteotomy sites are virtually planned and a cutting guide is generated. (*C*) A 3D computer-generated model of the fibula and tibia bone, with fibula cutting guide, which is to fit on the lateral border of the fibula. (*D*) Virtual fibula cutting guide seen from the medial showing planned osteotomies and cylinders for location of implant placement. (*E*) Cutting guide with slots for fibula (*green arrow*) and implant (*black arrow*) osteotomies. (*F*) A 3D computer-generated model of the reconstructed facial skeleton with ideal occlusion and primary placed appropriately angulated endosseous implants.

that is conducive for prosthetic rehabilitation on fibula bone, while avoiding conflict between the implant and transosseous screws holding the FFF in place[9,74–77] (**Fig. 6**). This plan makes fabrication and placement of a final prosthesis more efficient, and leads to higher rates of tertiary rehabilitation. The increased cost of VSP is offset by reduced operating time, fewer procedures, greater use of placed implants, reduced time for prosthesis delivery, higher rates of tertiary prosthetic rehabilitation, and improved patient satisfaction and QOL.[2,78]

FIBULA FREE FLAP AND IMPLANT PLACEMENT CONSIDERATIONS

As discussed earlier, generally endosseous implants can reliably be placed in FFF primarily (immediately at the time of fibula harvest) or secondarily (delayed by 6–12 months); they have similar implant survival and complication rates, and a comparable safety profile.[37,43,48,79] Less commonly, reconstruction can be performed using prefabricated flaps or single-stage complete maxillofacial reconstruction, also termed "Jaw in a day."[80] Each of these techniques has advantages and disadvantages, which are discussed here in detail.

Primary Implant Placement

Primary or one-stage implant placement (see **Fig. 5**) in FFF is safe to perform without having vascular compromise to the fibula bone. This procedure improves functional outcome and is cost effective because it reduces overall reconstruction time by reducing the number of procedures; it adds an extra hour to the total surgical time, and generally FFF warm ischemia time is less than 4 hours.[12,81] Advantages of immediate implant placement include easier access to the fibula bone, fewer surgical procedures, lower cost, early oral rehabilitation, and faster return to oral nutrition and prosthesis use; moreover it allows time for osseointegration of implants before starting radiation therapy, and potentially reduces the risk of implant loss and ORN.[67,79,81] Disadvantages include improper positioning of implants, potential interference with radiation therapy, alteration of local anatomy, and possibility of tumor recurrence at the implant placement site.[10,39,81] Because of the likelihood of recurrence, primary implant placement after malignant tumor extirpation is contraindicated.[19]

Secondary Implant Placement

Secondary implant placement is a 2-stage technique. In the first stage the defect is reconstructed with a FFF and reconstruction plate (**Fig. 7**) and then allowed to heal for 4 to 6 months. In the second stage, CAD/CAM technology is used to identify and guide the surgeon to the ideal location and angulation for implant placement. At the authors' institution, in malignant tumor defects treated with FFF and adjuvant radiation therapy, secondary placement of implants is delayed for 1 year after completion of therapy. Reconstructive hardware is removed at second-stage surgery if it interferes with placement of implants (**Fig. 8**). Debulking of the flap skin paddle, vestibuloplasty,

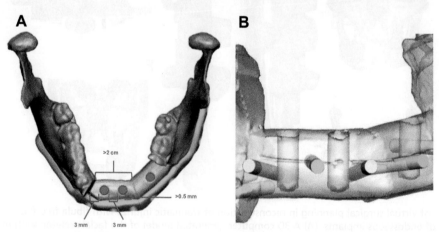

Fig. 6. Ideal placement of endosseous implants and fibula reconstruction hardware. (*A*) Occlusal view of a 3D computer-generated mandible from patient in **Fig. 5**, showing close adaptation of the reconstruction plate (*green*) to the native mandible and fibula segments. Demonstrated is a guide for ideal spacing of the implants in relation to other implants and surrounding fibula bone. (*B*) An anterior-posterior view of the same mandible showing use of virtual surgical planning in placement of implants in fibula bone while avoiding conflict with monocortical (*yellow*) and bicortical (*green*) transosseous screws.

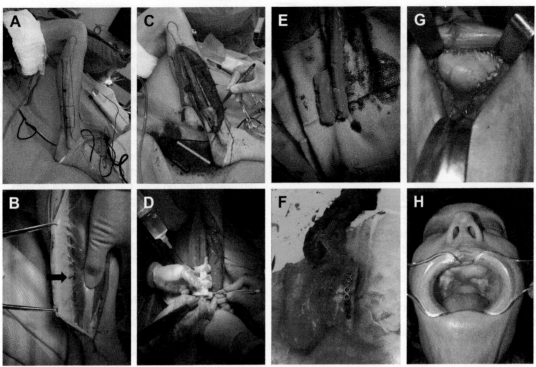

Fig. 7. Maxillary reconstruction using osteocutaneous fibula free flap. (*A*) Right lateral leg with marked surgical anatomy, skin perforators, and planned incisions. (*B*) Lateral leg anatomy, showing vascular perforators (*black arrow*) form the peroneal artery and vena comitans to the skin paddle. (*C*) Harvested osteocutaneous fibula free flap. (*D*) Making osteotomies through the patient-specific fibula cutting guide. (*E*) Closing osteotomies made on fibula bone. (*F*) Fibula osteotomies plated with titanium plate and monocortical transosseous screws. (*G*) Inset of the fibula skin paddle. (*H*) Four-month postoperative view of the skin paddle and surgical site.

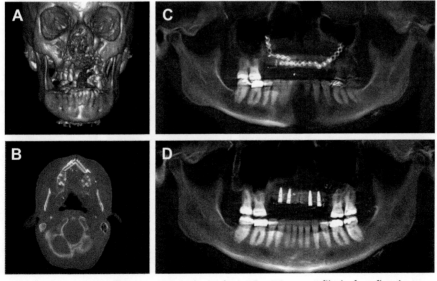

Fig. 8. Radiographs showing maxillary reconstruction using osteocutaneous fibula free flap (same patient as in Fig. 7). (*A*) A 3D rendering of computed tomography scan showing maxillary defect secondary to ballistic injury. (*B*) Axial view showing inset of fibula bone into the defect. (*C*) A panoramic radiograph showing the same. (*D*) Radiograph showing removal of maxillary hardware and placement of 4 endosseous bicortical implants into the fibula segments.

and grafting around the implant placement site can be done either at the time of implant placement or at the time of implant uncovering[47] (**Fig. 9**). Advantages of secondary implant placement include identifying patients motivated to undergo further prosthetic rehabilitation, shorter initial surgical procedure, verifying the viability of FFF, creating an ideal implant placement guide and prosthodontic plan, and allowing time to rule out local tumor recurrence.[35,39,67] Disadvantages include delay in oral rehabilitation, more trips to the operating room, and increased cost.

Prefabrication and Jaw in a Day

Data regarding reconstruction of the maxillofacial complex with prefabricated FFF with an endosseous implant-supported prosthesis is limited to case reports and small case series.[82–85] Major drawbacks of this technique are that it requires several trips to the operating room and incorporation of a skin paddle to reconstruct a concomitant soft-tissue defect.

The first case series of "Jaw in a day" was published in 2013 by Levine and colleagues,[80] who described one-stage reconstruction of maxillofacial defects using virtually planned guides for FFF and implant placement, and concomitant delivery of the dental prosthesis. This technique has obvious advantages of fewer visits to the operating room, and early restoration of deformity and return to function. Disadvantages include longer single general anesthetic, challenges in incorporating a skin paddle, and limited available data on long-term flap, implant, and prosthesis success rates.[86]

Both of these methods may be a good option for maxillofacial reconstruction in select patients, but long-term data on their efficacy are still lacking. It is noteworthy that owing to challenges in incorporating a skin paddle in these constructs, its use in previously irradiated recipient sites should be avoided. Furthermore, given its one-stage nature, its use for reconstruction of defects created by resection of malignant disease is contraindicated.

The Reconstruction Method

At the authors' institution, for both primary and secondary implant reconstruction, if possible VSP is preferentially used to evaluate the anatomy,

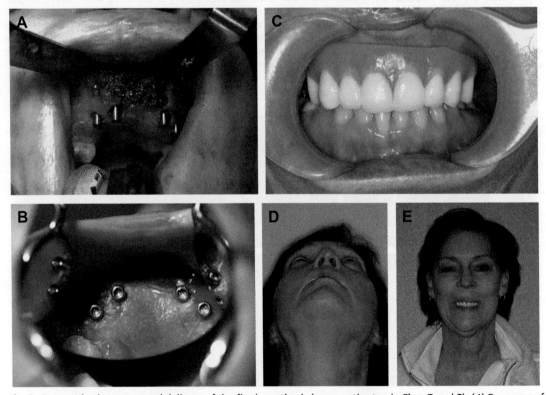

Fig. 9. Preprosthetic surgery and delivery of the final prosthesis (same patient as in **Figs. 7** and **8**). (*A*) Exposure of implants, placement of healing abutments, and maxillary labial vestibuloplasty. (*B*) Occlusal view of the implants before placement of temporary prosthesis. (*C*) Final prosthesis and occlusion. (*D*) Worm's-eye view showing good projection of the upper lip and competence. (*E*) Frontal view showing good tooth-to-lip relationship during smile.

ensure precise osteotomies in the recipient site and the FFF, and guide ideal placement of fibula segments, transosseous reconstruction plates, screws, and endosseous implants. **Figs. 10–13** show a case presentation of the technique routinely used at this center.

Fibula bone can have variations based on gender and specific location along its length.[87] Males have higher cross-section volume of fibula bone in comparison with females. Fibula bone is triangular in shape at the head, then becomes more quadrilateral in the middle and oval/irregular at the malleolus. For most reconstructed defects, to allow for a longer vascular pedicel length the distal fibula bone is used, which is generally quadrilateral in shape. If the shape is triangular, it may require trimming and flattening of the ridge before placement of the implant. The fibula bone should be placed in an ideal location to allow for appropriately angled implant placement while avoiding the screws from the reconstruction plate (see **Fig. 6**). Use of monocortical screws with reconstruction plates is preferred over multiple miniplate fixation. Adequate stability using a minimal number of screws is preferred.[19] Osteotomized fibula segments should ideally be kept larger than 2 cm, but segments as small as 1 cm can be

successfully used for reconstructions as long as periosteal blood supply can reliably be maintained.[88,89] Fibulas placed at the inferior border yield good facial esthetic results but, because of a lack of vertical "alveolar" height compared with a dentate adult patient, it requires the prosthesis to have a substantially taller suprastructure, leading to a poor emergence profile and increased loading forces on the implants.[15] To prevent this, the authors prefer to place their fibula segment 5 to 10 mm above the inferior border of the mandible (see **Fig. 10**).

Fibula bone segments and transosseous reconstruction plates should be placed in such a way that they do not interfere with implant placement and allow for prosthodontic rehabilitation. A minimum mouth opening of 15 mm at the incisal edge of anterior teeth[35] is necessary to make dental impressions, place implants, deliver a prosthesis, and allow for mastication and swallowing. While in maximal occlusion, a 20- to 25-mm space between superior edge of the reconstruction plate and occlusal edge of opposing dentition is desirable. A 10- to 15-mm space between the superior edge of the fibula to the occlusal edge of the opposing dentition[12] should be available to allow for appropriate

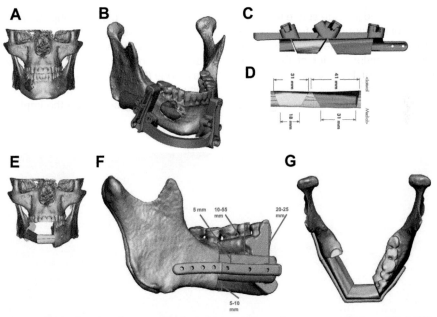

Fig. 10. Virtual surgical planning for mandibular reconstruction after tumor ablation. (*A*) A 3D computer-generated model of the facial skeleton showing right mandibular mass. (*B*) Mandible with patient-specific cutting guide allocating appropriate tumor margins. (*C*) Patient-specific fibula osteotomy guide. (*D*) Planned fibula osteotomies and dimensions. (*E*) Reconstructed model. (*F*) Right lateral view of the reconstructed mandible showing ideal placement of the reconstruction plate and fibula segments in relation to the native mandible and dentition. (*G*) Occlusal view of the reconstructed mandible with fibula graft and patient-specific reconstruction plate.

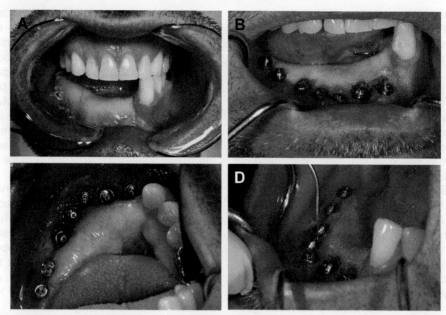

Fig. 11. Postoperative care (same patient as in **Fig. 10**). (*A*) Frontal view of the occlusion and skin paddle at 1 month postoperatively. The flap and skin paddle are allowed to integrate for 6 months, then the flap is debulked and implants are placed in the fibula bone and allowed to integrate for 4 months. Once implants are osseointegrated they are exposed, healing abutments are placed, vestibuloplasty is performed, and an implant-supported custom-fabricated compressive splint is applied. (*B*) Frontal view showing exposed implants after removal of the compressive splint and before placement of temporary prosthesis. (*C*) Occlusal view of the same. (*D*) Right lateral view showing the same along with use of a CO_2 laser for peri-implant tissue conditioning.

emergence profile, and provide space for fabrication of the implant-supported framework and suprastructure of the prosthesis. A distance of 5 mm from the superior border of the fibula to the superior border of the reconstruction plate should be maintained to allow for creation of a buccal vestibule and prevent interference of the

reconstruction plate during fabrication of the prosthesis (see **Fig. 10**).

Principles of implant placement in fibula bone are the same as those for placement in native jaw bone (**Fig. 14**), except owing to the high density of fibula bone, after completion of the implant drilling sequence the implant osteotomy

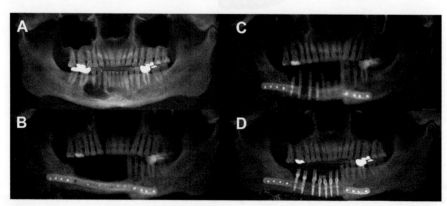

Fig. 12. Radiographs showing mandibular reconstruction using osteocutaneous fibula free flap (same patient as in **Figs. 10** and **11**). (*A*) Radiograph showing tumor in the right and anterior mandible. (*B*) Radiograph after tumor ablation and reconstruction of defect with an osteocutaneous fibula free flap. (*C*) Radiograph after flap debulking, exposure of integrated implants, vestibuloplasty, partial reconstruction plate removal, and placement of implant-supported custom-fabricated compressive splint. (*D*) Radiograph after delivery of temporary prosthesis.

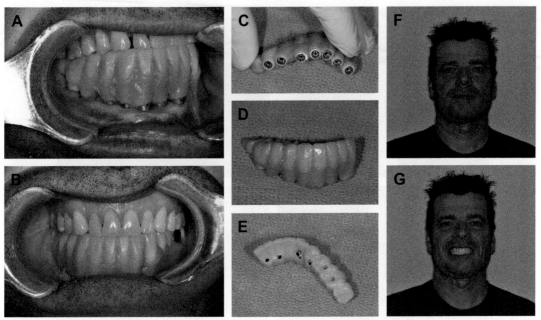

Fig. 13. Temporary and final prosthesis (same patient as in **Figs. 10–12**). (*A*) Right lateral view of the occlusion and labial vestibule with temporary prosthesis in place. (*B*) Frontal view of the occlusion with temporary prosthesis in place. (*C–E*) Final screw-retained prosthesis. (*F, G*) Frontal photos of the patient in smile and repose with final prosthesis in place.

site must be *tapped* to prevent fracture of the bone. Several soft-tissue management principles have to be kept in mind when planning for implant placement in vascularized bone grafts. For secondary implant placement, or when uncovering implants in an FFF with skin paddle, the incision to access the fibula bone should be designed not to damage perforators to the skin island. Given the unpredictability of revascularization of the skin paddle from the surrounding oral mucosa, the incision should be made on the lateral border of the paddle-mucosa interface if the perforators are emerging from the lingual; conversely, if the perforators are emerging from the lateral, the incision should be designed on the medial border to avoid accidentally injuring them and possibly devitalizing the skin paddle. Once fibula bone is exposed, *minimal* subperiosteal dissection should be performed to keep the bone-segment periosteal blood supply intact[10] (see **Fig. 14**).

A minimum of 10 mm of height and 5 mm of width in the fibula bone is required for endosseous implant placement.[54,76] Owing to lack of cancellous bone, bicortical placement of implants in FFF is important to achieve stability and attain higher removal torque values.[90] A maximum of 2 implants per 2-cm fibula segment should be planned. Segments should remain stabilized with

a reconstruction plate and 1 to 2 monocortical screws to maintain maximal bone vascularity.[12] For longer fibula segments, a minimum of 2 monocortical screws should be used to stabilize the segment, prevent micromovement at the osteotomy site, and avoid rotational forces on the segments. Minimum distance between 2 implants should be 3 mm,[91] distance between implant and lingual or buccal fibula bone cortical plate should be at least 0.5 mm, and distance of implant from the osteotomy site should be at least 3 mm (see **Fig. 6**). Implants should be parallel and angulation should be appropriate to allow for prosthetic rehabilitation. A maximum of 15° of divergence can be tolerated for prosthesis fabrication using angled abutments.[19,92] Minimal and maximal implant insertion torque should be 20 Ncm and 45 Ncm, respectively.[91]

To guide placement of endosseous implants in reconstructed bony segments, one may use a bone, mucosa, or tooth-borne virtually or conventionally planned and fabricated surgical guide. Teeth and bone supported implant placement guides are used in patients when there is insufficient vestibule to retain the guide. Use of implant placement guides allows one to precisely distance, angulate, and place implants within 1 mm margin of error from the plan.[76] If implant insertion torque is greater than or equal to 35 Ncm,[93] an

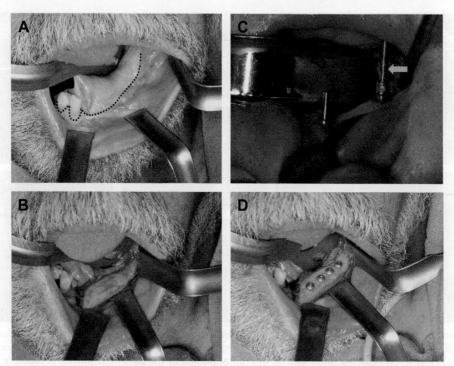

Fig. 14. Implant placement in fibula free flap. (*A*) Intraoral photograph of the left mandible showing incision markings. (*B*) Once the incision is made, minimal subperiosteal dissection over the fibula is performed to prevent devascularization of the segment. (*C*) Implants are placed in a standard fashion, making sure their angulation is correct using implant placement guide and paralleling pins (*green arrow*). (*D*) Implants in place with cover screws.

immediate screw-retained prosthesis can be delivered. If the insertion torque is less than 35 Ncm, a 2-stage protocol is used whereby the implants are buried after placement, then exposed and loaded 4 to 6 months later. At the time of implant exposure, osseointegration is checked by applying a reverse torque of 10 Ncm[47,91]

Timing of Implant Placement

For primary reconstruction, implants are placed at the time of FFF reconstruction. This technique has been well established, and noted to be safe and effective.[35,94] It has been proposed that detrimental effects of irradiation do not begin for 6 weeks *after* initiation of radiation therapy, thus allowing sufficient time for primarily placed implants to osseointegrate.[44]

For secondary reconstruction, implant placement is delayed for 4 to 6 months to allow for osteotomies to heal and soft tissues to integrate before starting oral prosthetic reconstruction.[35,39,95] Curi and colleagues[52] reported in 2018 that waiting longer than 6 months does not affect implant survival. In general, minimum time adopted for placement of implants after completion of irradiation is 6 months,[56]

although waiting 12 months after irradiation is ideal to avoid a likely higher risk of implant failure.[62]

Type of Implant

Brand of implant is not a factor in implant survival.[52] Most commercially available implant systems (Biomet 3i, Nobel Biocare, Astra tech, Straumann, and Ankylos) are equally compatible for restoration of FFF.[54] Implants with a treated surface have relatively fewer failures when compared with machined implants,[56] which is likely due to greater surface area and accelerated osseointegration in rough-surface implants. Compared with standard-size implants (10 mm or greater length), short implants have higher failure rates when placed in irradiated fields.[56] Based on these data and the authors' experience, a surface-treated implant that is at least 3.5 mm in width and 10 mm in length should be used for FFF reconstruction.[10]

SOFT-TISSUE MANAGEMENT

It has been established that oral function is strongly correlated with the size of soft-tissue defect and not the size of mandibular bony defect.[96] To reconstruct this soft-tissue defect, often a skin paddle is incorporated with the FFF harvest. This skin paddle provides necessary bulk and maintenance of integrity by separating the oral cavity from the neck, sinuses and nasal cavity. Appropriate management of oral soft tissues is critical for oral health, function, form, and long-term stability of the reconstructed area. Proper soft-tissue management includes thinning bulky or redundant tissue from the skin paddle, providing attached tissue around the implants to prevent peri-implantitis (**Fig. 15**), creation of buccal, labial, and lingual vestibules, allowing unrestricted tongue mobility, providing support for the lips, and improving cosmesis (**Fig. 16**).

As discussed earlier, access to the fibula bone or buried implants should be made in a way to avoid injury to the vascular pedicle and its perforators to the skin paddle (see **Figs. 14** and **15**). Once down to the periosteum, minimal subperiosteal dissection should be carried out to prevent devascularization of the fibula segment. On exposure of implants, several methods have been described to provide attached tissue around implants; these include debulking the flap skin paddle, placement of split- or full-thickness skin grafts, excising the skin paddle entirely and allowing the area to heal via secondary intention, and application of palatal mucosa grafts. Debulking of skin paddle and use of split-thickness skin grafts for providing keratinized tissues around implants has shown promising results, with no significant issues with formation of hyperplastic granulation tissue at the implant and skin interface[10,44] (see **Fig. 15**). Excision of skin paddle in a supraperiosteal plane and allowing it to heal via secondary intention is *not* a good option for patients with a history of irradiation.[44,97] Of all the choices, the palatal mucosa graft has been shown to be an ideal candidate because it provides keratinized attached mucosa that creates a seal around the

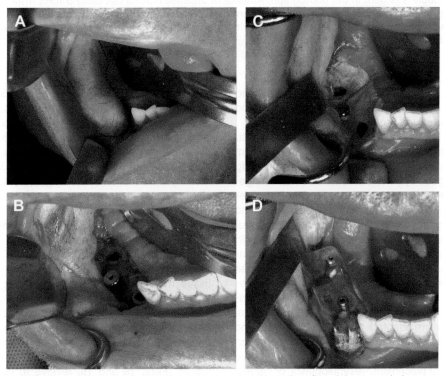

Fig. 15. Preprosthetic surgery in a patient with osteocutaneous fibula free flap. (A) Intraoral photograph of right mandible showing incision markings on the lingual of the skin paddle. Lingual incision was chosen because the perforators to the skin paddle originate from the buccal. (B) Incision is made, supraperiosteal dissection is performed, healing abutments are placed on select implants, and the skin paddle is debulked and lateralized to create a deeper vestibule. (C) A split-thickness skin graft is placed over the fibula to gain attached tissue around the implants. (D) An implant-supported custom-fabricated compressive splint is then placed over the graft and screwed in place for 6 to 8 weeks.

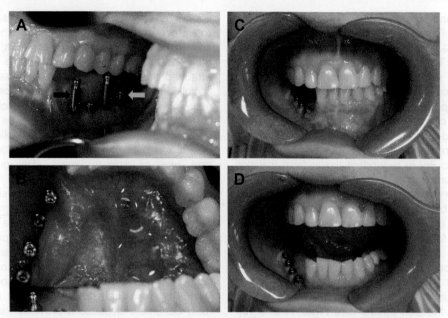

Fig. 16. Vestibuloplasty in a patient reconstructed with fibula free flap. (*A*) Right lateral view of the occlusion and buccal vestibule at the time of implant uncovering and impressions, showing implants with healing abutments (*blue arrow*) and impression copings (*black arrow*) in place. The sublingual gland is abutting behind the impression copings, which show a lack of attached lingual mucosa. (*B*) Occlusal view of the same patient. Again, lack of lingual vestibule is evident in this photograph. Absence of attached mucosa can cause chronic irritation around the implant-mucosa interface and lead to peri-implantitis. (*C*) Frontal view of the occlusion, buccal vestibule, and implants with healthy attached tissue surrounding them. (*D*) Photograph of the same patient showing good mobility of the tongue and a fair lingual vestibule.

implants, allows for appropriate hygiene, and prevents formation of granulation tissue and bone loss around the implants.[12,13,15,19,81,98,99]

Implants surrounded by mobile tissue leads to inflammation, which causes formation of exuberant granulation tissue and leads to peri-implantitis (**Fig 17**). With good hygiene and routine dental management, peri-implant soft-tissue hyperplasia decreases with time.[100] Furthermore, use of skin and mucosal grafts along with an implant-supported, custom-fabricated compressive splint lined with tissue conditioner inhibits granulation tissue formation around the abutments during the healing phase after implant exposure[101] (see **Fig. 15**). These splints can concomitantly be used for vestibuloplasty and should be left in place for 6 to 8 weeks, to allow for firm adaptation of graft to the underlying tissue and creation of a vestibule. Reconstruction plate and screws are removed if they interfere with implant placement, vestibuloplasty, or seating of the fabricated prosthesis (see **Fig. 8**).

PROSTHODONTIC CONSIDERATIONS

The goals of prosthetic reconstruction include mastication, speech, maintaining tongue mobility,

lip support, oral competence, and improving cosmesis. In FFF reconstructed patients, several factors are considered when deciding on implant-supported removable versus fixed prosthesis. These include height of the neoalveolar ridge, presence of labial and lingual vestibule, mobility and function of the tongue, number of implants present, hygiene, and cost.[51]

Factors that make the postablative patient a poor candidate for conventional (non–implant-supported) dentures are lack of bone and poor quality and quantity of soft tissue. Radiation therapy-related factors such as lack of soft-tissue mobility and xerostomia leading to poor suction, lack of denture retention, and ulceration from acrylic rubbing against the mucosa. Use of an endosseous implant-supported prosthesis in patients after oncology surgery and reconstruction provides stable, clinically comparable long-term results (**Figs. 18** and **19**) relative to healthy patients.[102] **Figs. 18** and **19** show a case of long-term stability of reconstructed mandibular segment.

Implant-supported removable dentures allow for better oral hygiene and require fewer implants (**Fig. 20**). Depending on the amount and type of

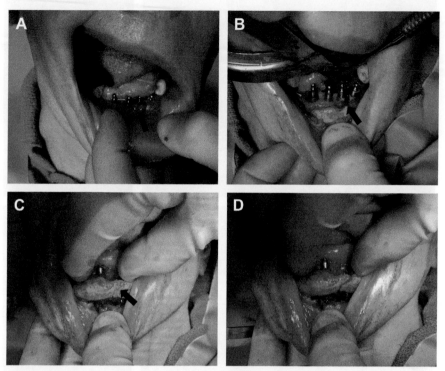

Fig. 17. Peri-implantitis. (*A*) Patient with mobile tissue around mandibular implants causing chronic inflammation and granulation tissue (*arrow*). (*B*) Exposure of the area shows peri-implantitis, significant bone loss (*arrow*), and mobility of implants. (*C*) Pathologic fracture (*arrow*) in the buccal cortex was noted. (*D*) Another photograph of the fracture site.

soft tissue present in the oral cavity, the prosthesis may be unstable and cause mechanical trauma to the surrounding tissue.[51] If this is the case, one should consider using bar connectors over ball-and-socket connectors, because the bar reduces micromovements of the implants and overcomes issues with misaligned or improperly placed implants. Ball-and-socket connectors in a removable implant-supported prosthesis have higher failure rates.[103] For implant-supported overdentures, the length and thickness of the prosthesis flange is based on the need for retention, allows unrestricted tongue mobility, and provides lip support. For edentulous patients being treated with implant-supported overdentures, a minimum of 4 implants should be placed per arch (**Fig. 21**). Kumar and colleagues[100,104] reported in 2016 that there was no difference in QOL in patients treated with overdentures based on 2 versus 4 implants, although the 2-implant system had higher marginal bone loss. An ideal removable implant-supported overdenture would be fabricated on and supported by 4 implants with bar attachments. Implant-supported fixed prostheses require longer abutments and long-term

maintenance, and are difficult to keep clean. A screw-retained fixed prosthesis is preferred in these patients because it allows for compensation of vertical discrepancy and removal of the prosthesis for maintenance and examination around the implants.

Causes of prosthetic rehabilitation failure include poor intermaxillary relationship, tumor recurrence, implant loss, microstomia, and lack of patient cooperation.[45] Implants with poor vectors, unaligned arches, long abutment, and increased distance between the fibula and opposing occlusal surface leads to a poor emergence profile, increased loading forces, and stress on the implants, which may jeopardize long-term implant survival.[8,105]

The reported rate of terminal rehabilitation with a prosthesis remains low, approximately 45%.[21,45] Higher rates of rehabilitation haven been reported from institutions that have secured funding for implant placement and prosthesis fabrication.[44] For the patients who have been rehabilitated, prosthesis survival rate is high, greater than 98%.[37,43] Cancer recurrence is the most common reason for not placing implants in FFF, and death is the main reason for not prosthetically

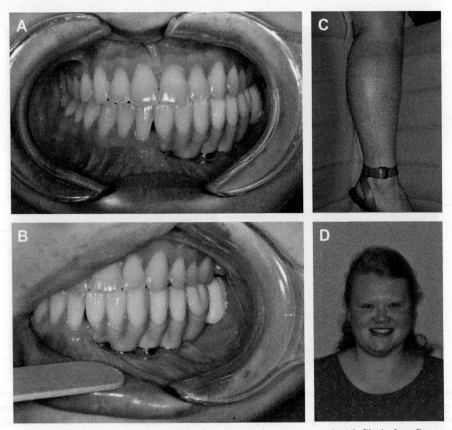

Fig. 18. Long-term outcome: a 10-year follow-up of a patient who was treated with fibula free flap and implant-supported prosthesis after resection of left mandibular mass. (*A*) Frontal view of the occlusion and prosthesis. (*B*) Left lateral view of the occlusion, prosthesis, and buccal vestibule. (*C*) Right leg surgical site showing good esthetics and minimal scarring. (*D*) Frontal view of face in smile.

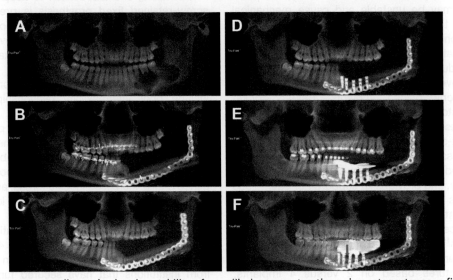

Fig. 19. Long-term radiographs showing stability of mandibular reconstruction using osteocutaneous fibula free flap and implant-supported prosthesis (same patient as in **Fig. 18**). (*A*) Radiograph showing left mandibular mass. (*B*) Immediate postoperative radiograph of left mandibular mass resection and reconstruction with fibula free flap. (*C*) Radiograph after consolidation of the graft and before implant placement. (*D*) Radiograph immediately after placement of endosseous implants. (*E*) Radiograph with interim prosthesis, and patient in orthodontic hardware. (*F*) Long-term follow-up (10 years) radiograph showing stable final prosthesis and mild marginal interproximal bone loss (*arrow*).

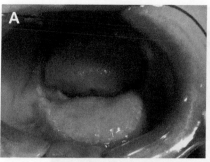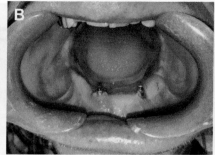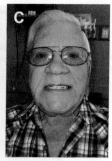

Fig. 20. Implant-supported removable prosthesis. (*A*) Photograph of anterior mandibular reconstruction site with bulky soft-tissue skin paddle. (*B*) Same patient after significantly debulking and excising the skin paddle and secondary reconstruction with 2 endosseous implants to support a removable overdenture. Note the significant debulking that was performed to create labial and lingual vestibules that would support the flanges of the implant-supported removable overdenture. (*C*) Frontal view of face in smile.

rehabilitating placed implants. Other reasons for not being able to prosthetically rehabilitate patients include trismus, compromised patient health, patient choice, financial constraint, poor placement of bone flap, peri-implantitis, and formation of hyperplastic granulation tissue at the implant-mucosa interface.[37,44]

Difficulties in reconstruction can also be due to lack of labial vestibule and lip length, bulky skin paddle (**Fig. 22**), limited bone volume, lack of bone height, and trismus. Ideal lip reconstruction requires appropriate lip length, bulk, height, texture, mobility, competence, passive stability, neural motor and sensory innervation, and supporting bony and prosthetic infrastructure.[35] It is most difficult to perform after free flap reconstruction and irradiation.

For maxillectomy patients, implant-supported obturators can be used to close off oronasal

fistula and improve speech and oral function, and allow for clinical examination in patients with a higher chance of recurrence.[31] In these patients there is no difference in oral function and QOL between implant-supported obturator versus free flap and implant-supported fixed prosthesis, but patients with obturators have poorer mental health and social life.[106] Patients with FFF and implant-supported overdentures do better than those without. When compared with no prosthesis or non–implant-supported prosthesis in postablative defects, statistically significant improvement in QOL was noted in patients reconstructed with FFF and implant-supported overdentures.[104]

Restorative options for these patients include implant-supported cement- or screw-retained bridge, overdenture, or hybrid prosthesis. An ideal option would be a fixed hybrid screw-retained

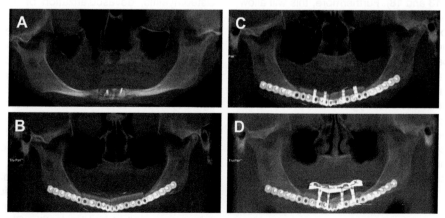

Fig. 21. Fibula free flap and implant-supported prosthesis in an edentulous patient with atrophic mandible. (*A*) Radiograph showing anterior mandibular lesion. (*B*) Radiograph after resection of the lesion and reconstruction with fibula free flap. (*C*) Radiograph taken immediately after placement of 4 endosseous implants. (*D*) Radiograph showing stable reconstruction with final hybrid prosthesis.

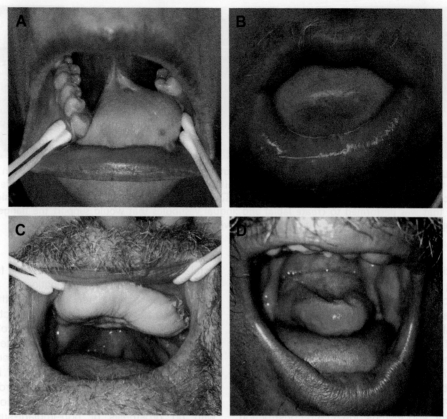

Fig. 22. Bulky skin paddles. (*A*) Photograph of skin paddle obliterating the labial and lingual vestibule. (*B*) Excess skin paddle bulk leading to lip incompetence. (*C*) Excess volume of fibula skin paddle used in reconstruction of the maxillary defect. (*D*) Another anterior mandibular skin paddle causing obliteration of the lingual vestibule and limiting tongue mobility.

prosthesis that does not derive any support from the mucosa, to decrease the chance of pressure necrosis and ulceration of the soft tissue[35,57,76] (see **Figs. 13** and **18**). Furthermore, this will allow for improved hygiene and prevent impaction of debris around the implants. Acrylic restoration and cement-retained prostheses should be avoided because they lead to granulation tissue formation around the implant and bone interface. A metal and ceramic final restoration is more appropriate to allow for hygiene and prevents tissue hyperplasia.[99,101] Because of its toughness, zirconia ceramic is advantageous for a prosthesis that will occlude against native teeth.[16] It is important to undertake good hygiene and routine maintenance of the prosthesis for long-term success.[35,49]

COMPLICATIONS

Most common complications associated with implant placement in FFF are peri-implantitis

(**Figs. 23** and **24**) and marginal bone loss[37] (see **Fig. 19**). Furthermore, peri-implantitis is the most common cause of implant loss in FFF.[35] Osteomyelitis, devascularization of fibula, fracture of fibula, ORN, and tumor recurrence at implant placement site have been reported.[35] Oral cancer can present around implants as peri-implantitis. There is no correlation established between oral cancer presenting at implant sites in patients with and without a history of malignancy. All cases of tumor recurrence at implant sites occurred in implants placed primarily.[71,107] Recurrence at primary implant sites can possibly be due to seeding of the implant placement bed, interference in radiation dosage from presence of metallic implant, and generally higher propensity of chronically irritated oral mucosa from long-term use of ethanol, tobacco, as well as peri-implantitis. Chronic peri-implantitis should be closely monitored, treated, and biopsied to rule out oral squamous cell carcinoma.[107] A linear fracture (parallel to the

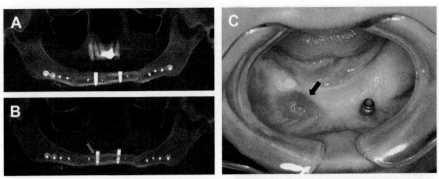

Fig. 23. Peri-implantitis in patient implant-supported removable overdenture. (*A*) Radiograph of patient reconstructed with fibula free flap and 2 endosseous implants. (*B*) Radiograph of the same patient taken on the day of presentation with peri-implantitis. Arrow points to bone loss around the implant. (*C*) Photograph of implant with peri-implantitis (*arrow*). Note lack of attached tissue around the implant which, combined with lack of labial vestibule, may be a factor leading to chronic irritation and inflammation.

long axis of the shaft) of the fibula can occur at the time of implant placement if the final osteotomy is not tapped all the way to the apex. If fracture occurs during implant placement, the implant and fibula segment can be salvaged by stabilization of the fibula segment using bicortical lag-screw fixation between implants (**Fig. 25**).

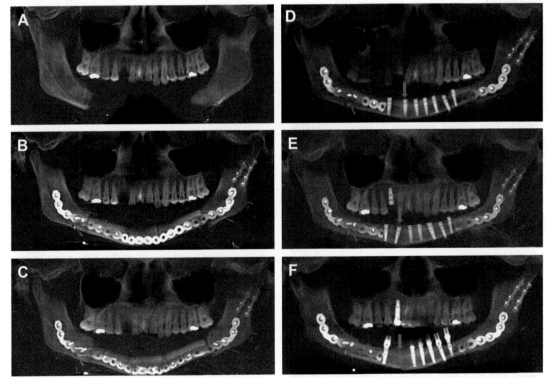

Fig. 24. Loss of implant before placement of prosthesis. (*A*) Radiograph of patient with extensive defect of hard and soft tissues of mandible. (*B*) Radiograph of the same patient taken immediately after reconstruction of the defect with osteocutaneous fibula free flap, and open reduction internal fixation of left subcondylar fracture. (*C*) Radiograph taken after allowing 6 months of consolidation for the fibula free flap. (*D*) Radiograph taken immediately after partial reconstruction plate removal and placement of 7 bicortical endosseous implants in the fibula bone. Arrow points to implant placed into the healed fibula osteotomy site. (*E*) Radiograph showing failure of the implant (*arrow*) in the osteotomy site. (*F*) Radiograph showing removal of failed implant, healed osteotomy site (*arrow*), and patient in temporary prosthesis.

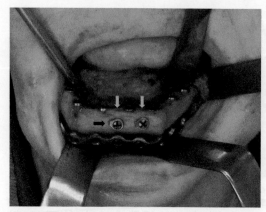

Fig. 25. Photograph of fibula bone showing healed osteotomy sites and placed endosseous implants. A linear fracture (*blue arrows*) of the fibula was noted during placement of implants in the anterior segment. To prevent further propagation of the fracture and loss of implants, the anterior fibula segment was stabilized by placing 2 bicortical lag screws with washers (*black arrow*).

SUMMARY

Maxillofacial subunit reconstruction using FFF and implant-supported prosthesis is a reliable and lasting option to provide integrity, function, and form to the patient while improving their QOL. Careful patient selection, planning, execution, and communication between the treating team is critical for achievement of optimal long-term outcomes. This review presents currently available data to aid in planning and treating patients with large and complex maxillofacial deformities using FFF and endosseous implant-supported prosthesis. At the authors' institution, if the cost of implant-supported prosthetic reconstruction and patient choice are not a factor, VSP is preferably used to guide primary placement of implants in FFF for all defects, except for those created by resection of malignant disease. Secondary implant reconstruction of patients who previously received therapeutic radiation after placement of FFF should be done with caution. Soft-tissue management should be performed as needed, and prosthodontic rehabilitation should ideally be done with a fixed hybrid metal ceramic screw-retained prosthesis. A motivated patient, meticulous hygiene, and long-term follow-up are important for maintenance and success of the reconstruction.

REFERENCES

1. Urken ML, Buchbinder D, Weinberg H, et al. Primary placement of osseointegrated implants in microvascular mandibular reconstruction. Otolaryngol Head Neck Surg 1989;101(1):56–73.

2. Chuka R, Abdullah W, Rieger J, et al. Implant utilization and time to prosthetic rehabilitation in conventional and advanced fibular free flap reconstruction of the maxilla and mandible. Int J Prosthodont 2017;30(3):289–94.

3. Ooi A, Feng J, Tan HK, et al. Primary treatment of mandibular ameloblastoma with segmental resection and free fibula reconstruction: achieving satisfactory outcomes with low implant-prosthetic rehabilitation uptake. J Plast Reconstr Aesthet Surg 2014;67(4):498–505.

4. Wallace CG, Chang YM, Tsai CY, et al. Harnessing the potential of the free fibula osteoseptocutaneous flap in mandible reconstruction. Plast Reconstr Surg 2010;125(1):305–14.

5. Wilkman T, Apajalahti S, Wilkman E, et al. A comparison of bone resorption over time: an analysis of the free scapular, iliac crest, and fibular microvascular flaps in mandibular reconstruction. J Oral Maxillofac Surg 2017;75(3):616–21.

6. Fujiki M, Miyamoto S, Sakuraba M, et al. A comparison of perioperative complications following transfer of fibular and scapular flaps for immediate mandibular reconstruction. J Plast Reconstr Aesthet Surg 2013;66(3):372–5.

7. Yilmaz M, Vayvada H, Menderes A, et al. A comparison of vascularized fibular flap and iliac crest flap for mandibular reconstruction. J Craniofac Surg 2008;19(1):227–34.

8. Politi M, Toro C. Iliac flap versus fibula flap in mandibular reconstruction. J Craniofac Surg 2012;23(3):774–9.

9. Brown JS, Lowe D, Kanatas A, et al. Mandibular reconstruction with vascularised bone flaps: a systematic review over 25 years. Br J Oral Maxillofac Surg 2017;55(2):113–26.

10. Kim DD, Ghali GE. Dental implants in oral cancer reconstruction. Oral Maxillofac Surg Clin North Am 2011;23(2):337–45.

11. Schardt C, Schmid A, Bodem J, et al. Donor site morbidity and quality of life after microvascular head and neck reconstruction with free fibula and deep-circumflex iliac artery flaps. J Craniomaxillofac Surg 2017;45(2):304–11.

12. Chana JS, Chang YM, Wei FC, et al. Segmental mandibulectomy and immediate free fibula osteoseptocutaneous flap reconstruction with endosteal implants: an ideal treatment method for mandibular ameloblastoma. Plast Reconstr Surg 2004;113(1):80–7.

13. Chang YM, Wallace CG, Tsai CY, et al. Dental implant outcome after primary implantation into double-barreled fibula osteoseptocutaneous free flap-reconstructed mandible. Plast Reconstr Surg 2011;128(6):1220–8.

14. He Y, Zhang ZY, Zhu HG, et al. Double-barrel fibula vascularized free flap with dental rehabilitation for

mandibular reconstruction. J Oral Maxillofac Surg 2011;69(10):2663–9.

15. Shen YF, Rodriguez ED, Wei FC, et al. Aesthetic and functional mandibular reconstruction with immediate dental implants in a free fibular flap and a low-profile reconstruction plate: five-year follow-up. Ann Plast Surg 2015;74(4):442–6.

16. Yoon H-I. Prosthetic rehabilitation after fibular free flap surgery of mandibular defects in a patient with oral squamous cell carcinoma. J Craniofac Surg 2016;27(7):e685–8.

17. Lee JH, Kim MJ, Choi WS, et al. Concomitant reconstruction of mandibular basal and alveolar bone with a free fibular flap. Int J Oral Maxillofac Surg 2004;33(2):150–6.

18. Lizio G, Corinaldesi G, Pieri F, et al. Problems with dental implants that were placed on vertically distracted fibular free flaps after resection: a report of six cases. Br J Oral Maxillofac Surg 2009;47(6):455–60.

19. Chang YM, Santamaria E, Wei FC, et al. Primary insertion of osseointegrated dental implants into fibula osteoseptocutaneous free flap for mandible reconstruction. Plast Reconstr Surg 1998;102(3):680–8.

20. Moscoso J, Keller J, Genden E, et al. Vascularized bone flaps in oromandibular reconstruction. A comparative anatomic study of bone from various donor sites to assess suitability for endosseous dental implants. Arch Otolaryngol Head Neck Surg 1994;120(1):36–43.

21. Van Gemert JTM, Van Es RJJ, Rosenberg AJWP, et al. Free vascularized flaps for reconstruction of the mandible: complications, success, and dental rehabilitation. J Oral Maxillofac Surg 2012;70(7):1692–8.

22. Frodel JLJ, Funk GF, Capper DT, et al. Osseointegrated implants: a comparative study of bone thickness in four vascularized bone flaps. Plast Reconstr Surg 1993;92(3):448–9.

23. Akkocaoglu M, Cehreli MC, Tekdemir I, et al. Primary stability of simultaneously placed dental implants in extraoral donor graft sites: a human cadaver study. J Oral Maxillofac Surg 2007;65(3):400–7.

24. Blake F, Bubenheim M, Heiland M, et al. Retrospective assessment of the peri-implant mucosa of implants inserted in reanastomosed or free bone grafts from the fibula or iliac crest. Int J Oral Maxillofac Implants 2008;23(6):1102–8.

25. Möhlhenrich SC, Kniha K, Elvers D, et al. Intraosseous stability of dental implants in free revascularized fibula and iliac crest bone flaps. J Craniomaxillofac Surg 2016;44(12):1935–9.

26. Beckers A, Schenck C, Klesper B, et al. Comparative densitometric study of iliac crest and scapula bone in relation to osseous integrated dental implants in microvascular mandibular reconstruction. J Craniomaxillofac Surg 1998;26(2):75–83.

27. Ling XF, Peng X, Samman N. Donor-site morbidity of free fibula and DCIA flaps. J Oral Maxillofac Surg 2013;71(9):1604–12.

28. Shpitzer T, Neligan PC, Gullane PJ, et al. The free iliac crest and fibula flaps in vascularized oromandibular reconstruction: comparison and long-term evaluation. Head Neck 1999;21(7):639–47.

29. Mertens C, Decker C, Engel M, et al. Early bone resorption of free microvascular reanastomized bone grafts for mandibular reconstruction–a comparison of iliac crest and fi bula grafts. J Craniomaxillofac Surg 2014;42(5):e217–23.

30. Kniha K, Möhlhenrich SC, Foldenauer AC, et al. Evaluation of bone resorption in fibula and deep circumflex iliac artery flaps following dental implantation: a three-year follow-up study. J Craniomaxillofac Surg 2017;45(4):474–8.

31. Otomaru T, Sumita YI, Aimaijiang Y, et al. Rehabilitation of a bilateral maxillectomy patient with a free fibula osteocutaneous flap and with an implant-retained obturator: a clinical report. J Prosthodont 2016;25(4):341–8.

32. Lonie S, Herle P, Paddle A, et al. Mandibular reconstruction: meta-analysis of iliac- versus fibula-free flaps. ANZ J Surg 2016;86(5):337–42.

33. Ferrari S, Copelli C, Bianchi B, et al. Rehabilitation with endosseous implants in fibula free-flap mandibular reconstruction: a case series of up to 10 years. J Craniomaxillofac Surg 2013;41(2):172–8.

34. Wijbenga JG, Schepers RH, Werker PMN, et al. A systematic review of functional outcome and quality of life following reconstruction of maxillofacial defects using vascularized free fibula flaps and dental rehabilitation reveals poor data quality. J Plast Reconstr Aesthet Surg 2016;69(8):1024–36.

35. Raoul G, Ruhin B, Briki S, et al. Microsurgical reconstruction of the jaw with fibular grafts and implants. J Craniofac Surg 2009;20(6):2105–17.

36. Jacobsen H-C, Wahnschaff F, Trenkle T, et al. Oral rehabilitation with dental implants and quality of life following mandibular reconstruction with free fibular flap. Clin Oral Investig 2016;20(1):187–92.

37. Parbo N, Murra NT, Andersen K, et al. Outcome of partial mandibular reconstruction with fibula grafts and implant-supported prostheses. Int J Oral Maxillofac Surg 2013;42(11):1403–8.

38. Attia S, Wiltfang J, Pons-Kühnemann J, et al. Survival of dental implants placed in vascularised fibula free flaps after jaw reconstruction. J Craniomaxillofac Surg 2018;46(8):1205–10.

39. Roumanas ED. Reconstructed mandibular defects: fibula free flaps and osseointegrated implants. Plast Reconstr Surg 1997;99(2):356–65.

40. Garrett N, Roumanas ED, Blackwell KE, et al. Efficacy of conventional and implant-supported mandibular resection prostheses: study overview and treatment outcomes. J Prosthet Dent 2006; 96(1):13–24.

41. Gbara A, Darwich K, Li L, et al. Long-term results of jaw reconstruction with microsurgical fibula grafts and dental implants. J Oral Maxillofac Surg 2007; 65(5):1005–9.

42. Chiapasco M, Colletti G, Romeo E, et al. Long-term results of mandibular reconstruction with autogenous bone grafts and oral implants after tumor resection. Clin Oral Implants Res 2008;19(10): 1074–80.

43. Jackson RS, Price DL, Arce K, et al. Evaluation of clinical outcomes of osseointegrated dental implantation of fibula free flaps for mandibular reconstruction. JAMA Facial Plast Surg 2016;18(3): 201–6.

44. Ch'ng S, Skoracki RJ, Selber JC, et al. Osseointegrated implant-based dental rehabilitation in head and neck reconstruction patients. Head Neck 2016;38(Suppl 1):E321–7.

45. Smolka K, Kraehenbuehl M, Eggensperger N, et al. Fibula free flap reconstruction of the mandible in cancer patients: evaluation of a combined surgical and prosthodontic treatment concept. Oral Oncol 2008;44(6):571–81.

46. Teoh KH, Huryn JM, Patel S, et al. Implant prosthodontic rehabilitation of fibula free-flap reconstructed mandibles: a Memorial Sloan-Kettering Cancer Center review of prognostic factors and implant outcomes. Int J Oral Maxillofac Implants 2005;20(5):738–46.

47. Sozzi D, Novelli G, Silva R, et al. Implant rehabilitation in fibula-free flap reconstruction: a retrospective study of cases at 1-18 years following surgery. J Craniomaxillofac Surg 2017;45(10): 1655–61.

48. Chiapasco M, Romeo E, Coggiola A, et al. Long-term outcome of dental implants placed in revascularized fibula free flaps used for the reconstruction of maxillo-mandibular defects due to extreme atrophy. Clin Oral Implants Res 2011;22(1):83–91.

49. Fang W, Liu Y, Ma Q, et al. Long-term results of mandibular reconstruction of continuity defects with fibula free flap and implant-borne dental rehabilitation. Int J Oral Maxillofac Implants 2015;30(1): 169–78.

50. Hakim SG, Kimmerle H, Trenkle T, et al. Masticatory rehabilitation following upper and lower jaw reconstruction using vascularised free fibula flap and endosseal implants—19 years of experience with a comprehensive concept. Clin Oral Investig 2015; 19(2):525–34.

51. Bodard AG, Salino S, Desoutter A, et al. Assessment of functional improvement with implant-supported prosthetic rehabilitation after mandibular reconstruction with a microvascular free fibula flap: a study of 25 patients. J Prosthet Dent 2015; 113(2):140–5.

52. Curi MM, Condezo AFB, Ribeiro KDCB, et al. Long-term success of dental implants in patients with head and neck cancer after radiation therapy. Int J Oral Maxillofac Surg 2018;47(6):783–8.

53. Chrcanovic BR, Albrektsson T, Wennerberg A. Dental implants in irradiated versus nonirradiated patients: a meta-analysis. Head Neck 2016;38(3): 448–81. Eisele DW.

54. Carbiner R, Jerjes W, Shakib K, et al. Analysis of the compatibility of dental implant systems in fibula free flap reconstruction. Head Neck Oncol 2012;4: 37.

55. Ernst N, Sachse C, Raguse JD, et al. Changes in peri-implant bone level and effect of potential influential factors on dental implants in irradiated and nonirradiated patients following multimodal therapy due to head and neck cancer: a retrospective study. J Oral Maxillofac Surg 2016;74(10):1965–73.

56. Smith Nobrega A, Santiago JF, de Faria Almeida DA, et al. Irradiated patients and survival rate of dental implants: a systematic review and meta-analysis. J Prosthet Dent 2016;116(6): 858–66.

57. Mancha De La Plata M, Gas LN, Dez PM, et al. Osseointegrated implant rehabilitation of irradiated oral cancer patients. J Oral Maxillofac Surg 2012; 70(5):1052–63.

58. Visch LL, Van Waas MAJ, Schmitz PIM, et al. A clinical evaluation of implants in irradiated oral cancer patients. J Dent Res 2002;81(12):856–9.

59. Esser E, Wagner W. Dental implants following radical oral cancer surgery and adjuvant radiotherapy. Int J Oral Maxillofac Implants 1997;12(4): 552–7.

60. Yerit KC, Posch M, Seemann M, et al. Implant survival in mandibles of irradiated oral cancer patients. Clin Oral Implants Res 2006;17(3):337–44.

61. Granström G. Osseointegration in irradiated cancer patients: an analysis with respect to implant failures. J Oral Maxillofac Surg 2005;63(5): 579–85.

62. Claudy MP, Miguens SAQ, Celeste RK, et al. Time interval after radiotherapy and dental implant failure: systematic review of observational studies and meta-analysis. Clin Implant Dent Relat Res 2015;17(2):402–11.

63. Zen Filho EV, Tolentino E de S, Santos PSS. Viability of dental implants in head and neck irradiated patients: a systematic review. Head Neck 2016; 38(S1):E2229–40. Eisele DW.

64. Sammartino G, Marenzi G, Cioffi I, et al. Implant therapy in irradiated patients. J Craniofac Surg 2011;22(2):443–5.

65. Salinas TJ, Desa VP, Katsnelson A, et al. Clinical evaluation of implants in radiated fibula flaps. J Oral Maxillofac Surg 2010;68(3):524–9.

66. Carr AB. Oral cancer therapy may influence survival of dental implants. J Evid Based Dent Pract 2011;11(3):124–6.

67. Burgess M, Leung M, Chellapah A, et al. Osseointegrated implants into a variety of composite free flaps: a comparative analysis. Head Neck 2017; 39(3):443–7.

68. Brasseur M, Brogniez V, Grégoire V, et al. Effects of irradiation on bone remodelling around mandibular implants: an experimental study in dogs. Int J Oral Maxillofac Surg 2006;35(9):850–5.

69. Friedrich RE, Manuel TA, Andreas K. Simulation of scattering effects of irradiation on surroundings using the example of titanium dental implants: a Monte Carlo approach. Anticancer Res 2010; 30(5):1727–30.

70. Korfage A, Raghoebar GM, Slater JJRH, et al. Overdentures on primary mandibular implants in patients with oral cancer: a follow-up study over 14 years. Br J Oral Maxillofac Surg 2014;52(9): 798–805.

71. De Ceulaer J, Magremanne M, Van Veen A, et al. Squamous cell carcinoma recurrence around dental implants. J Oral Maxillofac Surg 2010; 68(10):2507–12.

72. Friedrich RE, Todorovic M, Heiland M, et al. Scattering effects of irradiation on surroundings calculated for a small dental implant. Anticancer Res 2012;32(5):2043–6.

73. Schoen PJ, Raghoebar GM, Bouma J, et al. Rehabilitation of oral function in head and neck cancer patients after radiotherapy with implant-retained dentures: effects of hyperbaric oxygen therapy. Oral Oncol 2007;43(4):379–88.

74. Schepers RH, Raghoebar GM, Vissink A, et al. Accuracy of fibula reconstruction using patient-specific CAD/CAM reconstruction plates and dental implants: a new modality for functional reconstruction of mandibular defects. J Craniomaxillofac Surg 2015;43(5):649–57.

75. Rana M, Chin SJ, Muecke T, et al. Increasing the accuracy of mandibular reconstruction with free fibula flaps using functionalized selective laser-melted patient-specific implants: a retrospective multicenter analysis. J Craniomaxillofac Surg 2017;45(8):1212–9.

76. Cebrian-Carretero JL, Guinales-Diaz de Cevallos J, Sobrino JA, et al. Predictable dental rehabilitation in maxillomandibular reconstruction with free flaps. The role of implant guided surgery. Med Oral Patol Oral Cir Bucal 2014;19(6):e605–11.

77. Rude K, Thygesen TH, Sørensen JA. Reconstruction of the maxilla using a fibula graft and virtual planning techniques. BMJ Case Rep 2014;1:1–5.

78. Avraham T, Franco P, Brecht LE, et al. Functional outcomes of virtually planned free fibula flap reconstruction of the mandible. Plast Reconstr Surg 2014;134(4):628e–34e.

79. Menapace DC, Van Abel KM, Jackson RS, et al. Primary vs secondary endosseous implantation after fibular free tissue reconstruction of the mandible for osteoradionecrosis. JAMA Facial Plast Surg 2018;20(5):401–8.

80. Levine JP, Bae JS, Soares M, et al. Jaw in a day: total maxillofacial reconstruction using digital technology. Plast Reconstr Surg 2013;131(6): 1386–91.

81. Chang YM, Coskunfirat OK, Wei FC, et al. Maxillary reconstruction with a fibula osteoseptocutaneous free flap and simultaneous insertion of osseointegrated dental implants. Plast Reconstr Surg 2004; 113(4):1140–5.

82. Nazerani S, Behnia H, Motamedi MHK. Experience with the prefabricated free fibula flap for reconstruction of maxillary and mandibular defects. J Oral Maxillofac Surg 2008;66(2):260–4.

83. Freudlsperger C, Bodem JP, Engel E, et al. Mandibular reconstruction with a prefabricated free vascularized fibula and implant-supported prosthesis based on fully three-dimensional virtual planning. J Craniofac Surg 2014;25(3):980–2.

84. Nkenke E, Vairaktaris E, Schlittenbauer T, et al. Masticatory rehabilitation of a patient with cleft lip and palate malformation using a maxillary full-arch reconstruction with a prefabricated fibula flap. Cleft Palate Craniofac J 2016;53(6):736–40.

85. Rohner D, Bucher P, Kunz C, et al. Treatment of severe atrophy of the maxilla with the prefabricated free vascularized fibula flap. Clin Oral Implants Res 2002;13(1):44–52.

86. Qaisi M, Kolodney H, Swedenburg G, et al. Fibula jaw in a day: state of the art in maxillofacial reconstruction. J Oral Maxillofac Surg 2016;74(6): 1284e1–15.

87. Ide Y, Matsunaga S, Harris J, et al. Anatomical examination of the fibula: Digital imaging study for osseointegrated implant installation. J Otolaryngol Head Neck Surg 2015;44:1–8.

88. Hidalgo DA. Fibula free flap: a new method of mandible reconstruction. Plast Reconstr Surg 1989;84(1):71–9.

89. Bahr W. Blood supply of small fibula segments: an experimental study on human cadavers. J Craniomaxillofac Surg 1998;26(3):148–52.

90. Rohner D, Tay A, Chung SM, et al. Interface of unloaded titanium implants in the iliac crest, fibula, and scapula: a histomorphometric and biomechanical study in the pig. Int J Oral Maxillofac Implants 2004;19(1):52–8.

91. Maluf PSZ, Ching AW, Angeletti P, et al. Insertion torque of dental implants after microvascular

fibular grafting. Br J Oral Maxillofac Surg 2015; 53(7):647–9.

92. Bidez MW, Misch CE. Force transfer in implant dentistry: basic concepts and principles. J Oral Implant 1992;18(3):264–74.

93. Meloni SM, Tallarico M, De Riu G, et al. Guided implant surgery after free-flap reconstruction: Four-year results from a prospective clinical trial. J Craniomaxillofac Surg 2015;43(8):1348–55.

94. Urken ML, Buchbinder D, Costantino PD, et al. Oromandibular reconstruction using microvascular composite flaps: report of 210 cases. Arch Otolaryngol Head Neck Surg 1998;124(1):46–55.

95. Anne-Gaëlle B, Samuel S, Julie B, et al. Dental implant placement after mandibular reconstruction by microvascular free fibula flap: current knowledge and remaining questions. Oral Oncol 2011; 47(12):1099–104.

96. Iizuka T, Häfliger J, Seto I, et al. Oral rehabilitation after mandibular reconstruction using an osteocutaneous fibula free flap with endosseous implants: factors affecting the functional outcome in patients with oral cancer. Clin Oral Implants Res 2005;16(1): 69–79.

97. Kumar VV, Jacob PC, Kuriakose MA. Sub-periosteal dissection with denture-guided epithelial regeneration: a novel method for peri-implant soft tissue management in reconstructed mandibles. J Maxillofac Oral Surg 2016;15(4):449–55.

98. Chang YM, Chan CP, Shen YF, et al. Soft tissue management using palatal mucosa around endosteal implants in vascularized composite grafts in the mandible. Int J Oral Maxillofac Surg 1999; 28(5):341–3.

99. Chang YM, Pan YH, Shen YF, et al. Success of dental implants in vascularised fibular osteoseptocutaneous flaps used as onlay grafts after marginal mandibulectomy. Br J Oral Maxillofac Surg 2016; 54(10):1090–4.

100. Kumar VV, Ebenezer S, Peer WK, et al. Implants in free fibula flap supporting dental rehabilitation-implant and peri-implant related outcomes of a randomized clinical trial. J Craniomaxillofac Surg 2016;44:1849–58.

101. Ciocca L, Corinaldesi G, Marchetti C, et al. Gingival hyperplasia around implants in the maxilla and jaw reconstructed by fibula free flap. Int J Oral Maxillofac Surg 2008;37(5):478–80.

102. Kovács AF. The fate of osseointegrated implants in patients following oral cancer surgery and mandibular reconstruction. Head Neck 2000;22(2):111–9.

103. Brauner E, Cassoni A, Battisti A, et al. Prosthetic rehabilitation in post-oncological patients: report of two cases. Ann Stomatol (Roma) 2010;1(1): 19–25.

104. Kumar VV, Jacob PC, Ebenezer S, et al. Implant supported dental rehabilitation following segmental mandibular reconstruction- quality of life outcomes of a prospective randomized trial. J Craniomaxillofac Surg 2016;44(7):800–10.

105. Chiapasco M, Biglioli F, Autelitano L, et al. Clinical outcome of dental implants placed in fibula-free flaps used for the reconstruction of maxillomandibular defects following ablation for tumors or osteoradionecrosis. Clin Oral Implants Res 2006;17(2):220–8.

106. Wang F, Huang W, Zhang C, et al. Functional outcome and quality of life after a maxillectomy: a comparison between an implant supported obturator and an implant supported fixed prostheses in a free vascularized flap. Clin Oral Implants Res 2017;28(2):137–43.

107. Pinchasov G, Haimov H, Druseikaite M, et al. Oral cancer around dental implants appearing in patients with\without a history of oral or systemic malignancy: a systematic review. J Oral Maxillofac Res 2017;8(3):1–10.

Quad Zygoma
Technique and Realities

Rubén Davó, MD, PhD[a], Lesley David, DDS, DOMFS, FRCDC[b],*

KEYWORDS

- Zygomatic implants • Quad zygoma technique • Graftless implant solution • Atrophic maxilla
- Survival rates • Immediate loading

KEY POINTS

- Four zygomatic implants (quad zygoma) can be used in patients with severe maxillary atrophy as an alternative to bone grafting to reconstruct the maxilla. This approach is used as the first line of treatment or as a rescue solution for failed implants and severe bone loss.
- Initial stability of zygomatic implants is typically excellent; as such, immediate loading with a fixed bridge is often performed and different techniques can be employed to fabricate a provisional prosthesis.
- The technique of placing a zygomatic implant has evolved over the years. The evolution of this procedure takes into account the potential complications of the use of zygomatic implants and patients' anatomy (zygoma anatomy guided approach).
- The quad zygoma surgical procedure is technique sensitive and requires advanced surgical skill. The surgical procedure for the quad zygoma is described.
- Various complications can occur with the placement of zygomatic implants such as oral-antral communication, paresthesia, infection at the tip of the implant, tissue retraction, and more. Understanding the etiology of these complications will assist with prevention and management.

Complete maxillary rehabilitation has changed dramatically since the advent of osseointegration; treatment options have become more varied and less invasive procedures have emerged. This is timely as life expectancy has increased, resulting in more elderly patients seeking treatment.[1] Thus, severe maxillary atrophy can present relatively frequently in clinical practice. The quad zygoma concept addresses the severely atrophic maxilla by making use of 4 zygoma implants (**Fig. 1**). Two implants are placed bilaterally with appropriate anterior and posterior spread and inclination for prosthetic rehabilitation. Typically, a fixed prosthesis is provided although this implant solution may also be used to retain an overdenture.

Bone loss secondary to dental extractions occurs in a predictable manner. Many phenomena affect the alveolar bone leading to severe atrophy and a decrease in volume making it difficult to insert dental implants.[2] (**Fig. 2**) The timeline of progression to severe bone loss is variable among patients; however, with enough time and overlying compressive forces of a complete denture, the fate of edentulous jaws is predictable.

Rehabilitation of completely edentulous patients regardless of the degree of atrophy has historically involved the use of complete removable dentures. This approach, however, may not meet the functional, psychological, and social needs of each individual.[3]

Disclosure Statement: Both authors are global speakers for NobelBiocare.
[a] Department of Implantology and Maxillofacial Surgery, Medimar International Hospital, Padre Arrupe, 20, 5th floor, Alicante 03016, Spain; [b] Oral and Maxillofacial Surgery, Trillium Health Partners, University of Toronto, Private Practice, Toronto, Canada
* Corresponding author. Implant Surgical Care, 1849 Yonge Street, #302, Toronto, Ontario M4S 1Y2, Canada.
E-mail address: drdavid@implantsurgicalcare.com

Oral Maxillofacial Surg Clin N Am 31 (2019) 285–297
https://doi.org/10.1016/j.coms.2018.12.006
1042-3699/19/© 2019 Elsevier Inc. All rights reserved.

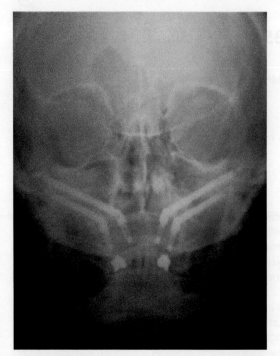

Fig. 1. Quad zygoma.

Over time options evolved:

1. Surgical reconstruction of the jaws involving bone grafting followed by secondary implant placement
2. Using implants in a tilted fashion to eliminate the need for bone grafting and engage available bone where possible with appropriate distribution of the implants for prosthetic rehabilitation
3. Using an alternate source of bone such as the zygoma or pterygoids for anchorage of implants[4,5]

When severe bone atrophy has occurred, the option of prosthetic reconstruction to compensate for the composite defect as opposed to surgical reconstruction (to rebuild lost anatomy) enables less invasive surgical interventions for patients (**Fig. 3**). The synergy between surgery and prosthetics is paramount. The quad zygoma combined

with prosthetic reconstruction can address patients' needs for esthetics and function similar to conventional treatments.[3] The reality of needing less surgery to rehabilitate the edentulous maxilla is one that beckons surgeons to examine their goals of treatment and work closely with prosthodontists to obtain successful outcomes. Inarguably, prosthetic reconstruction of lost anatomy eliminates the morbidity associated with surgical reconstruction.

Bone augmentation techniques are widely used and are supported by a great deal of scientific evidence. Nevertheless, clinical and biological limitations are inherent, preventing success rates from reaching those of the alternative approach based on extra-alveolar implants.[6] In clinical practice, the presence of hyperplastic maxillary sinuses with uncontrollable infectious processes, severe alveolar atrophy, or other clinical situations such as defects secondary to trauma or the treatment of pathology requiring severe resective surgeries may mean that the only possible treatment is by means of zygomatic implants.[7]

From a biological perspective, autologous bone grafts are considered the gold standard. However, morbidity at the donor site, bone resorption when subjected to loading, a prolonged treatment timeline, and problems that can arise with clinically challenging scenarios must be weighed in considering this treatment solution. In addition, the need to achieve adequate vascularization internally and externally makes the technique difficult to apply in cases of severe vertical atrophy. It is often impossible to achieve adequate internal and peripheral vascularization of the graft in large vertical reconstructions.[8] Furthermore, few studies have investigated the use of grafts (bone grafts or other biomaterials) to regenerate severe maxillary atrophy. A recent randomized clinical trial conducted with this profile of patients suggested that, although the use of biomaterials might be possible, rehabilitation takes an average of 430 days. Zygoma implants obtained better outcomes and constituted a much faster means of rehabilitation.[9]

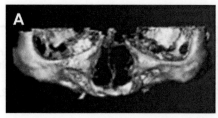 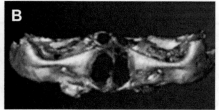

Fig. 2. (*A*) Cawood and Howell class V. (*B*) Cawood and Howell class VI.

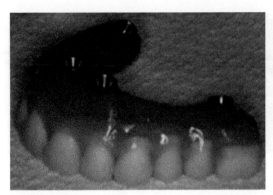

Fig. 3. Provisional bridge: acrylic compensating for lost anatomy.

Nonalveolar implants offer a predictable alternative to bone augmentation techniques in situations of severe alveolar atrophy. The placement of implants in bone of a different embryologic origin favors high survival rates derived from the absence of bone resorption and atrophy. In the authors' experience, bone resorption can be seen years later in grafted sites with implants; this is not typically seen in the malar bone (**Fig. 4**).

Zygomatic implants were introduced for the rehabilitation of patients with extensive bone loss derived from trauma, neoplasms, or congenital pathologies. These implants can be combined with intra-alveolar implants or may be used alone to support a prosthesis. Several anatomic studies have validated the good quality of zygomatic bone and have stressed the importance of the cortical portion of the zygomatic bone for anchoring implants. It has also been documented that the area of zygomatic bone used for implant insertion has wider and thicker trabecular bone. This may explain the excellent potential for primary stability of zygomatic implants and, thus, the suitability for immediate loading. This advantage of immediate loading with zygomatic implants normalizes patients' quality of life immediately.[3]

INDICATIONS AND CONTRAINDICATIONS

Indications include severe maxillary atrophy, in particular inadequate bone volume for the placement of even a single dental implant both anteriorly and posteriorly.[10] (**Fig. 5**). The quad zygoma is used as the first option of choice in these patients. It may also be used as a rescue implant in patients who previously had bone grafting and implants that failed.

The concept of using short implants anteriorly in conjunction with a zygoma implant posteriorly is controversial with few supporting studies in the literature. In the authors' experience, it is prudent to perform a quad zygoma whenever the bone loss anteriorly precludes placement of conventional implants of at least 10 mm in length.

The quad zygoma may be used for rehabilitation with either a fixed or removable prosthesis (**Fig. 6**).

Contraindications include:

- General contraindications to implant surgery
- Radiation to the head and neck region of more than 70 Gy
- Immunosuppressed or immunocompromised patients
- Intravenous amino-bisphosphonates use
- Untreated periodontal disease
- Poor oral hygiene and motivation
- Uncontrolled diabetes
- Pregnant or lactating women
- Addiction to alcohol or drugs
- Restricted mouth opening (<3 cm interarch measured anteriorly)
- Acute or chronic infection/inflammation in the area intended for implant placement
- Acute maxillary sinusitis
- Chronic maxillary sinusitis with obstruction of the osteomeatal complex
- Abnormalities in the malar bone

Pre-operative planning should include prosthetic work-up of the patient as per conventional full-mouth rehabilitation protocols.

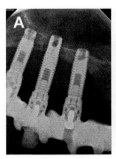
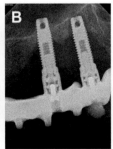
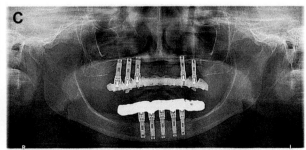

Fig. 4. (*A–C*) Bone loss around implants placed in grafted maxilla using iliac crest; 8 years prior.

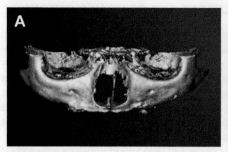
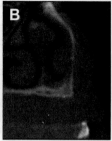
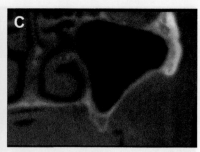

Fig. 5. (*A*) 3-dimensional reconstructed view of maxilla. (*B*) anterior area. (*C*) posterior area.

Factors to consider include:

- Vertical dimension
- Occlusion
- Smile line
- Smile curvature
- Teeth position
- Size of teeth
- Buccal corridors
- Opposing dentition
- Parafunctional habits
- Skeletal jaw relationship

In addition, other key factors must be considered such as the restoration of masticatory function, phonation, and aesthetics—all the criteria that traditionally ensure quality of any complete prosthesis.[11] Pre-operative prosthetic treatment planning is critical for success.

The quad zygoma procedure is a prosthetically driven technique in which the patient must undergo complete prosthetic preparation before implant placement. Once the provisional prosthesis has been made, a surgical guide with palatal support is prepared based on the assembly of the teeth and then used for implant placement. This is fabricated in transparent acrylic resin. It will also be used post-operatively to register implant positions for fabricating the definitive prosthesis in the laboratory.[12]

Radiographic Analysis

Plain film radiography in the form of a panoramic radiograph is suitable as a preliminary film only. Appropriate radiographic analysis and planning can only be done using a computed tomography (CT) scan.

Various implant planning software is available to enable 3-dimensional reconstruction of the atrophic maxilla and enable virtual implant placement. This facilitates determination of the implant lengths and appropriate positioning at the level of the alveolar process and the zygoma (**Fig. 7**). Using cone beam CT (CBCT), the anatomy of the zygomatic processes should be analyzed as well as the position, volume, and amount of the residual alveolar ridge, the health of the maxillary sinus, and patency of the osteomeatal complex bilaterally.

Surgical technique

The surgical technique has been described by several authors.[3,13,14] Intravenous sedation or general anesthesia is typically used with intraoral infiltrative local anesthesia in the surgical area facilitating hemostasis and reducing the amount of analgesia required. Pre-operative antibiotics are prescribed. The patient is prepared and draped such that a sterile field is present and the infraorbital rim, lateral orbital rim, and body of the zygoma can be palpated by the surgeon during the procedure.

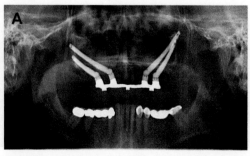
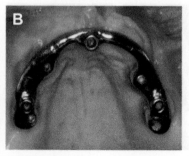

Fig. 6. (*A*) Quad zygoma supporting a bar for an overdenture. (*B*) Prosthetic bar.

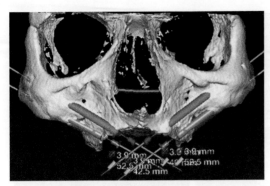

Fig. 7. Virtual planning of implants.

A full-thickness palatal-crestal incision is made on the alveolar ridge from first molar to first molar. The palatal incision design is to ensure that a good width of keratinized tissue surrounds the implants labially/buccally. Distal vertical releasing incisions are made bilaterally to enable good visualization of the surgical field by raising a mucoperiosteal flap. Subperiosteal dissection is also carried out superiorly following the path of the zygomatic buttress to the frontozygomatic notch. It is important to visualize several anatomic structures:

- The maxilla from the piriform apertures up to and including the zygomatic buttress
- The infraorbital foramen
- The malar bone
- The palate adjacent to the incision

Care must be taken to identify, preserve, and protect the infraorbital neurovascular bundle. Once the dissection is completed, an oblique osteotomy is made measuring approximately 0.5 × 1.5 to 2 cm in the lateral wall of the maxilla adjacent to the sinus. The Schneiderian membrane is dissected off the lateral wall of the sinus and the internal cortex of the zygomatic bone. This allows for visual and/or tactile access to the internal cortex of the zygoma. This window can be made using the surgeon's instrumentation typically used to perform a direct sinus lift.

Once the surgical field is appropriately exposed, a retractor is placed in the frontozygomatic notch to allow for good visualization of the malar bone during osteotomy preparation. This also enables the surgeon to appreciate the path of the osteotomy preparation.

Positioning of the implants takes into account the anatomy of the body of the zygoma and the maxilla. The goal is to place 2 zygoma implants into a finite space with appropriate prosthetic emergence and as midcrestal as possible. This is both a conceptual and digital exercise for the surgeon. In a cadaver study assessing the accuracy of drilling guides, it was demonstrated that 2 implants can indeed be placed at the level of the zygoma bone in the vast majority of cases given the height and width measurements of a typical malar bone.[15]

The anterior implants are placed first with emergence at the level of the canines or lateral incisors. Posterior implants emerge in the molar or premolar areas. The implants must be evenly distributed in the zygomatic bone and, ideally, be positioned so that they are spacially separated. The drilling sequence corresponds to the manufacturer's recommendations progressively increasing the diameter of the drills to avoid overheating the bone and to facilitate insertion of the implant. Drilling begins with a 2.9 mm round drill and continues with a 2.9 mm twist drill. Depending on the implant system one uses, the osteotomy may be widened with a final 3.5 mm diameter twist drill. Abundant irrigation is crucial at the crest but also equally important at the apex in the malar bone to avoid overheating. While drilling the osteotomy, palpating the malar bone extraorally is prudent. In preparing the osteotomy sites, the clinician must bear in mind the desire for immediate loading (as per the prosthetic plan) and ensure appropriate anchorage for this.

After implant insertion, abutments are placed (multi-unit or angulated as required) to support the prosthetic rehabilitation. The flap is co-apted ensuring an excellent collar of keratinized tissue around the implants (**Fig. 8**).

Prosthetic Phase

During the prosthetic phase, it is preferable for the patient to be fully conscious, whereby impressions are taken only a few hours after surgery. Impressions can also be taken while the patient is still unconscious (under intravenous sedation or general anesthesia), but this will be more difficult.

Following abutment placement, impression copings are attached to the implant abutments and the transparent surgical guide is used for impression transfer, placing and joining implants by means of general purpose acrylic resin. The same guide is used to register the patient's occlusion and jaw relationship. Once the occlusion has been registered and the guide secured, the space between the impression copings and the surgical guide is filled with fluid silicone. As soon as the material has hardened, the copings are removed in conjunction with the guide and the transepithelial abutments are covered with protective caps. The provisional prosthesis is fabricated in the conventional manner casting a

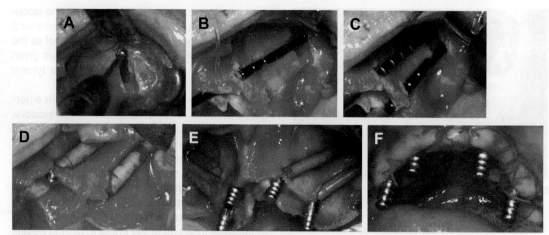

Fig. 8. (*A*) Window between the lateral wall of the maxilla and zygoma bone. (*B*) Preparation for the anterior implant. (C) Preparation for the posterior implant. (*D*) Two implants in place. (*E*) Impression copings in place on all 4 implants. (*F*) Site sutured and ready for fabrication of provisional.

model and connecting laboratory analogues (**Fig. 9**). If the patient already has a conventional denture that fulfills all the prosthetic requirements, this may be used as a guide for the surgical template and also be used in the conversion process to an all-acrylic bridge for immediate loading. Two or three of the impression copings are picked up in the mouth (**Fig. 10**). An impression is then made using an impression tray. The last implants are picked up on the model and the intaglio surface is filled in.

Six months after surgery, implant integration is verified and the soft tissues are assessed prior to fabricating the definitive prosthesis[3,16] (**Fig. 11**).

Surgical Techniques for Zygomatic Implant Placement

There is a lack of consensus in the literature as to the ideal surgical technique for the placement of zygomatic implants. All protocols involve similar incisions designed to expose the surgical site. However, the relationship between the portion of the implant not anchored in the zygoma and the sinus membrane, sinus cavity, and lateral

wall of the maxilla vary from one technique to another. Different approaches have evolved and developed in order to minimize potential sinus complications and improve the emergence of the implant at the alveolar crest without compromising the reported high survival rates. When it comes to the quad approach, crestal implant emergence is paramount for designing an appropriate prosthesis.

There are several zygoma implant placement techniques.

The classic Branemark approach

The implant passes through the maxillary sinus and the prosthetic platform is on the palatal crest of the alveolus.[16] The lateral antrostomy window perforates through the sinus permitting direct visibility of the roof of the sinus. The Schneiderian membrane is reflected classically.

Sinus slot approach

The slot made through the zygomatic buttress and the implant follows the path of the slot with minimal invasion into the sinus.[14] This is a more crestal position of the prosthetic platform.

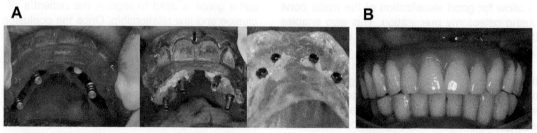

Fig. 9. (*A*) Taking impressions by using the surgical guide. (*B*) Provisional prosthesis.

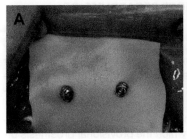 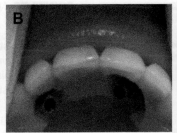 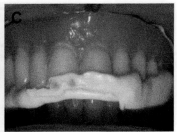

Fig. 10. (A) Beginning process of picking up (luting anterior 2 copings to the denture); temporary copings in place and rubber dam placed to prevent material flow into fresh wound. (B) Ensure no interferences. (C) Patient occluding while acrylic hardening.

Classic exteriorized approach

This approach was first introduced by Miglioranca and colleagues in 2006.[17] A spherical drill is used for the osteotomy penetrating the residual ridge near to the top of the crest from palatal to buccal. The ridge is then transfixed with the drill emerging in the buccal aspect of the ridge external to the sinus. A maxillary antrostomy is not necessary. Drilling continues along the outer aspect of the lateral wall of the sinus until reaching the lateral portion of the zygomatic bone, which is perforated, surpassing the bone's outer cancellous layer. Implants are placed outside the sinus (Fig. 12).

Extramaxillary approach

In 2008, Maló and colleagues modified the exteriorized approach and used an implant without threads on the coronal two-thirds of the implant.[18,19] The maxilla is prepared to allow burs direct access to the zygoma's inferior edge. The maxilla is not used for implant anchorage. The implant is anchored exclusively in the zygomatic bone which is the main conceptual difference between this approach and the others.

Extended sinus lift

Chow and colleagues (2010) proposed an approach to eliminate the risk of maxillary sinusitis. An extended sinus lift[20] (Fig. 13) is performed with a retained bone window. The aim is to keep the sinus membrane intact during zygomatic implant osteotomy preparation.

This procedure has potential advantages:

- Eliminates the risk of maxillary sinusitis
- Increases zygomatic implant stability by promoting bone formation adjacent to the elevated maxillary sinus membrane.

Zygoma Anatomy Guided Approach

In 2011, Aparicio[21] developed a classification system based on skeletal forms of the zygomatic buttress-alveolar crest complex and possible implant pathways related to these categories (Fig. 14). The zygoma anatomy guided approach, named ZAGA 0 to 4, is useful for classifying zygomatic implant cases in terms of operative planning.

The authors identified basic skeletal forms of the zygomatic buttress-alveolar crest complex and subsequent implant pathways among a sample of 100 patients:

- ZAGA 0 (anterior maxillary wall is flat, maxillary horizontal dimension maintained) 15%, of the patient sample
- ZAGA 1 (slightly concave wall, horizontal dimension maintained) 49%
- ZAGA 2 (concave wall, horizontal dimension maintained) 20.5%
- ZAGA 3 (very concave wall, horizontal dimension maintained) 29%

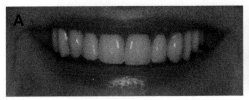 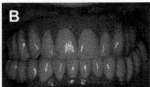 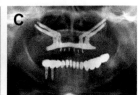

Fig. 11. (A) Smiling; final prosthesis. (B) Occlusion (C) Panoramic radiograph.

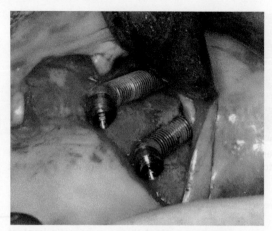

Fig. 12. Implants are exteriorized/extramaxillary.

- ZAGA 4 (extreme vertical and horizontal atrophy, horizontal dimension NOT maintained) 6.5%

Aparicio proposed different implant placement techniques for these 5 anatomic categories. In short, whether the implant runs completely or partially in the sinus, lateral to the sinus, or lateral to the maxilla is entirely dependent on the patient's anatomy. In theory, any of these techniques for placing zygomatic implants may be used in the quad zygoma approach. Typically quad zygoma treatment is reserved for severe maxillary atrophy. These patients often present with ZAGA 3 or ZAGA 4 anatomy. As such, often a significant portion of the implants will be exteriorized or extramaxillary.

POINTS TO NOTE REGARDLESS OF TECHNIQUE

Implants must be well distributed in the maxillary arch to obtain adequate anterior and posterior support. Implants should be positioned on the maxillary crest with stable anchorage in the zygomatic bone.

Quad zygoma represents a cross-arch stabilization system in which the provisional prosthesis offers implant stabilization immediately after surgery. Although insertion torque above 35Ncm for every single implant is always a goal, it is not mandatory.

Given that in many scenarios there is lack of implant integration at the crest, a slight bending (but not rotational) movement can be expected with some implants. This ceases as soon as the prosthesis is connected.

If adequate primary stability is not achieved (rare), the implants are submerged. Under no circumstances should the implants be loaded free standing.

POST-OPERATIVE CARE

Post-operative care is similar to that of any implant surgery. In addition, sinus instructions are given. Analgesics and anti-inflammatories are prescribed, as well as antibiotics for a 1 week course. Post-operative follow-up visits are scheduled 1 and 2 weeks after surgery and then at 2, 3 and 6 months after surgery. After 4 to 6 months of loading, the acrylic resin provisional prosthesis is removed to assess the

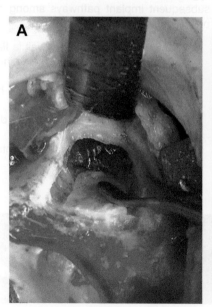
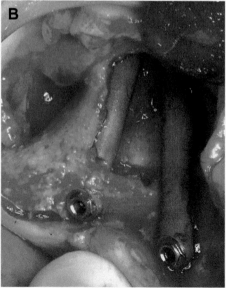

Fig. 13. (A) Extended sinus lift for the placement of 2 zygoma implants. (B) Implants in place.

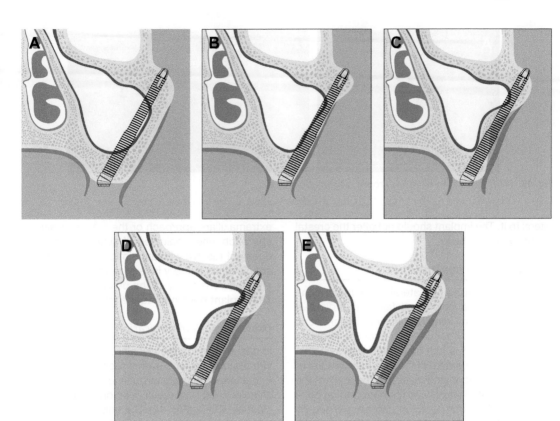

Fig. 14. Zygoma anatomic guided approach. (*A*) ZAGA 0 (*B*) ZAGA 1 (*C*) ZAGA 2 (*D*) ZAGA 3 (*E*) ZAGA 4.

implants and soft tissues prior to fabrication of the definitive prosthesis.

COMPLICATIONS OF ZYGOMATIC IMPLANTS
Penetration into the Orbital Cavity

It is possible to penetrate the orbital cavity especially in zygomatic bones less than 1.8 to 2 cm in height.[3] Damage to the orbital contents and surrounding musculature can ensue. Appropriate training and experience are required to perform zygomatic implants and in particular the quad zygoma technique. Pre-operative planning, adequate exposure, and an in-depth knowledge of the regional anatomy are fundamental to performing this procedure safely. Caution must be taken to avoid inappropriate positioning of the implants; some authors advocate having a 3-dimensional printed model from the patient's CT scan to enable appropriate study of the site as well as planning and rehearsal of the surgery.[22]

Peri-Implant Mucositis, Peri-Implantitis, and Retraction of Buccal/Labial Peri-Implant Tissue

These complications partly depend on the approach selected for implant placement. In a retrospective study, the classic intrasinus approach was compared with ZAGA.[23] Both procedures obtained similar clinical outcomes with respect to implant survival. Nevertheless, the ZAGA concept minimized the risk of maxillary sinus associated pathology and resulted in less bulky, more comfortable, and easier-to-clean prostheses. The relationship between the soft tissues, the bone, and the portion of the implant outside the malar bone remains controversial. Inflammation and tissue retraction can occur around zygomatic implants especially when the implant is placed on the crest without being surrounded by bone (**Fig. 15**). Zygoma implants without threads in the coronal two-thirds of the implant are available for use in these scenarios, with the goal to minimize soft tissue complications. Interestingly, it has been shown that there is normally gingival attachment at this level.[19] Some authors suggest the use of the buccal fat pad[24,25] to thicken the tissues at the crestal implant level to prevent retraction of the tissues in the extramaxillary technique. These reports need to be supported by scientific studies. The surgeon should bear in mind that if the patient's anatomy dictates an exteriorized or extramaxillary approach, it is critical that at the crestal level, the implant is actually embedded in the maxilla rather than lying truly

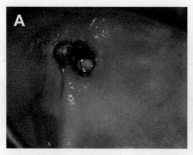
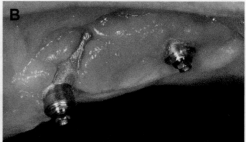

Fig. 15. (*A-B*) Retraction of tissue around zygomatic implant.

lateral to it. The implant should not alter the crestal anatomy and be bulky.

Infection at the Implant Apex

An extraoral swelling just lateral to the malar bone with or without a cutaneous fistula is indicative of an underlying infection in the malar bone (**Fig. 16**). This may occur years after the implants have been placed. It can be treated with systemic antibiotics, debridement of the area (via intraoral or extraoral approach), and resecting the apex of the implant so that it is flush with the surrounding bone as needed. This complication can be avoided by ensuring that the implant length is appropriate; the implant apex should engage the outer zygoma cortex but not extend much beyond it. In addition, lack of contamination and ensuring good irrigation of the area throughout the procedure and specifically prior to closure is important.

Sinusitis

Sinusitis is the most common complication of zygomatic implants historically.

The prevalence of sinus pathology associated with zygomatic implant surgery remains controversial. It would appear that the risk can be reduced by meticulously assessing the status of the sinuses before implant placement, treating any factors that will predispose the patient to sinus pathology, and by using the exteriorized or

extramaxillary approach or the extended sinus lift approach when indicated. If sinusitis occurs that does not resolve with antibiotics, functional endoscopic sinus surgery is required to clear the sinus and ensure patency of the osteomeatal complex. The implant does not require removal.

Oral-Antral Communication

In cases in which the alveolar bone is very thin or virtually nonexistent, even a slight overpreparation of the osteotomy site or bone loss over time at the alveolar crest may result in an oral-antral communication (OAC) (**Fig. 17**). Caution in preparing this area is crucial. Closure of the OAC in these cases are difficult. The use of the buccal fat pad has been reported.[25] A different approach to deal with this complication is the use of bone morphogenic protein.[26] There is no consensus on the best way to manage this negative outcome. Evidence in the literature is required to determine the most predictable method of resolution and prevention.

Paresthesia/Dysesthesia

Patients may experience temporary or permanent altered sensation in the distribution of the infraorbital nerve. Careful identification of this neurovascular bundle, preservation, and protection are crucial to prevent this complication. The zygomaticofacial nerve may also be injured resulting in loss of feeling over the cheek prominence.

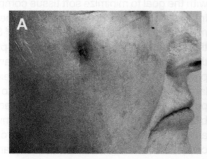
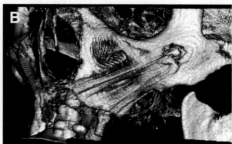

Fig. 16. (*A*) cutaneous fistula. (*B*) Bone loss at apex of zygomatic implant.

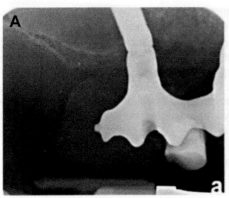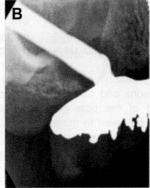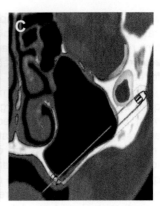

Fig. 17. (A, B) OAC. (C) minimal bone at crest; susceptibility to OAC.

Fracture of the Zygomatic Implant

Fracture of the zygomatic implant is due to inappropriate implant positioning resulting in overloading and biomechanical failure (**Fig. 18**). This is a rare complication.

Prosthetic Complications

These include loosening of the transepithelial abutments, loosening of the prosthesis fixation screws, and fracture of the prosthetic teeth or prosthetic structure.

SCIENTIFIC EVIDENCE FOR THE QUAD ZYGOMA

There is an abundance of literature to date supporting the use and high survival rates of zygomatic implants when combined with anterior implants. The quad zygoma concept came into clinical practice years after the single zygomatic implant (combined with conventional implants) proved itself. The literature in this regard is reflective of this timing. There are only a few studies on the quad zygoma procedure. This is certainly not reflective of the international use of this technique and the frequency of its use. The authors encourage others to report on this implant solution.

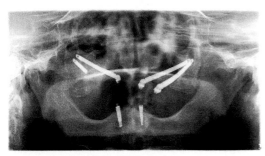

Fig. 18. Fractured zygoma implant.

In 2007, Duarte and colleagues[12] analyzed 12 patients who were treated with 4 zygomatic implants to address severe maxillary atrophy. Immediate loading was performed. Forty-eight zygomatic implants were placed. One implant failed to achieve osseointegration at the 6-month follow-up; integration was maintained for all other implants at 30 months. There were no prosthetic complications.

Stiévenart and Malevez[13] in 2010 reported on a clinical series of 20 patients with extremely resorbed maxillae rehabilitated with 4 zygomatic implants: 10 had 2-stage implant treatment and the remaining 10 had single stage implant treatment. The cumulative survival rate after 40 months was 96%.

In a 5-year prospective study, Davó and Pons[3] obtained high long-term survival rates (implants 98.5% and prosthesis 100%) with few complications. The oral health-related quality of life of these patients was found to be normal even with the passage of time.

A meta-analysis by Wang and colleagues[27] in 2015 revealed that the quad zygoma treatment solution is a reliable technique for maxillary rehabilitation. The zygomatic implant survival rate weighted mean was 96.7%.

A systematic review and meta-analysis by Aboul-Hosn Centenero and colleagues[28] evaluated the survival rates of 2 zygomatic implants combined with regular implants versus 4 zygomatic implants. No statistical differences were seen using 1 treatment over the other in terms of survival and failure rates.

A recent randomized clinical trial compared immediately loaded cross-arch maxillary prostheses supported by zygomatic implants to conventional implants placed in augmented bone. This study revealed that immediately loaded zygomatic implants are associated with significantly fewer prosthetic and implant failures (1 out of 36 patients with zygomatic implants, compared to 6 out of 37 patients with conventional implants) and a shorter time required for functional loading (1.3 days with zygomatic implants, compared with 444.3 days for conventional implants).[9]

All studies report some complications with the quad zygoma technique. Surgeons and patients must be aware and informed of the potential adverse outcomes; steps must be taken to minimize such occurrences. The evidence compiled to date suggests that implants placed in the quad zygoma format may still offer a better rehabilitation modality for the severely atrophic maxilla. Nevertheless, long-term data and more studies are needed to confirm or dispute these preliminary findings. There are no randomized controlled clinical trials comparing surgical techniques for the placement of zygomatic implants. It is the authors' opinion, however, that the prudent approach is one in which the patient's anatomy dictates the surgical technique as per Aparicio and colleagues.

Future developments needed in quad zygoma surgery encompass the ability to accurately transfer virtually planned implant positions clinically. To date, stereolithographic templates, either bone-supported or mucosa-supported, have been used to install zygomatic implants in the designated positions based on computer-assisted planning. However, there is no effective mechanism yet to physically control the drilling trajectory for zygomatic implants and ensure precision of placement. Therefore, deviation between the actual and planned implant position is inevitable. This is clearly less tolerable in circumstances of extreme resorption in which the quad zygoma approach is utilized. The exact position of both implants in the malar bone is critical. A novel device designed to increase the precision of guided surgical placement of zygomatic implants has recently been published.[29] To date, however, given the limited data in the literature, guided zygoma surgery should be considered experimental.

An alternative novel approach to achieving precision with zygoma placement entails surgical navigation. A recently published study examined the use of surgical navigation for zygomatic implant placement in patients with severe maxillary atrophy. The results seem to be promising.[30] More data in this regard will be most interesting.

SUMMARY

The quad zygoma provides a predictable and efficient way to rehabilitate the severely atrophic maxilla. It is an advanced surgical procedure that requires appropriate training, planning, and meticulous surgery. It is not without potential complications. If executed appropriately, however, these can be minimized. Provided that the surgeon has significant clinical experience, the use of 4 zygomatic implants with an immediate loading protocol is typically predictable. It enables implants to be placed in an alternate anchorage site, eliminating the need for more invasive and lengthy surgical reconstruction of the maxilla.

REFERENCES

1. Aparicio C, Manresa C, Francisco K, et al. Zygomatic implants: indications, techniques and outcomes, and the zygomatic success code. Periodontol 2000 2014;66(1):41–58.
2. Araújo MG, Sukekava F, Wennström JL, et al. Ridge alterations following implant placement in fresh extraction sockets: an experimental study in the dog. J Clin Periodontol 2005;32(6):645–52.
3. Davó R, Pons O. 5-year outcome of cross-arch prostheses supported by four immediately loaded zygomatic implants: a prospective case series. Eur J Oral Implantol 2015;8(2):169–74.
4. Aghaloo TL, Mardirosian M, Delgado B. Controversies in implant surgery. Oral Maxillofac Surg Clin North Am 2017;29(4):525–35.
5. Ahlgren F, Størksen K, Tornes K. A study of 25 zygomatic dental implants with 11 to 49 months' follow-up after loading. Int J Oral Maxillofac Implants 2006;21(3):421–5.
6. Becktor JP, Hallström H, Isaksson S, et al. The use of particulate bone grafts from the mandible for maxillary sinus floor augmentation before placement of surface-modified implants: results from bone grafting to delivery of the final fixed prosthesis. J Oral Maxillofac Surg 2008;66(4):780–6.
7. Jensen OT, Adams MW, Butura C, et al. Maxillary V-4: four implant treatment for maxillary atrophy with dental implants fixed apically at the vomer-nasal crest, lateral pyriform rim, and zygoma for immediate function. Report on 44 patients followed from 1 to 3 years. J Prosthet Dent 2015;114(6):810–7.
8. Khoury F, Doliveux R. The bone core technique for the augmentation of limited bony defects: five-year prospective study with a new minimally invasive technique. Int J Periodontics Restorative Dent 2018;38(2):199–207.
9. Davó R, Felice P, Pistilli R, et al. Immediately loaded zygomatic implants vs conventional dental implants in augmented atrophic maxillae: 1-year post-loading results from a multicentre randomised controlled trial. Eur J Oral Implantol 2018;11(2):145–61.
10. Davó R, Malevez C, Rojas J, et al. Clinical outcome of 42 patients treated with 81 immediately loaded zygomatic implants: a 12- to 42-month retrospective study. Eur J Oral Implantol 2008;9(2):141–50.

11. Kim HC, Paek J. Customized Locator abutment fabrication on inclined implants: a clinical report. J Prosthet Dent 2018;119(4):522–5.

12. Duarte LR, Filho HN, Francischone CE, et al. The establishment of a protocol for the total rehabilitation of atrophic maxillae employing four zygomatic fixtures in an immediate loading system–a 30-month clinical and radiographic follow-up. Clin Implant Dent Relat Res 2007;9(4):186–96.

13. Stiévenart M, Malevez C. Rehabilitation of totally atrophied maxilla by means of four zygomatic implants and fixed prosthesis: a 6-40-month follow-up. Int J Oral Maxillofac Surg 2010;39(4):358–63.

14. Stella JP, Warner MR. Sinus slot technique for simplification and improved orientation of zygomaticus dental implants: a technical note. Int J Oral Maxillofac Implants 2000;15:889–93.

15. Van Steenberghe D, Malevez C, Van Cleynenbreugel J, et al. Accuracy of drilling guides for transfer from three-dimensional CT-based planning to placement of zygoma implants in human cadavers. Clin Oral Implants Res 2003;14:131–6.

16. Branemark PI, Grondahl K, OhrnellL O, et al. Zygoma fixture in the management of advanced atrophy of the maxilla: technique and long-term results. Scand J Plast Reconstr Surg Hand Surg 2004;38:70–85.

17. Migliorança RM, Coppedê A, Dias Rezende RC, et al. Restoration of the edentulous maxilla using extrasinus zygomatic implants combined with anterior conventional implants: a retrospective study. Int J Oral Maxillofac Implants 2011;26(3):665–72.

18. Maló P, de Araújo Nobre M, Lopes A, et al. Extramaxillary surgical technique: clinical outcome of 352 patients rehabilitated with 747 zygomatic implants with a follow-up between 6 months and 7 years. Clin Implant Dent Relat Res 2015;17:153–62.

19. Maló P, Nobre Mde A, Lopes I. A new approach to rehabilitate the severely atrophic maxilla using extramaxillary anchored implants in immediate function: a pilot study. J Prosthet Dent 2008;100(5):354–66.

20. Chow J, Wat P, Hui E, et al. A new method to eliminate the risk of maxillary sinusitis with zygomatic implants. Int J Oral Maxillofac Implants 2010;25(6):1233–40.

21. Aparicio C. A proposed classification for zygomatic implant patient based on the zygoma anatomy guided approach (ZAGA): a cross-sectional survey. Eur J Oral Implantol 2011;4(3):269–75.

22. Dawood A, Kalavresos N. Management of extraoral complications in a patient treated with four zygomatic implants. Int J Oral Maxillofac Implants 2017;32(4):893–6.

23. Aparicio C, Manresa C, Francisco K, et al. Zygomatic implants placed using the zygomatic anatomy-guided approach versus the classical technique: a proposed system to report rhinosinusitis diagnosis. Clin Implant Dent Relat Res 2014;16(5):627–42.

24. Guennal P, Guiol J. Use of buccal fat pads to prevent vestibular gingival recession of zygomatic implants. J Stomatol Oral Maxillofac Surg 2018;119(2):161–3.

25. de Moraes EJ. The buccal fat pad flap: an option to prevent and treat complications regarding complex zygomatic implant surgery. Preliminary report. Int J Oral Maxillofac Implants 2012;27(4):905–10.

26. Jensen OT, Adams M, Cottam JR, et al. Occult peri-implant oroantral fistulae: posterior maxillary peri-implantitis/sinusitis of zygomatic or dental implant origin. Treatment and prevention with bone morphogenetic protein-2/absorbable collagen sponge sinus grafting. Int J Oral Maxillofac Implants 2013;28(6):e512–20.

27. Wang F, Monje A, Lin G, et al. Reliability of four zygomatic implant-supported prostheses for the rehabilitation of the atrophic maxilla: a systematic review. Int J Oral Maxillofac Implants 2015;30(2):293–8.

28. Aboul-Hosn Centenero S, Lázaro A, Giralt-Hernando M, et al. Zygoma quad compared with 2 zygomatic implants: a systematic review and meta-analysis. Implant Dent 2018. https://doi.org/10.1097/ID.0000000000000726.

29. Chow J. A novel device for template-guided surgery of the zygomatic implants. Int J Oral Maxillofac Surg 2016;45(10):1253–5.

30. Wang F, Bornstein MM, Hung K, et al. Application of real-time surgical navigation for zygomatic implant insertion in patients with severely atrophic maxilla. J Oral Maxillofac Surg 2018;76(1):80–7.

Managing the Posterior Maxilla with Implants Using Bone Grafting to Enhance Implant Sites

Peter E. Larsen, DDS[a],*, Kelly S. Kennedy, DDS, MS[b]

KEYWORDS

- Posterior maxilla • Implant placement • Onlay grafting

KEY POINTS

- There are some advantages to implant placement in the posterior maxilla, such as better phonetics, esthetics and hygiene, and biomechanical load distribution.
- There are limitations to implant placement in the maxilla resulting from ridge resorption and sinus pneumatization. Grafting the posterior maxilla can improve implant support.
- Traditional sinus floor augmentation (sinus lift) can be accomplished with direct or indirect approaches and constitute the mainstay for improving implant support in the posterior maxilla, particularly in the partially edentulous patient in whom there are teeth adjacent to the implant site.
- Less traditional grafting modalities such as simultaneous sinus floor grafting with concomitant LeFort 1 osteotomy or sinus floor augmentation along with onlay grafting may be necessary in more complex situations with greater osseous compromise.

INTRODUCTION

Since the introduction of dental implant therapy, the posterior maxilla has been a challenging site for implant placement. The quality of bone in the posterior maxilla is often not as good as other regions of the oral cavity. The mechanical forces created by occlusal function are greater in the posterior of either jaw. Finally, even in dentate patients, the sinus cavity can encroach on the alveolus, resulting in a significant lack of vertical bone height, even if implants are placed relatively soon following loss of a tooth. In addition, long-standing edentulism or traumatic extraction can further complicate the bony support by compromising the buccal-palatal dimension of bone.

Several strategies exist to address concerns raised above. They can be categorized as follows:

1. Altering the dimension of the implants being placed. This is primarily accomplished by placing shorter or narrower implants.
2. Altering the location of the implants. This includes maxillary tuberosity implants, zygomaticus implants, and, more recently, angling the posterior implant to maintain the posterior position of the platform while avoiding the sinus (the "all on four" technique).

Disclosure Statement: The authors have nothing to disclose.

[a] Division of Oral and Maxillofacial Surgery and Dental Anesthesiology, The Ohio State University College of Dentistry, Room 2131, Postle Hall, 305 West 12th Avenue, Columbus, OH 43210, USA; [b] Oral and Maxillofacial Surgery Residency Program, Division of Oral and Maxillofacial Surgery and Dental Anesthesiology, The Ohio State University College of Dentistry, Room 2131, Postle Hall, 305 West 12th Avenue, Columbus, OH 43210, USA
* Corresponding author.
E-mail address: larsen.5@osu.edu

Oral Maxillofacial Surg Clin N Am 31 (2019) 299–308
https://doi.org/10.1016/j.coms.2019.01.002
1042-3699/19/© 2019 Elsevier Inc. All rights reserved.

3. Grafting the maxilla to restore the bone to allow more traditional implant size/location.

There are indications for each of these techniques, and all have met with some success when applied appropriately. Perhaps some of the mainstream acceptance of various approaches is regional and is, of course, also driven by the expectations and preference of the restorative dentist. The purpose of this article is not to attempt to delineate all of the possible advantages/disadvantages and indications of each of these possible approaches. There are clear advantages and limitations of each approach (**Table 1**). Rather, the assumption will be made that a decision has already been made to use implants placed in the posterior maxilla. This is not to say that, in some of the example cases, other techniques could not have been used to either avoid the sinus or use implants with varying dimensions to also solve the treatment dilemma presented.

INDICATIONS FOR POSTERIOR MAXILLARY GRAFTING

Loss of 1 or 2 teeth with a short edentulous span, particularly if there is no distal tooth, thus ruling out a conventional prosthodontic solution, is an ideal situation for limited grafting of the posterior

maxilla. This may entail a localized sinus floor elevation and/or onlay grafting depending on the nature of the defect.

Large posterior edentulous defects where the plan is to maintain anterior teeth (canine to canine) and might benefit from grafting the sinus if there is inadequate vertical bone height. The presence of anterior dentition precludes the additional stability afforded by anterior implants, which is important to both the zygomaticus and "all on four" techniques.

Completely edentulous maxilla where both pneumatized sinuses and anterior bony atrophy are present may be best managed with sinus floor elevation and grafting. The zygomatic and "all on four" techniques require anterior implants. If the anterior maxillary atrophy is such that onlay grafting will be required, an approach which focuses on posterior implant restoration, avoiding anterior implants, has some advantages. Block grafting of the anterior maxilla may be less predictable and more costly than sinus floor augmentation. Allogeneic block grafts are more costly than particulate bone and require skeletal fixation with screws or plates. The overlying prosthesis must be worn with extreme caution or not at all. There are esthetic, phonetic, and hygiene considerations that are at times competitive. A smile line that exposes the implant/prosthesis interface must be managed esthetically, often leading to a "ridge

---

Table 1
Strategies for addressing bone loss in the posterior maxilla

Technique	Advantages	Limitations
Shorter or narrower implants	• No grafting needed • Shorter time to restoration • Less cost	• Cannot address extreme dimensional problems • Crown-to-root ratio compromised • Biomechanical limitations possible • Prosthodontic challenge if significant deviation from ideal platform dimension
Altered implant position	• No grafting needed in posterior maxilla • Shorter time to restoration	• These approaches are primarily for full arch restoration and do not lend themselves to single teeth or localized defects • Technique sensitive or require special training (zygomaticus) • Require anterior implants, which could include the need for grafting in that area • Implant support is concentrated in the anterior maxilla, which can create a hygiene or phonetic problem
Posterior grafting	• Applicable to full arch as well as localized defects, because once bone is restored, traditional implant techniques are used • Biomechanical advantage of placing implants more posterior in the fully edentulous case	• Requires additional time for grafting particularly if implants cannot be placed simultaneously • Additional cost • Risk of grafting in the maxillary sinus

lap" of the prosthesis, which if present in the region of the implant, can compromise hygiene. If esthetics are not of concern, and enough space is maintained in the anterior for hygiene around the implants, then a phonetic problem may result. By placing the implants in the posterior maxilla, adequate space can be allowed for hygiene. The prosthesis can be extended more facially and apically in the anterior for better esthetics and phonetics without implant compromise. The resulting anterior cantilever is biomechanically more favorable than a posterior cantilever (**Fig. 1**). This technique relies on robust posterior maxillary bone to support at least 2 implants on each side. Sinus floor elevation and grafting is often required in such cases.

Completely edentulous maxilla with both bony deficiency in all dimensions including pneumatized sinuses, and facial/palatal resorption or bone loss of the anterior and posterior maxilla is a complex problem. These defects may be the result of long-standing acquired edentulism, hereditary oligodontia, tumor ablation, or trauma. They may require sinus floor augmentation grafting, onlay grafting, and even osteotomy techniques.

PROCEDURES WITH ILLUSTRATIVE CASES

Pneumatized maxillary sinuses and/or unfavorable alveolar remodeling after tooth extraction may lead to reduced vertical bony dimensions in the posterior maxilla. This may preclude the placement of implants of traditional size, 10 mm or longer, required to support masticatory forces. As vertical augmentation of the alveolar ridge with onlay techniques has a guarded prognosis,

the workhorse procedure for increasing the vertical dimension of bone in the posterior maxilla is grafting of the sinus floor either by indirect (vertical) or direct (lateral) means. Augmenting the sinus floor has the benefits of a well-vascularized and protected environment, affording the surgeon a myriad of choices for grafting materials (autogenous, allogeneic, alloplastic). As with any grafting, considerations in choosing a graft material include the size of the defect, functional expectations of the grafted site, osteogenic capacity of the patient, and cost-benefit ratio.

Traditional Indirect Sinus Graft

The indirect, also referred to as vertical, approach is typically reserved for single edentulous sites in which 2–3 mm of bony augmentation is required for placement of an implant of traditional size. The sinus floor elevation and augmentation are both performed via the implant osteotomy followed by placement of the implant.

In an illustrative case, a 25-year-old healthy man presented for implant restoration of tooth no. 4 that was lost secondary to a vertical fracture. The patient's panoramic radiograph (**Fig. 2**A), displayed approximately 7 mm in the bony vertical dimension at the edentulous site. An implant 10 mm in length is ideal for this site with protected occlusion, and therefore an indirect sinus lift of 3 mm was required. Clinically, the initial drill was used to prepare the osteotomy to a depth at which the sinus floor was encountered (**Fig. 2**B); this depth was found to match the radiograph at approximately 7 mm. The osteotomy was widened with drills of progressive size to the final diameter. An osteotome was inserted into the osteotomy and the sinus floor was in-fractured approximately

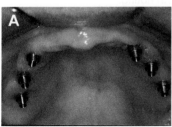
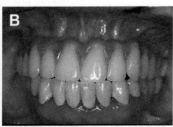
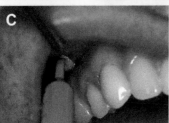

Fig. 1. (*A*) Posterior implants placed 25 years previously into bilaterally grafted sinuses. (*B*) Anterior incisor position is determined by lip position and phonetics without concern for hygiene access or implant position. (*C*) Posteriorly, the access for hygiene is maintained in an area where phonetics and esthetics are not compromised.

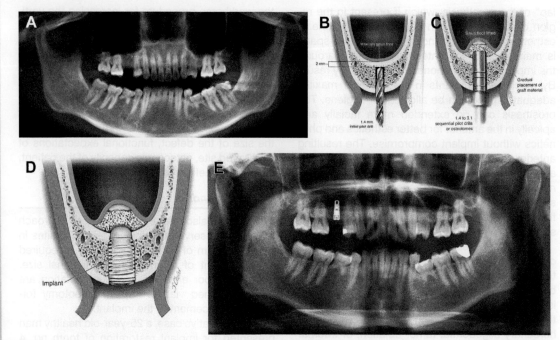

Fig. 2. (*A*) Non-calibrated panoramic radiograph demonstrating approximately 7 mm of bone available below the maxillary sinus. (*B*) Coronal cross-section through the maxillary sinus; pilot drill stopped at the sinus floor. (*C*) The final osteotome is used to tap the sinus floor up along with graft placement. (*D*) The implant is placed helping to tent the sinus membrane superiorly. (*E*) Immediate post-operative panoramic radiograph taken after indirect sinus lift and implant placement. The film demonstrates a 10-mm implant with the elevated sinus floor following the implant apex. (*From [B–E]* Louis PJ. The maxillary sinus lift. In: Kademani D, Tiwana P, editors. Atlas of oral & maxillofacial surgery. St Louis (MO): Elsevier; 2016; with permission.)

3 mm. A small amount of allograft was inserted into the apical portion of the osteotomy and the implant was placed (**Fig. 2**C, D) The post-operative panoramic radiograph (**Fig. 2**E) demonstrates the elevated cortical lining of the right maxillary sinus following the apical contour of the implant.

Lateral Approach Sinus Floor Graft

The direct, or lateral, approach is indicated when multiple implants are being placed into a region that requires augmentation greater than 3 mm.

The sinus floor to be augmented is accessed by surgically creating a window in the maxillary bone just lateral to the site (**Fig. 3**A). The sinus membrane is elevated with the use of curettes to create a space that coordinates with the size of the area to be augmented. The graft material is placed into the space created under the membrane (**Fig. 3**B). Several clinical variations of this technique are worth noting.

Simultaneously with tooth extraction

A 55-year-old healthy woman presented for evaluation of non-restorable tooth no. 3 with

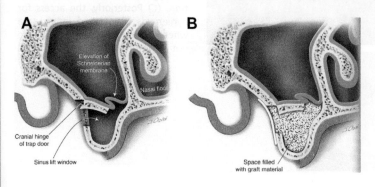

Fig. 3. (*A*) A coronal cross-section through the maxillary sinus; lateral maxillary sinus lift, showing a crestal incision and lateral osteotomy; in-fracture of the lateral sinus window with sinus membrane elevation. (*B*) Particulate bone graft in place.

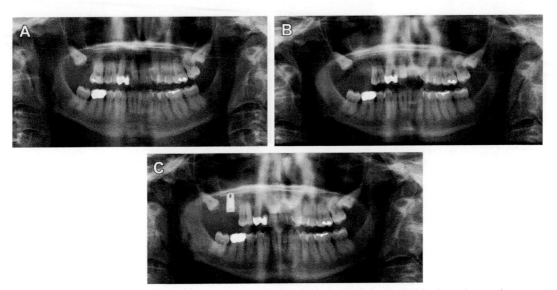

Fig. 4. (*A*) Evaluation of future implant site no. 3 demonstrates significant distal alveolar bone loss and pneumatization of the maxillary sinus. This combination will yield very little alveolar bone after extraction. Also, the roots of no. 3 do not appear to perforate the sinus floor. (*B*) Radiograph 5 months status post-extraction of no. 3 with socket preservation and direct sinus augmentation demonstrating ample vertical bone for implant placement. (*C*) 13 mm implant in place.

concomitant distal bone loss (**Fig. 4**A). The patient desired an implant restoration. Even with good results from a socket preservation graft, it was likely that, because a combination of bone loss and a low sinus floor, there would not be enough vertical bone for successful long-term implant restoration. Therefore, a direct sinus augmentation with an allograft was performed at the time of extraction of tooth no. 3 (**Fig. 4**B). The site was allowed to heal for 5 months and then re-entered to place a 6 × 13-mm implant (**Fig. 4**C).

Simultaneously with implant placement
A healthy 32-year-old woman presented for implant evaluation of edentulous site no. 3. The calibrated panoramic radiograph demonstrated approximately 5 mm of residual alveolar height. Although this is not enough bone and the sinus would need augmentation, 4 mm of bone is generally accepted as suitable

for primary stability of the implant and simultaneous direct augmentation. In this case the direct access to the sinus floor and membrane elevation was completed first. Then, with the membrane elevated, the implant osteotomy was prepared to final dimensions. Before placing the implant, an allograft was placed in the medial recess of the area under the elevated membrane. Then the implant was fully seated and the allograft was placed on the remaining exposed surfaces of the implant under the membrane. The post-operative radiograph demonstrates the implant and sinus augmentation (**Fig. 5**).

Staged before implant placement
In cases where the need for a direct sinus augmentation is obvious but there is not enough residual alveolar bone for simultaneous implant placement, a staged-surgical approach is required. The next case is that of a 57-year-old woman who required

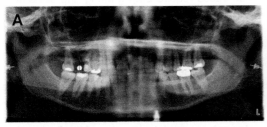
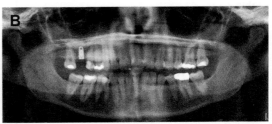

Fig. 5. (*A*) Calibrated panoramic radiograph demonstrating approximately 5 mm of bone below the sinus at edentulous site no. 3, (*B*) Post-operative radiograph demonstrating an 11.5-mm implant and direct sinus augmentation extending beyond the apex.

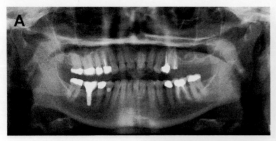
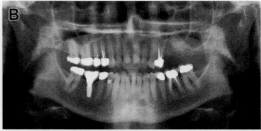
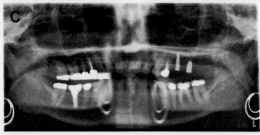

Fig. 6. (*A*) Pre-operative panoramic radiograph demonstrating non-restorable tooth no. 13 and severely pneumatized left maxillary sinus with approximately 2–3 mm of alveolar bone remaining at the proposed site for implant no. 14. (*B*) Radiograph 5 months status post-extraction of no. 13 and direct sinus augmentation of the left maxillary sinus with ample bone for implant placement. (*C*) Direct sinus augmentation yielded enough bone to allow restoring the posterior maxilla with 10- and 13-mm implants.

extraction of tooth no. 13 and implant placement to restore missing teeth nos 13 and 14. She had approximately 3 mm of residual alveolar bone at the site of implant no. 14 (**Fig. 6**A). Extraction of tooth no. 13 and direct sinus augmentation with allograft of the left maxillary sinus was performed (**Fig. 6**B). Implants of adequate length were placed approximately 5 months later (**Fig. 6**C).

A number of options for direct and indirect grafting with or without immediate implant placement have been described. **Table 2** helps identify when these techniques may be most reliably used.

As an alternative, some may choose to place short implants in the posterior maxilla and avoid sinus augmentation altogether. Complications cited with short implants include an increased crown-implant ratio, occlusal overload, and failure in the type IV bone common to the posterior maxilla.[1,2]

Despite these complications, current data on short implants are looking positive,[3] but there are no long-term data or comparative studies that support this technique. This is in contrast to the well-documented long-term success and low morbidity of sinus augmentation and placement of implants of traditional size.[4]

Combined Posterior Maxillary Augmentation with Sinus Grafting and Onlay Grafting for Severe Atrophy

Whether the result of acquired edentulism or hereditary oligodontia/anodontia, osseous defects that result in such cases can be dramatic. In cases where maxillary denture function has been primarily opposing natural teeth, the resulting resorption can be quite severe. Hereditary absence of teeth is often accompanied by concomitant hypoplasia of alveolar bone, resulting in nothing but basal bone. Such cases require both grafting and sinus floor augmentation if implants are to be placed in the posterior maxilla.

In an illustrative case (**Fig. 7**), a 19-year-old man with a medical history that included ectodermal dysplasia presented with long-standing oligodontia and maxillary and mandibular resorption. The cone beam computed tomography revealed substantial vertical and lateral bony deficiency (**Fig. 8**).

In such cases, determination of the final vertical dimension is the critical key first element in all treatment planning decisions. The determination

Table 2 Surgical decision making in sinus floor elevation		
Amount of Residual Alveolar Bone Height (mm)	Approach for Sinus Augmentation	Option to Place Implant Simultaneously
7–8	Indirect	Yes
4–6	Direct	Yes
<4	Direct	No

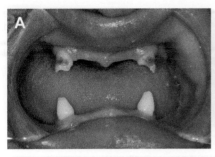
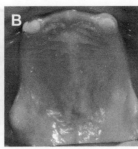

Fig. 7. (*A, B*) Clinical photographs of ectodermal dysplasia patient with oligodontia and severe skeletal hypoplasia.

of the vertical dimension will allow assessment of the anterior/posterior skeletal relationship. Often these patients present with a pseudo-prognathism that resolves when the proper vertical dimension is established. Identification of the proper vertical dimension also allows assessment of the likely post-restorative inter-arch space. This directly impacts the crown-to-root ratio and the biomechanical forces that will be placed on the final prosthesis and implants. This can help with the final design of the prosthesis relative to number and location of implants as well as grafting require-ments. A lateral cephalometric radiograph can be valuable in assessing vertical facial proportions. In this case, the lateral cephalometric film revealed that the patient was over-closed. A provisional removable denture was fabricated in what was determined to be the ideal vertical dimension. This must be assessed for esthetics and function before developing a final plan (**Fig. 9**). Once it is confirmed that the provisional prosthesis is both esthetic and functional, it is used as the guide for future planning.

In this patient's case, the substantial vertical and palatal/facial bony deficiency required both onlay grafting and sinus floor augmentation. Large uni-cortical blocks of iliac crest and cancellous bone were used to graft the lateral aspect of the maxilla along with traditional lateral approach sinus floor augmentation. Some key elements to this approach are outlined in **Table 3**.

Autogenous bone grafting is not required, but has the advantage of providing a large quantity of bone. Allogeneic block grafts could be used as well, but they are supplied in preset sizes that can reduce some flexibility. Allogeneic grafts require a longer period of time for incorporation, and, because of the relatively high proportion admixture of devital bone long term, are prone to micro-damage from use. Autogenous block grafts will heal quite well, but can remodel significantly leading to resorption early, at 3 to 4 months, and sometimes late term after implant placement. So care must be taken to place implants optimally, that is, in a timely fashion in consideration of the stability and integrity of the graft. Following 3 months of healing, the autogenous onlay block grafts and sinus floor augmentation generally re-sults in adequate bone healing for the placement of implants, as shown in **Fig. 10**. In this patient, 6 maxillary implants were placed and a component type prosthesis was used for the final restoration (**Fig. 11**).

Treatment options for this patient may have also included an "all on four" technique or zygomatic implant with anterior implants. His maxillary ante-rior osseous anatomy would have also required grafting of this site.

Posterior Grafting of the Maxillary Sinus in Conjunction with Lefort 1 Osteotomy

As mentioned in the previous section, long-standing edentulism, particularly that which results from congenital absence of teeth, may be accom-panied by severe osseous skeletal hypoplasia. In

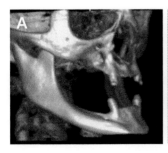
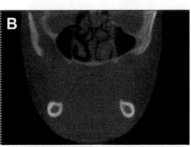

Fig. 8. (*A*) 3D reconstruction showing the large posterior maxil-lary defect, which is also shown in coronal sections (*B*).

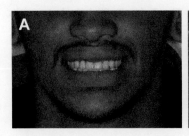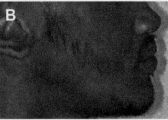

Fig. 9. (*A, B*) When a removable provisional prosthesis was placed at the ideal vertical dimension, good esthetic and functional outcome was obtained.

Table 3
Critical technical elements when performing onlay grafting of the posterior maxilla

Technical Considerations	Rationale
Close adaptation of the block to the recipient bed	Necessary for efficient vascular ingrown and incorporation of the graft
Perforate the cortical bone of the recipient bed using the same drill that will be used to drill the holes for the skeletal fixation	Drilling holes in denser cortical bone improves vascular ingrowth and using the same drill as the skeletal fixation decreases the chances that a screw will inadvertently be placed into a hole that is too large resulting in it being loose
Solid anchorage with 2 or more screws	Movement will inhibit vascular ingrowth
Location and size of bony window for traditional sinus graft	Large windows can interfere with location and stabilization of the onlay graft(s)
Tension free primary closure	Exposure of the graft may compromise successful incorporation or result in resorption
Limited prosthetic wear. If grafting is only on the facial and floor of the sinus, the prosthesis may be modified to remove the labial flange	Pressure from function can result in graft exposure or mobility

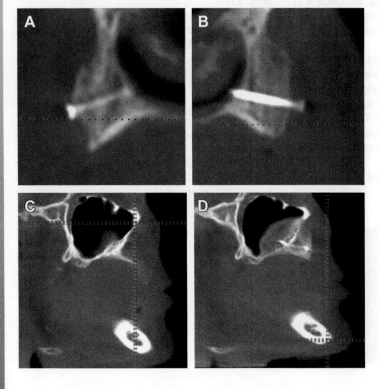

Fig. 10. (*A, B*) Large block grafts from the iliac crest were used to augment the lateral aspect of the maxilla bilaterally. Simultaneously, sinus floor elevation was used to augment the vertical height of the posterior maxilla. (*C*) The pre-grafting sagittal view of the right maxillary sinus and (*D*) the results of the sinus grafting.

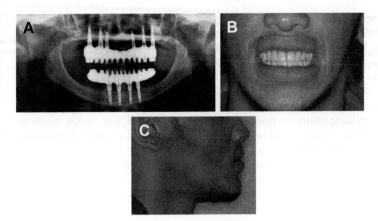

Fig. 11. (*A–C*) Clinically the final restoration has adequate bony support for proper esthetics and function while allowing access for hygiene.

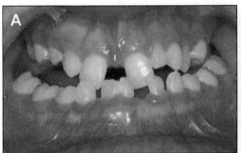
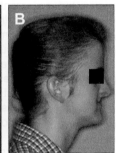

Fig. 12. (*A*) The patient's dentition when opened to the ideal vertical. A significant skeletal malocclusion remains indicating the likely need for a Lefort 1 osteotomy to advance the maxilla in conjunction with her implant restorative process. (*B*) Even when in ideal vertical, there is esthetic compromise owing to the significant maxillary AP hypoplasia.

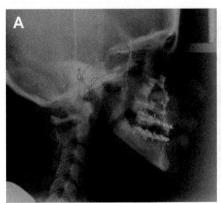
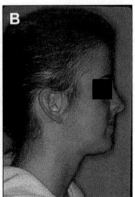

Fig. 13. Following Lefort 1 osteotomy with advancement, the AP relationship is improved relative to the desired osseous position for implants (*A*) and esthetically (*B*).

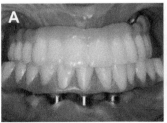
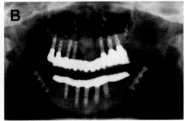

Fig. 14. (*A*) The post-treatment restoration with maxillary and mandibular hybrid type prosthesis. Posterior maxillary implants were placed into the grafts that were done at the time of the Lefort 1. (*B*) A panoramic of the patient's implants at 10-year follow-up. There is no bone loss or evidence of soft tissue defect around any of the maxillary implants.

many cases, the patient has the appearance of maxillary deficiency (pseudo-prognathism), which resolves with establishment of the ideal vertical dimension. In other cases, however, there is true maxillary deficiency. These patients may benefit from advancement of the maxilla via traditional Lefort 1. Some modification of the technique might be required in patients with multiple missing teeth to allow ideal positioning of the maxilla during surgery. Complete description of these techniques is beyond the scope of this article. However, if the maxillary skeletal anteroposterior (AP) deficiency requires a Lefort 1, consideration should be given to immediately augmenting the maxillary sinus if there is pneumatization of the sinus in an area that will subsequently require implant placement.

Previous authors[5,6] have described simultaneous grafting of the edentulous maxilla with a block of bone to facilitate implant placement. Traditional Lefort 1 surgery, when the positioning of the maxilla involves significant anterior or vertical movement, has used block grafting for improved stability. When the maxilla is repositioned anteriorly with a Lefort 1, the floor of the maxillary sinus can be grafted with cancellous bone. Other grafting options such as allogeneic bone or bone morphogenic protein, have not been used in this setting and it is unclear if they would be successful. In a representative case, an 18-year-old woman with oligodontia presented with maxillary AP hypoplasia even after the correct vertical dimension was obtained (**Fig. 12**). A Lefort 1 osteotomy was performed to advance the maxilla based on cone beam computed tomography with a provisional denture placed in the ideal position overlying the maxillary ridge. This allowed for determination of the magnitude of the advancement. Following down-fracture, and before skeletal fixation, the sinus membrane was removed from the inferior aspect of the maxillary sinus bilaterally, and cancellous bone was compressed into the sinus floor to approximately 1 cm. A fibrin glue was used to help consolidate the graft and prevent movement. Skeletal fixation was placed in the normal fashion with the maxilla in the planned post-surgical position. The Lefort 1 osteotomy created an improved skeletal relationship (**Fig. 13**) and improved bony support for implants. The non-restorable teeth were removed and implants were subsequently placed and restored (**Fig. 14**).

Advantages of this technique are that grafting can be accomplished at the same time as the Lefort surgery, allowing the procedure to be accomplished in a sterile OR setting, which aids in the use of autogenous bone. The direct visualization of the sinus for grafting allows efficient placement of the graft with more consistent density. Generally, this is reserved only for severe atrophy, and simultaneous implants would not be possible. However, even if the native bone is adequate for simultaneous implant placement, the unpredictable resorption of the graft and the possibility of vascular compromise due to the Lefort surgery would make simultaneous placement less predictable.

SUMMARY

There are clinical situations in which implant placement in the posterior maxilla is either required or desirable. The posterior maxilla poses challenges to implant placement because of frequent sinus pneumatization, poor quality of bone, and increased biomechanical forces. This article compares some of the advantages of grafting in the posterior maxilla when a variety of clinical conditions present. Advantages and limitations of various approaches have been reviewed.

REFERENCES

1. Thoma DS, Cha MK, Jung UW. Treatment concepts for the posterior maxilla and mandible: short implants versus long implants in augmented bone. J Periodontal Implant Sci 2017;47:2–12.
2. Telleman G, Raghoebar GM, Vissink A, et al. A systematic review of the prognosis of short (<10mm) dental implants placed in the partially edentulous patient. J Clin Periodontol 2011;38:667–76.
3. Bechara S, Kubilius R, Veronesi G, et al. Short (6mm) dental implants versus sinus floor elevation and placement of longer (>10mm) dental implants: a randomized controlled trial with a 3-year follow-up. Clin Oral Implants Res 2017;28(9):1097–107.
4. Aghaloo TL, Moy PK. Which hard tissue augmentation techniques are the most successful in furnishing bony support for implant placement? Int J Oral Maxillofac Implants 2007;22(Suppl):49–70.
5. Muñoz-Guerra MF, Naval-Gías L, Capote-Moreno A. Lefort 1 and simultaneous block graft for implants. J Oral Maxillofac Surg 2009;67(3):613–8.
6. Jensen OT, Ringeman JL, Cottam JR, et al. Orthognathic and osteoperiosteal flap augmentation strategies for maxillary dental implant reconstruction. Oral Maxillofacial Surg Clin N Am 2011;23:301–19.

Titanium Mesh Grafting Combined with Recombinant Human Bone Morphogenetic Protein 2 for Alveolar Reconstruction

Alan S. Herford, DDS, MD*, Isaac Lowe, MPH, DDS,
Paul Jung, DDS

KEYWORDS

- Titanium mesh • Membrane • Guided bone regeneration • Bone morphogenic protein
- Dental implant • Preprosthetic augmentation

KEY POINTS

- Guided bone regeneration (GBR) is the most common procedure for alveolar ridge augmentation.
- Titanium mesh is highly biocompatible and offers predictable results.
- The most common complication for titanium mesh augmentation is mesh exposure.
- Titanium mesh is compatible with recombinant human bone morphogenetic protein 2 enhancement of bone grafting.

INTRODUCTION

One of the more common oral and maxillofacial surgery procedures is alveolar ridge augmentation to correct for vertical and/or horizontal bone defects in preparation for dental implants, prosthetics, or even for major reconstruction cases.[1] Utilization of a titanium mesh to regenerate these defects in combination with growth factors and resorbable membranes has been successful.

BONE GRAFTING PHYSIOLOGY

Bone grafting procedure success depends on several factors: type of bone grafting materials used, location of the grafting site, patient health and social history, and the physiologic conditions of the grafting site itself. Physiologically, bone grafting success is a function of both graft integration and neovascularization.

For autogenous bone grafting, the incorporation process differs depending on the type of bone graft being placed (cortical vs cancellous bone). These 2 types of bone grafts primarily differ in the rate of both neovascularization and incorporation to the grafting site in that cortical grafts take longer and cancellous bone grafts tend to be more rapid[2] (**Table 1**). This is due to the number of endosteal cells surviving the transplant process, differences in density of the grafts, and the amount of graft necrosis that occurs during the neovascularization process.[2]

Autogenous grafting is beneficial due to the near impossibility of graft rejection. Host grafting tissue provides the benefit of housing natural growth factors and signaling proteins that produce an

Disclosure: The authors have nothing to disclose.
Department of Oral and Maxillofacial Surgery, Loma Linda University School of Dentistry, 11092 Anderson Street, Loma Linda, CA 92350, USA
* Corresponding author. Department of Oral and Maxillofacial Surgery, Loma Linda University School of Dentistry, 11092 Anderson Street, Room 3306, Loma Linda, CA 92350, USA.
E-mail address: aherford@llu.edu

Oral Maxillofacial Surg Clin N Am 31 (2019) 309–315
https://doi.org/10.1016/j.coms.2018.12.007

Table 1
Physiologic differences between cortical and cancellous bone grafts

Cortical Bone Graft	Cancellous Bone Graft
• More dense and requires initial osteoclastic activity necessary before osteoblastic/neovascularization steps • Revascularization starts later (~1 wk) • Revascularization takes longer • More necrotic bone impedes graft incorporation	• More porous, allowing more rapid vascular incorporation • Osteoprogenitor cells more rapidly gain access to graft • More rapid vascular invasion leads to less necrotic bone needing to be replaced

osteogenic effect instead of merely acting as a scaffold for bone infill seen with allografts and xenografts.[2] The demineralization phase, particularly in cortical bone, is necessary before bony incorporation can start, increasing the time it takes for grafts to be fully integrated into the site, which can delay further surgical or restorative treatment.[2] Despite these relative disadvantages, autografting is highly successful and is the current standard for bone grafting procedures.[2]

Grafting with other materials, such as bovine-derived materials or cadaver-derived bone products, benefits from the lack of a secondary surgical site and thus forgoes the associated complications: donor site morbidity, infection, pain, inadequate ambulation, hematoma, and fracture.[3,4] Using nonautogenous materials also has the benefit of not being limited by the amount of grafting material available at donor sites.[3,4] The trade-off for allografting and xenografting, however, is that these materials are not osteoinductive and thus require osteogenic cell recruitment. Nonautogenous grafts have delayed graft material turnover and even when incorporated persist as an admixture of nonvital bone. In addition, the decalcifying phase can be uncoupled, that is, resorptive without replacement of vital bone, leading to a reported greater rate of failure when used to repair larger segmental defects.[3,4]

Growth factors, cytokines, and signaling proteins also play a critical role in bone grafting success. The literature shows that the transforming growth factor ß superfamily, including recombinant human bone morphogenic protein 2 (rhBMP-2), plays an important role in mediating osteogenesis and the bone repair through recruiting and differentiation of osteoblasts as well as osteoclast cells, which start the initial process of bone graft incorporation. Osteogenic cells, extracellular matrix production, alkaline phosphate production, type I collagen deposition, and angiogenesis are all important aspects of the bone healing cascade.[2,5] Although other factors like insulinlike growth factor, platelet-derived growth

factor, and vascular endothelial growth factor also play roles in grafting procedures and osseous repair, overall their roles are less profound.[2,5]

WHY ALVEOLAR RECONSTRUCTION IS IMPORTANT

Tooth loss is the leading cause of alveolar bone loss, which has far-reaching implications.[6] Alveolar reconstruction is merely 1 part in the rehabilitation of most complicated dental cases. Often, alveolar reconstruction is needed to restore vertical and/or horizontal bone dimension to provide more ideal support and retention for dentures and/or implants.[6] Patients that require alveolar reconstruction may also require long-term procedures, such as replacement of teeth through implants and crowns or prosthetics, re-establishing a centric relationship or another occlusal scheme in an unstable environment, and re-establishing vertical dimension of occlusion.[7] Thus, the need for interdisciplinary cooperation and communication is critical in treating these cases to minimize overtreating or undertreating, which serve to complicate cases and may even subject patients to multiple unnecessary procedures. The alveolar reconstruction process can take years but serves to help prevent further bone loss, nutritional deficiencies, reduce the psychological impact of lost teeth, prevent collapse of the vertical dimension of the face, and reduce the risk of jaw fracture.[6]

ALVEOLAR RECONSTRUCTION PROCEDURES

Alveolar ridge augmentation, like other prepros-thetic augmentation procedures, needs to be restorative driven.[6–8] Surgical augmentation needs to restore osseous shape and volume to accommodate the most ideal treatment plan. If well executed surgical procedures are followed, then successful outcomes will ensure the availability of as many restorative treatment options as possible.[6–8]

One of the most common procedures for alveolar ridge augmentation is guided bone regeneration, which can reliably provide 3 mm to 5 mm of bone in the horizontal and vertical dimensions when titanium mesh or nonresorbable membranes are used.[9] Titanium mesh was first documented successfully by Boyne for repair of continuity defects in the mandible.[10] Titanium mesh has been shown to be ideal for this procedure due to its inherent characteristic of acting as a wall or guide for formation of bone. Its biocompatibility prevents host reaction to the barrier function. Mesh maintains space to prevent collapse due to its rigidity, prevents soft tissue invasion into the grafting material because it is nonresorbable, prevents compression of mucosal tissues through its elasticity, features a smooth surface to prevent bacterial adherence to the material, and is plastic enough to allow for modification intraoperatively as needed.[6,11] Postoperatively, patients can be placed on chlorhexidine mouth rinse for 2 weeks to 4 weeks.[6,12,13]

The main disadvantages of titanium mesh are the need for a second surgery to remove the mesh and the risk of early mesh exposure (**Tables 2** and **3**).[6,11] Mesh exposure has been documented to occur in 27% of cases, with some case studies documenting early exposure occurring as high as 50% of the time.[11] Although high, these adverse events are relative—often treated by simply removing the portion of the exposed mesh. This usually is enough to resolve the issue without an increased risk of infection or reduced graft success.[6,11] Mesh exposure leads to slightly less bone formation if the exposure is late in the healing course. Early mesh exposure leads to a worse prognosis for the graft, including the possibility of complete loss of the graft.[14]

Table 2
Advantages and disadvantages of titanium mesh for alveolar reconstruction

Advantages	Disadvantages
• Predictable results • Biocompatible • Rigid to prevent graft collapse • Nonresorbable to prevent soft tissue invasion • Elastic to prevent soft tissue compression • Smooth surface to prevent bacterial colonization • Plastic to allow for modifications intraoperatively	• Cost • High rate of mesh exposure • Requires second surgery

Table 3
Overall complication rates for rhBMP-2 use in comparison with local and distant autogenous harvesting sites

Advantages	Disadvantages
RhBMP-2 with titanium mesh • Alveolar ridge augmentation: <1%	Autografting ramus: 5.6%–21% • Mandibular symphysis: 16%–76% • Iliac crest: 15%–56% • Tibial: 1.3%–3.8% • Coronoid process: <1%

Data from Refs.[15–23]

Procedure

The procedure is initiated with a full-thickness flap elevated to expose the defect or graft site (**Fig. 1**). Grafting material is placed in the site (autograft, allograft, or xenograft) and a titanium mesh is placed over the grafting material and fixed with short titanium or resorbable screws typically on the buccal aspect. A collagen membrane is often placed over the mesh to thicken the tissue and prevent exposure of the mesh. This is especially important in thin tissue biotypes, where dehiscence of the mesh is a common consequence. Lastly, the site is sutured closed with resorbable sutures to allow for healing via primary intention.[6–8,12,24] An important factor in achieving success for this procedure is to obtain tension-free closure; any tension over the suture line likely results in early exposure of the mesh.

Approximately 6 months after this procedure is completed and graft integration is confirmed via panoramic radiograph or cone beam computed tomography, the site is reopened using a crestal full-thickness flap for mesh removal.[6–8,12,24] At this time the site may be further augmented to facilitate restorative procedures like implant placement or complete/partial denture(s).[6,9,13,24,25] If sufficient bone augmentation exists, dental implants can be placed at this time.

Management of Titanium Mesh Exposure

If the titanium mesh becomes exposed, the patient should irrigate the area with saline and be placed on a chlorhexidine rinse to locally manage the exposure. Because the risk of infection is low after titanium mesh exposure, the mesh is typically not removed to allow the graft to integrate.[26] After exposure, a variable amount of bone formation occurs. This is inversely proportional to the timing of mesh exposure; the earlier the exposure, the less likely bone will form.[14]

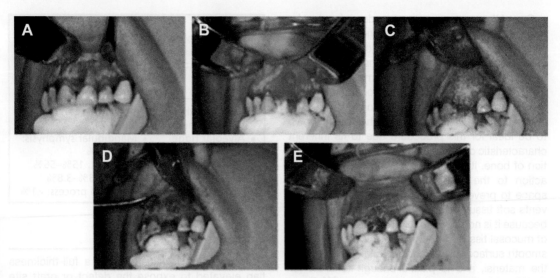

Fig. 1. (*A*) Full-thickness flap reflected to appreciate the 3-walled osseous defect at tooth #9. (*B*) Atraumatically extracted tooth #9. (*C*) Bone graft with rhBMP-2 placed and packed into the alveolus. (*D*) Adapted titanium mesh fixated with 2 titanium screws to the buccal aspect. (*E*) Primary closure.

Titanium Mesh with Biomimetic Enhancements

Recombinant human bone morphogenic protein 2

Bone morphogenic proteins (BMPs) are one of the type of cytokines within the superfamily of growth factors, called transforming growth factor ß.[27,28] They have integral roles in our natural physiology through angiogenesis, cell apoptosis, inflammation, osteogenesis and the development and maintenance of many other processes throughout the body.[27,28] Currently, rhBMP-2 is successfully used for complex maxillofacial reconstruction like critical continuity defects and more simple cases, such as local alveolar grafting, sinus lifts, and even cleft palate defects using autografting, allografting, and xenografting materials.[1,29,30]

The purpose of including rhBMP-2 in grafting procedures is to introduce osteoinductive properties, seen exclusively in autografting, to strictly osteoconductive materials in the hopes of safely providing more rapid, reliable, and consistent results and to reduce the need for secondary harvesting operations and their associated morbidities.[15,29] rhBMP-2 for bone grafting procedures has been shown to improve bone grafting procedures by enhancing bone and cartilage formation through osteogenic cell chemotaxis, osteoblastic and osteoclastic differentiation, and osteoblastic and osteoclastic maturation and stimulate production of extracellular matrix, alkaline phosphate, and type I collagen.[29]

Currently, titanium mesh with rhBMP-2 is used, in an off-label fashion, with the Infuse (Medtronic,

Minneapolis, Minnesota) system, which uses an absorbent collagen sponge to transport liquid rhBMP-2 to grafting sites.[29,31] It is critical to break the collagen sponge down into smaller parts to be mixed with the grafting material before placement into the grafting site to ensure the osteogenic properties are distributed evenly throughout. As with the other grafting techniques, the titanium mesh serves to stabilize the grafting material, prevent soft tissue invasion into the grafting site, and maintain shape in a dynamic environment to prevent site collapse.

rhBMP-2 with an absorbent collagen sponge, allograft, or xenograft and titanium mesh has been shown successful for reconstructing alveolar defects in both jaws for both horizontal and vertical dimensions across all sizes of defects.[30,32] Literature also reports that these bone grafting sites produce stable and predictable results, enough to successfully proceed to dental implant placement.[29,32–34] Because rhBMP-2 allows for successful bone grafting for larger continuity defects in the jaw, the upper limit of alveolar ridge augmentation has not yet been defined. Currently, the literature reports consistent results, ranging from 5 mm to 6 mm to in excess of 10 mm of vertical dimension. For sinus grafting, 9.5 mm to 11.3 mm of gain have been reported.[30,32,34]

For alveolar ridge augmentation with rhBMP-2, orofacial edema and erythema are the most commonly reported complications due to the inherent role of BMP in inflammation.[27] These events tend to resolve spontaneously without the need for intervention.[15–17] Because

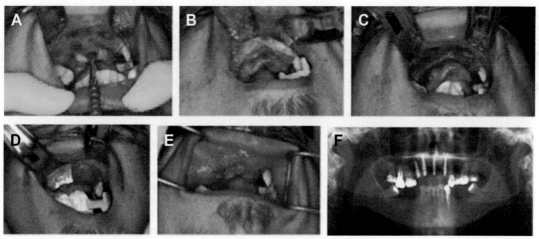

Fig. 2. (*A*) Critical maxillary anterior alveolar defect spanning teeth #3 to #11. (*B*) Full-thickness flap reflected and collagen sponge carrying rhBMP-2 mixed with allograft was placed in the alveolar defect. (*C*) Prefabricated titanium mesh adapted, placed, and secured via 3 titanium screws on the buccal surface. (*D*) Membrane placed over the titanium mesh to further prevent soft tissue invasion. (*E*) Primary closure via 3.0 chromic sutures. (*F*) Panoramic at 1-year follow-up post–implant placement with osseointegration.

the inflammatory response seen in patients tends to be dose-dependent, airway security should be a concern, especially in pediatric cases, but this tends to be isolated to complex craniofacial reconstruction cases.[15–17] Using rhBMP-2 for alveolar ridge augmentation is considered off-label from a Food and Drug Administration standpoint but is still considered an acceptable, successful, and safe product to use for alveolar ridge augmentation.[35] Airway complications that have been reported were limited to anterior cervical fusions using excessive doses of biomimetic product. BMP has been used successfully in a variety of osseous grafting procedures throughout the human skeleton, with the transient edema generally resolving without complication (**Fig. 2**).[18,36]

Pediatric patients are a particularly susceptible patient population due to natural differences in physiology and size, which can lead to simple complications, rapidly turning severe and life threatening. The major concern with using rhBMP-2 and Infuse on pediatric patients is only for cervical spine surgery and is not presently a significant increased risk for complication or morbidity for maxillofacial procedures.[18] The complications and complication rate for pediatric patients are similar to those seen in the adult population and are most commonly associated with profound edema.[18] Repeated exposure is not associated with increased risks for complications.[18] Using BMP also features an overall lower complication or adverse event rate compared with autografting techniques (see **Table 1**). Thus, although rhBMP-2 with titanium mesh represents

a safe alternative to autografting techniques, thorough patient evaluation and standard precautions are enough to ensure patient safety and excellent clinical outcomes. As with the adult patient population, precautions should be taken to ensure rapid identification of complications associated with profound edema or erythema and that the patient airway is secure or is able to be immediately secured.

SUMMARY

Although there are several alternatives to use for maxillary and mandibular alveolar reconstruction toward achieving orthoalveolar form, bone grafting procedures remain the most commonly used. Titanium mesh as an adjunct to bone grafting works favorably due to its improved resistance to deformation, preventing collapse and thus providing predictable outcomes. Although titanium mesh features a high incidence of exposure, this is usually resolved with minor intervention and rarely requires complete mesh removal. Biomimetic enhancement to the grafting procedure itself with rhBMP-2 has proved successful in combination with titanium mesh technology.

The addition of a growth factor, such as rhBMP-2, creates an osteoinductive graft and increases the amount of vital bone formation. It also improves soft tissue healing, likely due to the recruitment of cytokines and osteogenic stem cells to the area. Resorbable membranes placed over the mesh may prevent or at least delay exposure of the titanium mesh. The membrane also delays oral contaminate access to the developing osteoid and derives a net increased bone formation compared with early exposure of the titanium mesh without a membrane.

REFERENCES

1. Boyne PJ, Cole MD, Stringer D, et al. A technique for osseous restoration of deficient edentulous maxillary ridges. J Oral Maxillofac Surg 1985;43:87.
2. Herford AS, Dean JS. Complications in bone grafting. Oral Maxillofac Surg Clin North Am 2011; 23:433.
3. Sittitavornwong S, Gutta R. Bone graft harvesting from regional sites. Oral Maxillofac Surg Clin North Am 2010;22:317.
4. Herford AS, Dean J. Recombinant human bone morphogenic protein-2 (rhBMP-2) use in maxillofacial surgery. J Oral Maxillofac Surg 2008;16:1.
5. Katanec D, Granić M, Majstorović M, et al. Use of recombinant human bone morphogenetic protein (rhBMP2) in bilateral alveolar ridge augmentation: case report. Coll Antropol 2014;38:325.
6. Isaksson S, Alberius P. Maxillary alveolar ridge augmentation with onlay bone-grafts and immediate endosseous implants. J Craniomaxillofac Surg 1992;20:2.
7. Waasdorp J, Reynolds MA. Allogeneic bone onlay grafts for alveolar ridge augmentation: a systematic review. Int J Oral Maxillofac Implants 2010;25:525.
8. Her S, Kang T, Fien MJ. Titanium mesh as an alternative to a membrane for ridge augmentation. J Oral Maxillofac Surg 2012;70:803.
9. Rakhmatia YD, Ayukawa Y, Furuhashi A, et al. Current barrier membranes: Titanium mesh and other membranes for guided bone regeneration in dental applications. J Prosthodont Res 2013;57:3.
10. Haggerty CJ, Vogel CT, Fisher GR. Simple bone augmentation for alveolar ridge defects. Oral Maxillofac Surg Clin North Am 2015;27:203.
11. Wu YY, Xiao E, Graves DT. Diabetes mellitus related bone metabolism and periodontal disease. Int J Oral Sci 2015;7:63.
12. Louis PJ. Bone grafting the mandible. Dent Clin North Am 2011;55:673.
13. Misch CM. Maxillary autogenous bone grafting. Oral Maxillofac Surg Clin North Am 2011;23:229.
14. Lizio G, Corinaldesi G, Marchetti C. Alveolar ridge reconstruction with titanium mesh: a three-dimensional evaluation of factors affecting bone augmentation. Int J Oral Maxillofac Implants 2014; 29:1354.
15. Schliephake H. Bone growth factors in maxillofacial skeletal reconstruction. Int J Oral Maxillofac Surg 2002;31:469.
16. Shah MM, Smyth MD, Woo AS. Adverse facial edema associated with off-label use of recombinant

17. Ribeiro Filho SA, Francischone CE, Oliveira JC Do, et al. Bone augmentation of the atrophic anterior maxilla for dental implants using rhBMP-2 and titanium mesh: histological and tomographic analysis. Int J Oral Maxillofac Surg 2015;44:1492.
18. Riederman BD, Butler BA, Lawton CD, et al. Recombinant human bone morphogenetic protein-2 versus iliac crest bone graft in anterior cervical discectomy and fusion: dysphagia and dysphonia rates in the early postoperative period with review of the literature. J Clin Neurosci 2017;44.
19. Hammoudeh JA, Fahradyan A, Gould DD, et al. A comparative analysis of rhBMP-2/DBM vs. ICBG for secondary alveolar bone grafts in patients with cleft lip and palate: review of 501 cases. Plast Reconstr Surg 2017;140(2).
20. Reddi AH. Bone morphogenetic proteins and skeletal development : the kidney-bone connection. Review Article. Pediatr Nephrol 2000;8:598.
21. Herford AS, Boyne PJ. Reconstruction of mandibular continuity defects with bone morphogenetic protein-2 (rhBMP-2). J Oral Maxillofac Surg 2008;66:616.
22. Cicciù M, Herford AS, Stoffella E, et al. Protein-signaled guided bone regeneration using titanium mesh and Rh-BMP2 in oral surgery: a case report involving left mandibular reconstruction after tumor resection. Open Dent J 2012;6:51.
23. McKay WF, Peckham SM, Badura JM. A comprehensive clinical review of recombinant human bone morphogenetic protein-2 (INFUSE Bone Graft). Int Orthop 2007;31:729.
24. Oppenheimer AJ, Tong L, Buchman SR. Craniofacial bone grafting : Wolff ' s law revisited. Craniomaxillofac Trauma Reconstr 2008;1:49.
25. Funaki K, Takahashi T, Yamauchi K. Horizontal alveolar ridge augmentation using distraction osteogenesis: comparison with a bone-splitting method in a dog model. Oral Surgery. Oral Med Oral Pathol Oral Radiol Endodontol 2009;107:350.
26. Louis PJ, Gutta R, Said-Al-Naief N, et al. Reconstruction of the maxilla and mandible with particulate bone graft and titanium mesh for implant placement. J Oral Maxillofac Surg 2008;66:235–45.
27. Louis PJ. Vertical ridge augmentation using titanium mesh. Oral Maxillofac Surg Clin North Am 2010;22: 353.
28. Patel N, Kim B, Zaid W, et al. Tissue engineering for vertical ridge reconstruction. Oral Maxillofac Surg Clin North Am 2017;29:27.
29. Herford AS, Nguyen K. Complex bone augmentation in alveolar ridge defects. Oral Maxillofac Surg Clin North Am 2015;27:227.
30. Bottino MC, Thomas V, Schmidt G, et al. Recent advances in the development of GTR/GBR membranes

for periodontal regeneration - a materials perspective. Dent Mater 2012;28:703.

31. Elsalanty ME, Genecov DG. Bone grafts in craniofacial surgery. Craniomaxillofac Trauma Reconstr 2009;2:125.

32. FDA warning for infuse bone graft risks in kids. Available at: https://www.schmidtlaw.com/fda-warning-for-infuse-bone-graft-risks-in-kids/. Accessed January 17, 2018.

33. Stiel N, Hissnauer TN, Rupprecht M, et al. Evaluation of complications associated with off-label use of recombinant human bone morphogenetic protein-2 (rhBMP-2) in pediatric orthopaedics. J Mater Sci Mater Med 2016;27:184.

34. Lindley TE, Dahdaleh NS, Menezes AH, et al. Complications associated with recombinant human bone morphogenetic protein use in pediatric craniocervical arthrodesis. J Neurosurg Pediatr 2011;7:468.

35. Balaji SM. Use of recombinant human bone morphogenetic protein (rhBMP-2) in reconstruction of maxillary alveolar clefts. J Maxillofac Oral Surg 2009;8:211.

36. Davies SD, Ochs MW. Bone morphogenetic proteins in craniomaxillofacial surgery. Oral Maxillofac Surg Clin North Am 2010;22:17.

Managing Bone Grafts for the Mandible

Patrick J. Louis, DDS, MD*, Somsak Sittitavornwong, DDS, DMD, MS

KEYWORDS

- Mandible • Bone grafting • Onlay • Inlay • Guided bone regeneration

KEY POINTS

- Various graft materials and membrane barriers used for alveolar ridge reconstruction will be discussed.
- The authors will compare and contrast the various bone grafting techniques by reviewing the current literature.
- Onlay versus inlay bone grafting will be discussed.
- Autogenous versus allogenous, xenogenous, and other bone graft materials will be compared.

INTRODUCTION

Bone grafting has become an integral part of implant dentistry. To achieve a predictable long-term outcome for osseointegrated implants, a sufficient volume and quality of alveolar bone must be present at implant recipient sites. Resorption of the alveolar ridge and postsurgical or post-traumatic defects of the residual alveolar bone can prevent ideal placement of a dental implant, resulting in compromised esthetics and function. Thus, in many cases, alveolar bone grafting is the real challenge in implant reconstruction.[1] Alveolar ridge reconstruction can be achieved with various graft materials and membrane barriers to prevent soft tissue ingrowth.

This article will discuss the various techniques and graft materials for alveolar ridge reconstruction of the mandible (**Box 1**). It also compares and contrasts these techniques by reviewing the current literature (**Box 2**). The use of growth factors will not be discussed in this article.

INDICATIONS AND CONTRAINDICATIONS

The initial presentations for most patients is because of a desire for teeth or implants. All patients most undergo a thorough history and focused physical examination to determine if bone grafting is indicated. A cone beam computerized tomogram, CBCT, is an essential part of the patient evaluation. The height and width of the alveolar ridge can be measured to determine if bone grafting is needed prior to implant placement. The indications for each grafting technique will be presented in the appropriate section. Contraindications are presented in **Box 3**. Implants can be placed in patients with conditions that are listed in the relative contraindications section; however, the surgeon should have a thorough discussion with the patient to inform him or her of the potential increased risk of failure.

RECONSTRUCTION TECHNIQUES
Socket Grafting

Socket grafting is a particulate graft, comprised of autogenous, allogenous, xenogenous, and alloplastic materials. Indications include maintaining horizontal and vertical dimensions of the ridge. Healing time for bone consolidation is 3 to 4 months. Advantages include reduction of early alveolar bone loss after tooth extraction and

Disclosure Statement: P.J. Louis is a consultant for BioHorizons Implant Company. S. Sittitavornwong has nothing to disclose.
Department of Oral and Maxillofacial Surgery, University of Alabama at Birmingham, School of Dentistry, 1919 7th Avenue South SDB 419, Birmingham, AL 35294-0007, USA
* Corresponding author.
E-mail address: plouis@uab.edu

Oral Maxillofacial Surg Clin N Am 31 (2019) 317–330
https://doi.org/10.1016/j.coms.2018.12.008
1042-3699/19/© 2018 Elsevier Inc. All rights reserved.

minimal risks by using allografts. Disadvantages include inability to gain more height or width than tooth socket size and slow bone remodeling of graft material. Complications include graft infection, loss of graft material, and loss of alveolar ridge width or height.

The technique is shown in **Fig. 1**. To preserve facial and lingual bone, an atraumatic extraction of the tooth must be performed. This sometimes requires the use of periotomes to aid in the extraction. After successful extraction of the tooth, the socket is curetted and irrigated. The socket is then filled with particulate graft material and densely packed. The socket is covered with a collagen plug, membrane, or an epithelial graft.

Clinical results in the literature

Tan and colleagues reported that 6 months after tooth extraction, the horizontal bone loss and vertical alveolar bone loss were 29% to 63% and 11% to 22% respectively.[2] There was a great amount of alveolar bone resorption demonstrated in the first 3 months after tooth extraction, which continues changing up to 1 year, reducing approximately 50% of the bucco-lingual dimension. Most of this resorption occurs on the buccal bone plate.[3,4] Several studies show bovine xenograft will resorb slower than the cancellous allograft after bone grafting of the jawbone.[5–12] Grafting the alveolar ridge with hydroxyapatite and beta-tricalcium

phosphate (TCP) will preserve alveolar dimension more than deproteinized bovine bone mineral. TCP will interrupt and slow the normal healing process. It may delay implant placement.[13] The most efficacious socket graft material for maintaining bone height and width were freeze-dried bone with a membrane and autogenous bone marrow, respectively.[14]

Onlay Technique

The onlay technique is a block graft from autogenous, allogenous, and xenogenous materials. Indications include horizontal or vertical defects. Healing time for bone consolidation is 3 to 6 months. Advantages include bone gain in vertical and horizontal directions and avoidance of injury of the inferior alveolar nerve. Disadvantages include association with donor sight morbidity, more surgical time, and limited bone sources. Additionally, screw fixation is required, as well as tension-free primary closure. Complications include risk of wound dehiscence and graft loss.

The technique is described in **Fig. 2**. Segmental defects and the atrophic edentulous arch can be exposed through a crestal or vestibular incision, depending on surgeon preference. For horizontal defects, the authors generally make a crestal incision, and for vertical defects, they usually make a vestibular incision. A subperiosteal dissection is used to expose the alveolus. The block graft must be well adapted to the native bone. This sometimes requires contouring the bone block

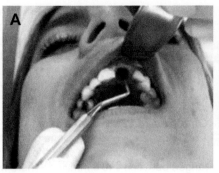
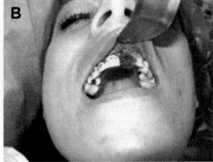

Fig. 1. Socket grafting. (*A*) Empty extraction socket #9. (*B*) Extraction socket #9 filled with bone graft material.

and mortising the alveolar ridge at the recipient site for more intimate contact between the 2 surfaces. Once good bone adaptation is achieved between the graft and recipient site, the graft is secured with titanium screws using the lag screw technique. Any gaps between the recipient site and the bone graft are filled with particulate bone graft, usually allograft or xenograft, and covered with a resorbable membrane. To achieve a tension-free primary closure of the wound, the periosteum of the flap is released. This is achieved by placing a horizontal incision just through the periosteum under the flap. This allows the flap to stretch and permits primary closure without wound tension.

Clinical results in the literature

There is a mean increase in horizontal and vertical dimension of 4.4 mm and 3.7 mm respectively.[15] Several articles reported favorable outcomes of ridge augmentation by adding growth factors in onlay bone grafting.[16,17] There were no differences in implant survival and peri-implant bone level compared with implants in native alveolar bone and onlay block grafting. This includes both horizontal and vertical grafts.[18–20] Six months after onlay bone grafts, bone resorption is reported between 20% and 50%.[21] Rates of graft resorption in horizontal and vertical dimension were 10% to 50%[22–25] and 29% to 42%,[26] respectively, depending on the choice of bone harvest site. Wound dehiscence and total graft loss were 3.3% and 1.4%, respectively.[22,23,25]

Inlay Technique

The inlay technique is usually performed with a block graft. Indications include horizontal or vertical defects. A minimum of 4 mm of alveolar width and 5 to 6 mm of bone above the inferior alveolar nerve is required to perform the osteotomy. Healing time for bone consolidation is 3 to 4 months. Advantages include maintenance of vascularity, faster vascularization of the graft, and less resorption of the graft. Disadvantages include the fact that it is technically difficult, especially in the atrophic mandible, and there is a risk of mandibular fracture. Additionally, the lingual flap could restrict the range of vertical augmentation because of limitation of the soft tissue and blood supply.[27] Complications include mandibular nerve injury and mandibular fracture.

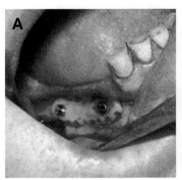
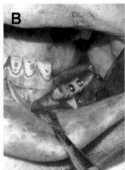
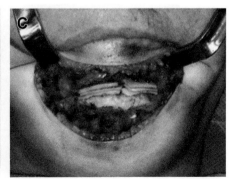

Fig. 2. Onlay bone grafts. (*A, B*) Autogenous onlay bone grafts to the right and left posterior mandible harvested from the ramus of the mandible. (*C*) Autogenous bone graft to the edentulous mandible harvested from the cranium.

The surgical technique is described in **Fig. 3**. For the anterior and posterior mandibular edentulous areas, the full-thickness vestibular incision is made at the anterior or posterior lower vestibule, respectively, below 10 to 12 mm from the crestal bone, avoiding the emergence of the mental nerves. The mucoperiosteal flap is carefully elevated toward the alveolar crest, gaining visibility of the alveolar bone and preserving blood supply to the alveolar crest. A minimum bone height of 5 to 6 mm above the inferior alveolar nerve is needed to avoid mandibular nerve injury and fracture of the mandible or transport segment.[27–32] Two oblique osteotomy and 1 horizontal osteotomy are performed through the buccal and lingual cortex and cancellous bone by using a reciprocal saw or piezosurgery to obtain a 4 mm height transport segment. This allows the application of fixation screws without a fracture risk.[27,33] In the anterior edentulous mandible, the 2 oblique cuts are placed approximately 2 mm from the adjacent teeth. The horizontal osteotomy is performed at least 2 mm above the inferior alveolar canal.[27] The osteotomy of the lingual cortex can be completed by using a small chisel. It is important to avoid injury or perforation of the lingual flap. After completion of the osteotomy, the transport bone segment, which should be 4 mm or more in height, is lifted in the coronal direction, preserving the lingual flap and blood supply. At this point, the planned autogenous or allogenous bone block is harvested, contoured, and placed properly in the interpositional graft site between the transport and basilar segments. The transport bone segment can be raised 5 to 8 mm as needed to level the alveolar plane.[27] The gaps between the inlay graft can be filled with particulate bone graft materials. Particulate bone grafts provide a low capacity of resistance for stabilization of the transport bone segment. In the case of particulate bone, a titanium miniplate and screws are necessary to immobilize the transport segment vertically. The gaps between the coronal segment and mandibular basal bone are filled with particulate bone graft materials. The grafted areas are secured with a resorbable membrane. A tension-free 2-layered closure is performed.

Clinical results in the literature

The postoperative vertical bone gain of the posterior edentulous mandible with the inlay technique ranged between 4 to 8 mm.[27–41] There was no histologic difference between autogenous and homologous bone grafts with well vascularized grafts after 6 weeks.[42] The alveolar bone of the interpositional osteotomies healed with rapid vascularization and bone remodeling. The difference between the interpositional grafts and adjacent native bone was almost indistinguishable after 12 weeks.[43,44] Bone resorption was reported between 0 to 1 mm at a follow-up of 1 to 4 years.[30] The inlay bone grafts showed less bone resorption than the onlay bone grafting, because the graft material was encircled by basal bone and periosteum, accommodating and ensuring blood circulation to the enclosing tissue.[27,42,45–49]

Several studies have demonstrated rapid bone incorporation when the grafted materials were placed between the upper and lower corticocancellous portions of the mandible.[44,45,50] There was good stability of the vertical augmentation when this technique was used in the posterior mandible.[42,51–54] The most common reported complication of the inlay technique in the posterior edentulous mandible was transient hypoesthesia, which has ranged from 20% to 54%.[27,38,55–58]

Guide Bone Regeneration

Guide bone regeneration is a particulate type of bone graft. Indications include horizontal and

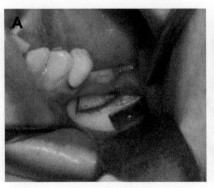
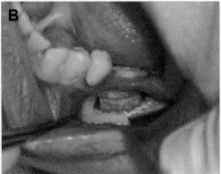

Fig. 3. Inlay bone graft. (*A*) Osteotomy of the alveolar ridge of the posterior mandible. Note the minimal soft tissue reflection. (*B*) Autogenous block graft placed between the basal segment and the crestal (transport) segment for a vertical augmentation.

vertical defects. Healing time for bone consolidation is 6 to 8 months. An advantage is that it can be adapted to any type of ridge defect.

Disadvantages include that membranes can be expensive. Additionally, nonresorbable membranes require removal, and titanium mesh and polytetrafluoroethylene (PTFE) membranes can result in higher exposure risk. Complications include that rigid membranes can result in a higher incidence of wound dehiscence, and early mesh exposure can sometimes result in loss of the graft.

Surgical technique is described in **Fig. 4**. An incision is made in the depth of the mandibular vestibule just anterior to the retromolar pad extending anteriorly across the midline. After the mental nerves are identified and protected, a subperiosteal dissection is performed. The subperiosteal dissection is carried over the crest of the ridge and onto the lingual surface of the mandible in a subperiosteal fashion. The lingual extent of the dissection anteriorly is to the genial tubercles. Once the mandible is exposed, a nonresorbable membrane is chosen and contoured. With partial defects, PTFE or titanium mesh are options. In the edentulous mandible, titanium mesh comes in preformed ridge shapes and are rigid. The mesh is contoured and trimmed to fit over the defect. The mesh is filled with the bone graft and secured into position with at least 2 screws on the facial surface. A 2-layered tension-free closure is performed.

Clinical results in the literature

Autogenous bone mixed with allogenous or xenogenous bone has been utilized in guided bone regeneration procedures with vertical bone gain between 2 to 7 mm.[59–63] Guided bone regeneration can employ occlusive membranes that prevent soft tissue ingrowth.[64,65]

Bone substitutes and a membrane can allow for bone regeneration.[66] Guided bone regeneration by using bone substitutes with a collagen membrane

has shown successes in maintaining alveolar ridge width and height.[67] Roccuzzo and colleagues[68] and Antoun and colleagues[69] showed the onlay osseous graft protected by titanium mesh and nonresorbable membranes displayed significantly less bone resorption compared with the onlay bone graft alone. Soft tissue dehiscence in titanium mesh cases did not seem to affect the outcome of implant placement.[68,70–73] Deproteinized bovine bone (BioOss), combined with hydroxyapatite and beta-tricalcium phosphate (Bone Ceramic), was twice as effective in protecting alveolar ridge width. However, hydroxyapatite and beta-tricalcium phosphate (Bone Ceramic) can impede the normal healing process of alveolar bone.[13] Both demineralized freeze-dried bone allograft (DFDBA) and mineralized freeze-dried bone allograft (FDBA) are osteoconductive and contain bone morphogenic proteins (BMP). Only DFDBA has been shown to be osteoinductive. FDBA may be a better scaffold for osteoconduction.[67] The disadvantages of GBR are membrane collapse and premature membrane exposure, causing bone graft infection and at times failure.[74,75] After GBR, alveolar ridge resorption occurs once the membrane is removed or resorbed.[76–78] Several studies recommend leaving the membranes in place prior to placing dental implants for 9 months.[62,79–81] Generally, only particulate bone grafting materials can augment the small vertical alveolar defects. In cases of 3-dimensional bone reconstruction, the titanium mesh techniques can provide scaffold and stability.[82] Titanium mesh has a high incidence of exposure rates, ranging 0% to 80%.[83–85] The bone formation is difficult to predict if the metallic mesh becomes exposed after placement, resulting in poor bone augmentation. Louis and colleagues reported utilizing flexible mesh with smaller pores in the posterior mandible with better outcome.[86] Some studies reported that titanium mesh exposure did not make the final outcome

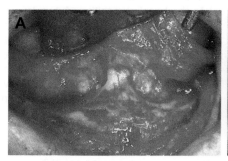 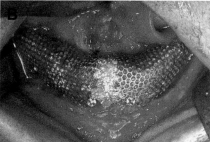

Fig. 4. (*A*) Preoperative mandible with severe atrophy. (*B*) Bone graft in place covered with pre-formed titanium mesh.

different and allowed for implants in the desired area.[68,70–73] Early wound dehiscence of titanium mesh in the first week was associated with a negative outcome on bone regeneration compared with a late dehiscence. A tension-free wound closure over the titanium mesh can decrease the risk of premature wound exposure.[79,83,87,88] The amount of vital bone was significant higher in DFDBA cases.[89] However, the effect on alveolar ridge preservation is not much different for mineralized freeze-dried bone allograft (FDBA).

Alveolar Distraction Osteogenesis

The direction of ridge augmentation for alveolar distraction osteogenesis is vertical. Healing time for bone consolidation is 4 months after the last activation of the distraction osteogenesis. An advantage of this technique is that no graft material is required. Disadvantages include daily activation, compromised speech, eating, and appearance, as well as risks of infection and loss of fixation.

Complications can occur during the intraoperative phase, the alveolar distraction osteogenesis (ADO) phase, the consolidation phase, or for other reasons.[90]

Complications during the intraoperative phase include

- Basal bone or segment fracture (2%)
- Excessive bleeding (4%)

Complications during the ADO phase include

- Infection (6%)
- Skin (chin) perforation (2%)
- Mucosal dehiscence (8%)
- Change of distraction vector: lingually orientated rotation (100%)

Complications during the consolidation phase include

- Basal bone or segment fracture (17%)
- Sensory disturbances (28%)
- Sagging chin (13%)

Other complications include[31,91]

- Partial relapse of initial bone height (8%)
- Change of distraction vector (8%)
- Basal bone or segment fracture (3%)
- Fracture of distraction device (2%)
- Incomplete distraction (2%)
- Transient paresthesia (2%)
- Total failure (1%)

Surgical technique is described in **Fig. 5**. The incision and alveolar osteotomy for ADO are similar to the inlay bone grafting technique. An

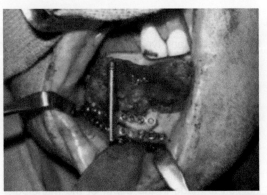

Fig. 5. Distraction osteogenesis. Posterior mandible with distractor in place after the osteotomy.

intraoral incision is made in the buccal vestibule of the mandible. The full-thickness vestibular incision is made at the anterior or posterior lower buccal vestibule 10 to 12 mm from the crestal bone, avoiding the emergence of the mental nerves depending on the site of reconstruction. The mental nerve is identified and secured. Subperiosteal dissection is carefully performed preserving blood supply toward the alveolar crest on the buccolingual aspect and alveolar bone segment that will be osteotomized. The distraction device is secured into position with screws, and the planned osteotomy is marked with a sterile pencil. The device is removed and set aside. With a piezo-osteotome, oscillating saw or fissure bur, the alveolar bone segment to be vertically distracted is cut to obtain at least a 5 mm height transport segment from the basal bone. A minimum bone height of 6 to 7 mm above the inferior alveolar nerve is required to avoid mandibular nerve injury and fracture of the mandible or transport segment. This allows applying microscrews for a distraction device without a fracture risk. The transport segment is gently mobilized to ensure the osteotomies are complete. The distraction device is placed back into position using the original screw holes and screws. The distraction device is activated to ensure it will move along the planned path. The device is brought back into the baseline position. A two-layered tension free closure is performed. The distractor device is activated after a waiting period of 1 week. A distraction of 1 mm per day is divided into 2 activations of 0.5 mm every 12 hours until the desired height of distraction is achieved. The alveolar distractor is kept in place for 3 to 4 months for a consolidation period.

Clinical results in the literature
The success rate was 95.5%,[31,92] and there was a vertical bone and soft tissue gain of 3 to

20 mm.[31,90,93] Results are similar when distraction osteogenesis was compared with the inlay technique in the posterior mandible.[28] The inlay technique is better with a single stage of surgery, while the distraction osteogenesis has an advantage of a greater vertical height of the transport bone.[28] A consolidation period of 5 days per millimeter space created should be respected as a minimum before device removal and implant placement.[26]

Postoperative Care

After the procedure is complete, the initial management should focus on hemostasis. However, the other areas that must be addressed include antibiotics, wound care, diet, follow-up visits, and temporization.

Intraoperative techniques can have a significant impact on postoperative hemostasis. Hemostasis can be achieved with judicious use of cautery and good wound closure. Pressure is usually the first technique employed postoperatively, but may be contraindicated, depending on the augmentation technique used. Pressure can be used over well-secured block grafts but may displace a particulate graft. A relined denture or partial denture can beneficial, but must be well adjusted, to avoid ischemia and wound breakdown.

Antibiotics should be used for 7 to 10 days. Amoxicillin or clindamycin provide excellent coverage against oral flora. Wound care should include mouth rinse and tooth-brushing. Chlorhexidine mouth rinse for 2 to 4 weeks can reduce the risk of infection. If a wound dehiscence develops, the patient should be maintained on chlorhexidine mouth rinse until the second-stage surgery. Appropriate cleaning should include use of a soft toothbrush to remove any plaque or debris and wound irrigation.

Follow-up visits are usually at 2 weeks, 1 month, and 3 months postoperatively. The second-stage surgery should be planned for 4 to 6 months postoperatively. The hardware is usually removed at second-stage surgery when implants are placed.

Temporization varies primarily based on if the patient is partially dentate. Most patients with some teeth can undergo immediate temporization using a partially or completely tooth-born prosthesis. Edentulous patients could undergo immediate temporization by relining an existing denture. To avoid pressure on the wound, for patients in whom hardware has been place, a period of rest is usually indicated to minimize the risk of wound dehiscence. The temporization could be delayed 2 to 4 weeks.

In general, patients should be on a soft diet. In patients with atrophic mandibles that have undergone complete or segmental osteotomies, a strict nonchew diet for 6 to 8 weeks is recommended to minimize the risk of fracture. In dentate patients, diet can be customized to the number of teeth present and location of the graft.

DISCUSSION
Onlay Versus Inlay Bone Grafts

The technique of interpositional bone graft was developed years ago. In 1966, Pasteur reported a 2-stage technique for interpositional bone grafting in the posterior mandible.[94] Three weeks after the first stage, the upper bone segment was elevated with a bovine allograft or plaster of Paris graft interpositional graft.[52,94,95] In 1976, Schettler reported the sandwich osteotomy technique with interpositional bone grafting for vertical augmentation of the anterior edentulous mandible by maintaining the integrity of the lingual periosteum.[42,45,96] Subsequently, this technique has been modified to accommodate vertical and horizontal movements.[51–54]

In this technique, it is necessary to maintain the integrity of the lingual flap, which could restrict the range of the vertical augmentation because of limitation of soft tissue and blood supply. The technique of interpositional grafting is to place the bone graft between the upper transport bone and lower basal bone segments by creating a horizontal osteotomy. By doing so, the internal cancellous will provide blood supply and allow bone graft incorporation.[43,50] Studies have demonstrated rapid bone incorporation when the grafted materials were placed between the upper and lower corticocancellous portions of the mandible.[44,45]

Schettler and Holtermann reported there was no histologic difference between the autogenous and homologous bone grafts after 6 weeks.[42] Frame and colleagues reported similar outcomes with the interpositional bone graft technique.[43,44,50] The alveolar bone of the interpositional osteotomies healed with rapid vascularization and bone remodeling. There were nearly indistinguishable differences between the interpositional grafts and adjacent native bone after 12 weeks.[44]

The onlay bone graft technique in the posterior mandible with intraoral bone harvest provided a mean bone gain between 2.4 and 4.6 mm.[21,97] Felice and colleagues stated the higher bone gain in the inlay technique may relate to the greater amount of bone harvested such as from the iliac crest.[29] They reported the postoperative vertical bone gain of the posterior edentulous mandible with inlay technique ranged between 4 and 8 mm. Jensen and colleagues[33] and Robiony and colleagues[34] reported the augmentation by interpositional osteotomies in the posterior edentulous mandible achieved up to 8 mm. These results were consistent with several studies.[27–33,38–41,98] Inlay bone grafting showed less bone resorption than onlay bone grafting, because the grafting material is encircled by basal bone and periosteum ensuring blood circulation to the enclosing tissue. Therefore, the interpositional grafting technique has great capability of bone graft incorporation with low final bone resorption.[27,42,45–49,96] Bone resorption was reported between 0 and 1 mm at a follow-up of 1 to 4 years. Marchetti and colleagues reported similar results, using autogenous cancellous particulate bone as the graft.[30] Compared with the onlay technique, Felice and colleagues reported there was 40% bone resorption from the obtained bone gain using the onlay bone grafting. However, once the dental implants were placed, the outcomes were not different in terms of both bone grafting techniques and maintenance of vertical bone.

However, the major challenge of vertical bone augmentation at the posterior mandible is the handling of the soft tissue. Vertically repositioning the transport bone segment can compromise the blood supply by strain on the lingual soft tissue pedicle causing wound breakdown, graft loss, and resorption.[27] The most common complication of the inlay technique in the posterior edentulous mandible was the postoperative transient hypoesthesia, which ranged from 20% to 54%.[27,38,55–58] There were no major complications reported for the inlay grafting technique to the anterior and posterior mandible.[33,48]

By understanding the physiologic limitations of bone and soft tissue healing, avoiding blood supply compromise, utilizing the concepts of osteointegration and fixation, and achieving the consolidation phase, interpositional bone grafting is a safe predictable technique that allows gain of 5 to 8 mm of vertical augmentation and early dental implant placement in the posterior mandible.[27] Between inlay and onlay bone grafts, the inlay technique has less bone resorption and more predictable results. However, it does require a skilled surgeon, because it is technically difficult. In contrast, the onlay technique shows more bone resorption and needs an oversized block graft to compensate for resorption but is less technically demanding. However, once a dental implant has been placed in either onlay or inlay graft sites, there was no difference in the outcomes.[27,38]

These results are also comparable between the inlay technique and distraction osteogenesis in the posterior mandible. There were no differences in the outcomes of dental implant osseointegration and prosthetic results between the distraction osteogenesis, inlay technique, and native bone. Bianchi and colleagues recommended the inlay technique as better because of a single-stage surgery, while distraction osteogenesis has an advantage for greater vertical height of the transport bone.[28,99] The personal skill and experience of individual surgeons should determine the bone grafting technique to be used in the mandible[27] (**Table 1**).

Autogenous Versus Allogenous, Xenogenous, and Other Bone Graft Materials

Particulate

Autogenous bone has long been considered the gold standard as a grafting material. However, improvements in the processing and development of new products have led to their use as an alternative to, or in combination with autogenous grafting. Bone graft materials are chosen based on reliability, safety, and ease of use. It is debatable as to what graft material is most reliable in producing bone. In a systematic review and network meta-analysis of parallel and cluster randomized controlled trials comparing the effectiveness of natural and synthetic bone grafts in oral and maxillofacial surgery, Papageorgiou reported on trends that appear to favor autogenous bone. Autografts presented the highest percentage of new bone, followed by synthetic grafts, xenografts, and allografts.[100] Autografts presented the lowest percentage of residual graft particles, followed by xenografts, synthetic grafts, and allografts. Autografts presented the lowest percentage of connective tissue, followed by allografts, xenografts, and synthetic grafts. Although particulate autogenous bone appeared to outperform other types of graft materials, there were no statistically significant differences found in the percentage of new bone from pairwise comparisons between any 2 bone grafts. In a systematic review, Troeltzsch and colleagues reported on the clinical efficacy of grafting materials in alveolar ridge augmentation.[82] The authors showed that horizontal gain was significantly higher for mixtures of autogenous bone with allogeneic/xenogeneic grafting materials (4.5 plus or minus 1.0 mm) compared with the use of synthetic grafting materials (2.2 plus or. minus 1.2 mm). The vertical gain varied without significant difference, from 3.6 plus or minus 1.0 mm in mixtures of autogenous bone with allogeneic/xenogeneic grafting materials to 3.9 plus or minus 1.7 mm for particulate autogenous grafts derived from mandibular bone. Thus,

Table 1
Mean bone gains achieved with various bone graft techniques

Grafting Technique	Potential Horizontal Gain (mm)	Potential Vertical Gain (mm)
Onlay block graft	4.5 ± 1.2	5.8 ± 2.8
Autogenous (distant)	~4.6	9.4 ± 3.1
Autogenous (local)	~4.6	5.3 ± 1.6
Allogenous	4.6 ± 1.2	2.9 ± 1.3
Xenogenous	3.7	
Inlay graft		4–8
Autogenous (distant)	8.6 ± 4.3	9.4 ± 3.1
Autogenous (local)	4.4 ± 1.9	5.3 ± 1.6
Allogenous	2.2 ± 3.5	2.9 ± 1.3
Xenogenous	6.5 ± 4.3	
Guided bone regeneration (particulate + membrane)	3.7 ± 1.2	3.7 ± 1.4
Autogenous	~3.5	3.9 ± 1.7
Autogenous + Xeno/Allo	4.5 ± 1.0	3.6 ± 1.0
Alloplast	2.2 ± 1.2	
Membrane differences		
Titanium mesh	~4.5	6.0 ± 2.3
Collagen membrane	~3.5	3.9 ± 1.9
PTFE membrane	~3.3	~4.0
Distraction osteogenesis		3–20

Data compiled from review articles listed below.

Data from Chiapasco M, Consolo U, Bianchi A, et al. Alveolar distraction osteogenesis for the correction of vertically deficient edentulous ridges: a multicenter prospective study on humans. Int J Oral Maxillofac Implants 2004;19(3):399–407; and Troeltzsch M, Troeltzsch M, Kauffmann P, et al. Clinical efficacy of grafting materials in alveolar ridge augmentation: a systematic review. J Craniomaxillofac Surg 2016;44(10):1618–29.

autogenous particulate bone in combination with other graft materials appears to offer some advantages over allogenous, xenogenous, and synthetic graft materials alone. Use of space-maintaining barriers, such as titanium, resulted in greater vertical gains than collagen-based membranes.

Block

In the same article, Troeltzsch reported that block grafts were able to achieve higher gains in the horizontal dimensions than particulate materials with weighted means between 3.7 mm for xenogeneic and 4.6 plus or minus 1.4 mm for allogeneic blocks, with an overall weighted mean of 4.5 plus or minus 1.2 mm. Vertical gains were significantly increased for autogenous bone blocks from the iliac crest and the calvarium (9.4 plus or minus 3.1 mm) compared with autogenous bone grafts from the mandible (5.3 plus or minus 1.6 mm) and allogenous blocks (2.9 plus or minus 1.3 mm).[82] Autogenous block grafts harvested from distant sites appear to outperform allogeneic and xenogenic block grafts and particulate grafts as onlay grafts (**Table 2**).

Table 2
Comparison between autogenous bone grafts and bone graft substitutes

Autogenous Bone	Bone Substitutes
Advantages	Advantages
Osteoinductive	Osteoinductive
Osteoconductive	Osteoconductive
Osteogenic	Unlimited amount
No disease	No donor site
transmission	Disadvantages
Disadvantages	Less predictable?
Nerve Injury	Disease transmission
Infection	Immune response
Hematoma	
Fracture	
Tooth injury	
Limited graft size	

SUMMARY

There are multiple techniques that can be used to reconstruct alveolar defects in the mandible. These techniques can be simple, as in the case of socket grafting and GBR techniques. However, when choosing a technique for mandibular reconstruction, the clinician must first determine the magnitude of the height and/or the width required to achieve a successful outcome. The overall health of the patient must be determined and whether there are any contraindications to performing a bone graft procedure. The clinician must be familiar with the advantages and disadvantages of the various bone grafting procedures and possess the surgical skills to properly perform the indicated procedure.

REFERENCES

1. Louis PJ. Bone grafting the mandible. Dent Clin North Am 2011;55(4):673–95.

2. Tan WL, Wong TL, Wong MC, et al. A systematic review of post-extractional alveolar hard and soft tissue dimensional changes in humans. Clin Oral Implants Res 2012;23(Suppl 5):1–21.

3. Schropp L, Kostopoulos L, Wenzel A. Bone healing following immediate versus delayed placement of titanium implants into extraction sockets: a prospective clinical study. Int J Oral Maxillofac Implants 2003;18(2):189–99.

4. Araujo MG, Sukekava F, Wennstrom JL, et al. Ridge alterations following implant placement in fresh extraction sockets: an experimental study in the dog. J Clin Periodontol 2005;32(6):645–52.

5. Vance GS, Greenwell H, Miller RL, et al. Comparison of an allograft in an experimental putty carrier and a bovine-derived xenograft used in ridge preservation: a clinical and histologic study in humans. Int J Oral Maxillofac Implants 2004;19(4):491–7.

6. Wang HL, Misch C, Neiva RF. "Sandwich" bone augmentation technique: rationale and report of pilot cases. Int J Periodontics Restorative Dent 2004; 24(3):232–45.

7. Wallace SS, Froum SJ, Cho SC, et al. Sinus augmentation utilizing anorganic bovine bone (Bio-Oss) with absorbable and nonabsorbable membranes placed over the lateral window: histomorphometric and clinical analyses. Int J Periodontics Restorative Dent 2005;25(6):551–9.

8. Scarano A, Pecora G, Piattelli M, et al. Osseointegration in a sinus augmented with bovine porous bone mineral: histological results in an implant retrieved 4 years after insertion. A case report. J Periodontol 2004;75(8):1161–6.

9. Burchardt H. The biology of bone graft repair. Clin Orthop Relat Res 1983;(174):28–42.

10. Goldberg VM, Stevenson S. The biology of bone grafts. Semin Arthroplasty 1993;4(2):58–63.

11. Sbordone C, Toti P, Guidetti F, et al. Volume changes of iliac crest autogenous bone grafts after vertical and horizontal alveolar ridge augmentation of atrophic maxillas and mandibles: a 6-year computerized tomographic follow-up. J Oral Maxillofac Surg 2012;70(11):2559–65.

12. Sbordone L, Levin L, Guidetti F, et al. Apical and marginal bone alterations around implants in maxillary sinus augmentation grafted with autogenous bone or bovine bone material and simultaneous or delayed dental implant positioning. Clin Oral Implants Res 2011;22(5):485–91.

13. De Coster P, Browaeys H, De Bruyn H. Healing of extraction sockets filled with BoneCeramic(R) prior to implant placement: preliminary histological findings. Clin Implant Dent Relat Res 2011;13(1):34–45.

14. Iocca O, Farcomeni A, Pardinas Lopez S, et al. Alveolar ridge preservation after tooth extraction: a Bayesian Network meta-analysis of grafting materials efficacy on prevention of bone height and width reduction. J Clin Periodontol 2017;44(1):104–14.

15. Jensen SS, Terheyden H. Bone augmentation procedures in localized defects in the alveolar ridge: clinical results with different bone grafts and bone-substitute materials. Int J Oral Maxillofac Implants 2009;24(Suppl):218–36.

16. De Angelis N, Scivetti M. Lateral ridge augmentation using an equine flex bone block infused with recombinant human platelet-derived growth factor BB: a clinical and histologic study. Int J Periodontics Restorative Dent 2011;31(4):383–8.

17. Simion M, Rocchietta I, Dellavia C. Three-dimensional ridge augmentation with xenograft and recombinant human platelet-derived growth factor-BB in humans: report of two cases. Int J Periodontics Restorative Dent 2007;27(2):109–15.

18. Sbordone L, Toti P, Menchini-Fabris G, et al. Implant survival in maxillary and mandibular osseous onlay grafts and native bone: a 3-year clinical and computerized tomographic follow-up. Int J Oral Maxillofac Implants 2009;24(4):695–703.

19. Sbordone L, Toti P, Menchini-Fabris G, et al. Implant success in sinus-lifted maxillae and native bone: a 3-year clinical and computerized tomographic follow-up. Int J Oral Maxillofac Implants 2009;24(2):316–24.

20. Sbordone L, Toti P, Menchini-Fabris GB, et al. Volume changes of autogenous bone grafts after alveolar ridge augmentation of atrophic maxillae and mandibles. Int J Oral Maxillofac Surg 2009; 38(10):1059–65.

21. Cordaro L, Amade DS, Cordaro M. Clinical results of alveolar ridge augmentation with mandibular

block bone grafts in partially edentulous patients prior to implant placement. Clin Oral Implants Res 2002;13(1):103–11.

22. Chiapasco M, Casentini P, Zaniboni M. Bone augmentation procedures in implant dentistry. Int J Oral Maxillofac Implants 2009;24(Suppl):237–59.

23. Chiapasco M, Felisati G, Maccari A, et al. The management of complications following displacement of oral implants in the paranasal sinuses: a multicenter clinical report and proposed treatment protocols. Int J Oral Maxillofac Surg 2009;38(12): 1273–8.

24. Chiapasco M, Zaniboni M. Methods to treat the edentulous posterior maxilla: implants with sinus grafting. J Oral Maxillofac Surg 2009;67(4):867–71.

25. Chiapasco M, Zaniboni M. Clinical outcomes of GBR procedures to correct peri-implant dehiscences and fenestrations: a systematic review. Clin Oral Implants Res 2009;20(Suppl 4):113–23.

26. Bernstein S, Cooke J, Fotek P, et al. Vertical bone augmentation: where are we now? Implant Dent 2006;15(3):219–28.

27. Felice P, Pistilli R, Lizio G, et al. Inlay versus onlay iliac bone grafting in atrophic posterior mandible: a prospective controlled clinical trial for the comparison of two techniques. Clin Implant Dent Relat Res 2009;11(Suppl 1):e69–82.

28. Bianchi A, Felice P, Lizio G, et al. Alveolar distraction osteogenesis versus inlay bone grafting in posterior mandibular atrophy: a prospective study. Oral Surg Oral Med Oral Pathol Oral Radiol Endod 2008;105(3):282–92.

29. Felice P, Marchetti C, Piattelli A, et al. Vertical ridge augmentation of the atrophic posterior mandible with interpositional block grafts: bone from the iliac crest versus bovine anorganic bone. Eur J Oral Implantol 2008;1(3):183–98.

30. Marchetti C, Trasarti S, Corinaldesi G, et al. Interpositional bone grafts in the posterior mandibular region: a report on six patients. Int J Periodontics Restorative Dent 2007;27(6):547–55.

31. Chiapasco M, Consolo U, Bianchi A, et al. Alveolar distraction osteogenesis for the correction of vertically deficient edentulous ridges: a multicenter prospective study on humans. Int J Oral Maxillofac Implants 2004;19(3):399–407.

32. Hwang SJ, Jung JG, Jung JU, et al. Vertical alveolar bone distraction at molar region using lag screw principle. J Oral Maxillofac Surg 2004; 62(7):787–94.

33. Jensen OT. Alveolar segmental "sandwich" osteotomies for posterior edentulous mandibular sites for dental implants. J Oral Maxillofac Surg 2006; 64(3):471–5.

34. Robiony M, Costa F, Politi M. Alveolar sandwich osteotomy of the anterior maxilla. J Oral Maxillofac Surg 2006;64(9):1453–4 [author reply: 1454–5].

35. Felice P, Barausse C, Pistilli R, et al. Guided "sandwich" technique: a novel surgical approach for safe osteotomies in the treatment of vertical bone defects in the posterior atrophic mandible: a case report. Implant Dent 2014;23(6):738–44.

36. Felice P, Cannizzaro G, Checchi V, et al. Vertical bone augmentation versus 7-mm-long implants in posterior atrophic mandibles. Results of a randomised controlled clinical trial of up to 4 months after loading. Eur J Oral Implantol 2009;2(1):7–20.

37. Felice P, Checchi L, Pistilli R, et al. The modified "sandwich" technique: a novel surgical approach to regenerative treatment of horizontal bone defects in the posterior atrophic mandible. A case report. Implant Dent 2014;23(3):232–8.

38. Block MS, Haggerty CJ. Interpositional osteotomy for posterior mandible ridge augmentation. J Oral Maxillofac Surg 2009;67(11 Suppl):31–9.

39. Yeung R. Surgical management of the partially edentulous atrophic mandibular ridge using a modified sandwich osteotomy: a case report. Int J Oral Maxillofac Implants 2005;20(5):799–803.

40. Felice P, Corinaldesi G, Lizio G, et al. Implant prosthetic rehabilitation of posterior mandible after tumor ablation with inferior alveolar nerve mobilization and inlay bone grafting: a case report. J Oral Maxillofac Surg 2009;67(5):1104–12.

41. Felice P, Iezzi G, Lizio G, et al. Reconstruction of atrophied posterior mandible with inlay technique and mandibular ramus block graft for implant prosthetic rehabilitation. J Oral Maxillofac Surg 2009; 67(2):372–80.

42. Schettler D, Holtermann W. Clinical and experimental results of a sandwich-technique for mandibular alveolar ridge augmentation. J Maxillofac Surg 1977;5(3):199–202.

43. Frame JW, Brady CL. Augmentation of an atrophic edentulous mandible by interpositional grafting with hydroxylapatite. J Oral Maxillofac Surg 1984; 42(2):89–92.

44. Frame JW, Brady CL, Browne RM. Augmentation of the edentulous mandible using bone and hydroxyapatite: a comparative study in dogs. Int J Oral Surg 1981;10(Suppl 1):88–92.

45. Canzona JE, Grand NG, Waterhouse JP, et al. Autogenous bone grafts in augmentation of the edentulous canine mandible. J Oral Surg 1976; 34(10):879–86.

46. Sugg KB, Rosenthal AH, Ozaki W, et al. Quantitative comparison of volume maintenance between inlay and onlay bone grafts in the craniofacial skeleton. Plast Reconstr Surg 2013;131(5):1014–21.

47. Stellingsma C, Raghoebar GM, Meijer HJ, et al. Reconstruction of the extremely resorbed mandible with interposed bone grafts and placement of endosseous implants. A preliminary report on

outcome of treatment and patients' satisfaction. Br J Oral Maxillofac Surg 1998;36(4):290–5.

48. Choi BH, Lee SH, Huh JY, et al. Use of the sandwich osteotomy plus an interpositional allograft for vertical augmentation of the alveolar ridge. J Craniomaxillofac Surg 2004;32(1):51–4.

49. Stoelinga PJ, Blijdorp PA, Ross RR, et al. Augmentation of the atrophic mandible with interposed bone grafts and particulate hydroxylapatite. J Oral Maxillofac Surg 1986;44(5):353–60.

50. Frame JW, Browne RM, Brady CL. Biologic basis for interpositional autogenous bone grafts to the mandible. J Oral Maxillofac Surg 1982;40(7): 407–11.

51. Politi M, Robiony M. Localized alveolar sandwich osteotomy for vertical augmentation of the anterior maxilla. J Oral Maxillofac Surg 1999;57(11): 1380–2.

52. Egbert M, Stoelinga PJ, Blijdorp PA, et al. The "three-piece" osteotomy and interpositional bone graft for augmentation of the atrophic mandible. J Oral Maxillofac Surg 1986;44(9):680–7.

53. Haers PE, van Straaten W, Stoelinga PJ, et al. Reconstruction of the severely resorbed mandible prior to vestibuloplasty or placement of endosseous implants. A 2 to 5 year follow-up. Int J Oral Maxillofac Surg 1991;20(3):149–54.

54. Moloney F, Stoelinga PJ, Tideman H, et al. Recent developments in interpositional bone-grafting of the atrophic mandible. J Maxillofac Surg 1985; 13(1):14–23.

55. Bormann KH, Suarez-Cunqueiro MM, von See C, et al. Sandwich osteotomy for vertical and transversal augmentation of the posterior mandible. Int J Oral Maxillofac Surg 2010;39(6): 554–60.

56. Kawakami PY, Dottore AM, Bechara K, et al. Alveolar osteotomy associated with resorbable non-ceramic hydroxylapatite or intra-oral autogenous bone for height augmentation in posterior mandibular sites: a split-mouth prospective study. Clin Oral Implants Res 2013;24(9):1060–4.

57. Lopez-Cedrun JL. Implant rehabilitation of the edentulous posterior atrophic mandible: the sandwich osteotomy revisited. Int J Oral Maxillofac Implants 2011;26(1):195–202.

58. Scarano A, Carinci F, Assenza B, et al. Vertical ridge augmentation of atrophic posterior mandible using an inlay technique with a xenograft without miniscrews and miniplates: case series. Clin Oral Implants Res 2011;22(10):1125–30.

59. Tonetti MS, Hammerle CH, European Workshop on Periodontology Group C. Advances in bone augmentation to enable dental implant placement: Consensus Report of the Sixth European Workshop on Periodontology. J Clin Periodontol 2008;35(8 Suppl):168–72.

60. Esposito M, Grusovin MG, Worthington HV, et al. Interventions for replacing missing teeth: bone augmentation techniques for dental implant treatment. Cochrane Database Syst Rev 2006;(1): CD003607.

61. Chiapasco M, Romeo E, Casentini P, et al. Alveolar distraction osteogenesis vs. vertical guided bone regeneration for the correction of vertically deficient edentulous ridges: a 1-3-year prospective study on humans. Clin Oral Implants Res 2004; 15(1):82–95.

62. Simion M, Trisi P, Piattelli A. Vertical ridge augmentation using a membrane technique associated with osseointegrated implants. Int J Periodontics Restorative Dent 1994;14(6):496–511.

63. Canullo L, Trisi P, Simion M. Vertical ridge augmentation around implants using e-PTFE titanium-reinforced membrane and deproteinized bovine bone mineral (bio-oss): A case report. Int J Periodontics Restorative Dent 2006;26(4):355–61.

64. Keestra JA, Barry O, Jong L, et al. Long-term effects of vertical bone augmentation: a systematic review. J Appl Oral Sci 2016;24(1):3–17.

65. Lang NP, Hammerle CH, Bragger U, et al. Guided tissue regeneration in jawbone defects prior to implant placement. Clin Oral Implants Res 1994; 5(2):92–7.

66. Rocchietta I, Fontana F, Simion M. Clinical outcomes of vertical bone augmentation to enable dental implant placement: a systematic review. J Clin Periodontol 2008;35(8 Suppl):203–15.

67. Wang RE, Lang NP. Ridge preservation after tooth extraction. Clin Oral Implants Res 2012;23(Suppl 6):147–56.

68. Roccuzzo M, Ramieri G, Bunino M, et al. Autogenous bone graft alone or associated with titanium mesh for vertical alveolar ridge augmentation: a controlled clinical trial. Clin Oral Implants Res 2007;18(3):286–94.

69. Antoun H, Sitbon JM, Martinez H, et al. A prospective randomized study comparing two techniques of bone augmentation: onlay graft alone or associated with a membrane. Clin Oral Implants Res 2001;12(6):632–9.

70. von Arx T, Wallkamm B, Hardt N. Localized ridge augmentation using a micro titanium mesh: a report on 27 implants followed from 1 to 3 years after functional loading. Clin Oral Implants Res 1998; 9(2):123–30.

71. Roccuzzo M, Ramieri G, Spada MC, et al. Vertical alveolar ridge augmentation by means of a titanium mesh and autogenous bone grafts. Clin Oral Implants Res 2004;15(1):73–81.

72. Proussaefs P, Lozada J, Kleinman A, et al. The use of titanium mesh in conjunction with autogenous bone graft and inorganic bovine bone mineral (Bio-Oss) for localized alveolar ridge

augmentation: a human study. Int J Periodontics Restorative Dent 2003;23(2):185–95.

73. Bahat O, Fontanesi FV. Complications of grafting in the atrophic edentulous or partially edentulous jaw. Int J Periodontics Restorative Dent 2001;21(5):487–95.

74. Chiapasco M, Abati S, Romeo E, et al. Clinical outcome of autogenous bone blocks or guided bone regeneration with e-PTFE membranes for the reconstruction of narrow edentulous ridges. Clin Oral Implants Res 1999;10(4):278–88.

75. Nystrom E, Ahlqvist J, Kahnberg KE, et al. Autogenous onlay bone grafts fixed with screw implants for the treatment of severely resorbed maxillae. Radiographic evaluation of preoperative bone dimensions, postoperative bone loss, and changes in soft-tissue profile. Int J Oral Maxillofac Surg 1996;25(5):351–9.

76. Rasmusson L, Meredith N, Kahnberg KE, et al. Effects of barrier membranes on bone resorption and implant stability in onlay bone grafts. An experimental study. Clin Oral Implants Res 1999;10(4):267–77.

77. Jensen OT, Greer RO Jr, Johnson L, et al. Vertical guided bone-graft augmentation in a new canine mandibular model. Int J Oral Maxillofac Implants 1995;10(3):335–44.

78. Gordh M, Alberius P, Johnell O, et al. Osteopromotive membranes enhance onlay integration and maintenance in the adult rat skull. Int J Oral Maxillofac Surg 1998;27(1):67–73.

79. Artzi Z, Dayan D, Alpern Y, et al. Vertical ridge augmentation using xenogenic material supported by a configured titanium mesh: clinicohistopathologic and histochemical study. Int J Oral Maxillofac Implants 2003;18(3):440–6.

80. Wilson TG Jr, Buser D. Advances in the use of guided tissue regeneration for localized ridge augmentation in combination with dental implants. Tex Dent J 1994;111(7):5, 7-10.

81. Tinti C, Parma-Benfenati S. Vertical ridge augmentation: surgical protocol and retrospective evaluation of 48 consecutively inserted implants. Int J Periodontics Restorative Dent 1998;18(5):434–43.

82. Troeltzsch M, Troeltzsch M, Kauffmann P, et al. Clinical efficacy of grafting materials in alveolar ridge augmentation: a systematic review. J Craniomaxillofac Surg 2016;44(10):1618–29.

83. von Arx T, Kurt B. Implant placement and simultaneous ridge augmentation using autogenous bone and a micro titanium mesh: a prospective clinical study with 20 implants. Clin Oral Implants Res 1999;10(1):24–33.

84. von Arx T, Kurt B. Implant placement and simultaneous peri-implant bone grafting using a micro titanium mesh for graft stabilization. Int J Periodontics Restorative Dent 1998;18(2):117–27.

85. Lizio G, Corinaldesi G, Marchetti C. Alveolar ridge reconstruction with titanium mesh: a three-dimensional evaluation of factors affecting bone augmentation. Int J Oral Maxillofac Implants 2014;29(6):1354–63.

86. Louis PJ, Gutta R, Said-Al-Naief N, et al. Reconstruction of the maxilla and mandible with particulate bone graft and titanium mesh for implant placement. J Oral Maxillofac Surg 2008;66(2):235–45.

87. Corinaldesi G, Pieri F, Sapigni L, et al. Evaluation of survival and success rates of dental implants placed at the time of or after alveolar ridge augmentation with an autogenous mandibular bone graft and titanium mesh: a 3- to 8-year retrospective study. Int J Oral Maxillofac Implants 2009;24(6):1119–28.

88. Watzinger F, Luksch J, Millesi W, et al. Guided bone regeneration with titanium membranes: a clinical study. Br J Oral Maxillofac Surg 2000;38(4):312–5.

89. Wood RA, Mealey BL. Histologic comparison of healing after tooth extraction with ridge preservation using mineralized versus demineralized freeze-dried bone allograft. J Periodontol 2012;83(3):329–36.

90. Perdijk FB, Meijer GJ, Strijen PJ, et al. Complications in alveolar distraction osteogenesis of the atrophic mandible. Int J Oral Maxillofac Surg 2007;36(10):916–21.

91. Saulacic N, Zix J, Iizuka T. Complication rates and associated factors in alveolar distraction osteogenesis: a comprehensive review. Int J Oral Maxillofac Surg 2009;38(3):210–7.

92. Ugurlu F, Sener BC, Dergin G, et al. Potential complications and precautions in vertical alveolar distraction osteogenesis: a retrospective study of 40 patients. J Craniomaxillofac Surg 2013;41(7):569–73.

93. Chiapasco M, Zaniboni M, Boisco M. Augmentation procedures for the rehabilitation of deficient edentulous ridges with oral implants. Clin Oral Implants Res 2006;17(Suppl 2):136–59.

94. Barros-Saint-Pasteur J. Plastic restoration of the alveolar crest of the mandible. Acta Odontol Venez 1966;4(1):3–21 [in Spanish].

95. Barros Saint Pasteur J. Plastic reconstruction of the alveolar crest. Clinico-surgical investigation. Acta Odontol Venez 1970;8(2):168–82 [in Spanish].

96. Schettler D. Long time results of the sandwich-technique for mandibular alveolar ridge augmentation. Dtsch Stomatol 1991;41(10):376–8 [in German].

97. Chiapasco M, Zaniboni M, Rimondini L. Autogenous onlay bone grafts vs. alveolar distraction osteogenesis for the correction of vertically deficient edentulous ridges: a 2-4-year prospective study

on humans. Clin Oral Implants Res 2007;18(4): 432–40.

98. Felice P, Piattelli A, Iezzi G, et al. Reconstruction of an atrophied posterior mandible with the inlay technique and inorganic bovine bone block: a case report. Int J Periodontics Restorative Dent 2010; 30(6):583–91.

99. Rocchietta I, Simion M, Hoffmann M, et al. Vertical bone augmentation with an autogenous block or particles in combination with guided bone

regeneration: a clinical and histological preliminary study in humans. Clin Implant Dent Relat Res 2016; 18(1):19–29.

100. Papageorgiou SN, Papageorgiou PN, Deschner J, et al. Comparative effectiveness of natural and synthetic bone grafts in oral and maxillofacial surgery prior to insertion of dental implants: systematic review and network meta-analysis of parallel and cluster randomized controlled trials. J Dent 2016; 48(5):1–8.

Guided Bone Regeneration in Alveolar Bone Reconstruction

Istvan A. Urban, DMD, MD, PhD[a,b,*], Alberto Monje, DDS, MS[c]

KEYWORDS

- Guided bone regeneration • Reconstructive therapy • Alveolar bone • Bone reconstruction

KEY POINTS

- Guided bone regeneration for alveolar bone reconstruction is effective and less invasive than other techniques, such as block grafting.
- Reconstructive therapy for atrophic ridges can be achieved following the biological principle of compartmentalization.
- Graft and membrane stability dictates success for regenerative purposes.
- The success of guided bone regeneration relies on flap management to ensure tension-free primary closure.

INTRODUCTION

Although the integrity of the jawbone is preserved through the stimulus of chewing, tooth loss caused by disease or trauma leads to alveolar bone resorption (**Figs. 1** and **2**). In order to compensate for ideal three-dimensional implant placement, numerous techniques and modifications have been proposed, conditioned to the clinical scenario involved. Traditionally, autologous block grafting was advocated as the gold standard for the horizontal and/or vertical reconstruction of edentulous ridges. However, advances in biomaterials and clinical techniques have led to the incorporation of guided bone regeneration (GBR) as a potential alternative in challenging cases.

GBR reflects the concept of compartmentalization, proposed in the late 1970s.[1] Briefly, it consists of preventing the migration of undesired cells through the adaptation of a barrier membrane to the area that is intended to be reconstructed. The barrier membrane provides stability to the bone graft, prevents soft tissue from collapsing into the defect, prevents competing nonosteogenic cell migration into the site, and accumulates growth factors.[2]

In terms of the composition of the membranes, synthetic materials have been used, such as nonresorbable polytetrafluoroethylene (PTFE), as well as resorbable synthetic materials such as a combination of polyglycolic acid and trimethylene carbonate.[3] At present, resorbable materials of xenogeneic origin, such as collagen, are the most commonly used option in GBR. One of the first membranes developed specifically for GBR was the nonresorbable, titanium-reinforced, expanded PTFE membrane. Reinforcement with a titanium frame stabilizes the form of the membrane. The use of these membranes has been well documented, and they are currently considered the gold standard for GBR. More recently, resorbable membranes have been developed that are not form stable. Accordingly, membranes can also be

Disclosure: Dr. Urban received honoraria and he is a consultant of Geistlich Pharma, Nobel Biocare, Osteogenics.

[a] Graduate Implant Dentistry, Loma Linda University, Loma Linda, CA, USA; [b] Urban Regeneration Institute, Pitypang utca 7, Budapest 1025, Hungary; [c] Department of Periodontology, Universitat Internacional de Catalunya, Barcelona, Spain

* Corresponding author. Pitypang utca 7, Budapest 1025, Hungary.

E-mail address: istvan@implant.hu

Oral Maxillofacial Surg Clin N Am 31 (2019) 331–338
https://doi.org/10.1016/j.coms.2019.01.003
1042-3699/19/© 2019 Elsevier Inc. All rights reserved.

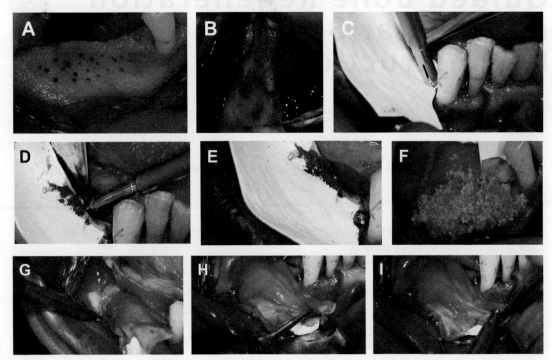

Fig. 1. Treatment of a representative case of the sausage technique in the posterior mandible using a natural collagen membrane. (*A, B*) Labial and occlusal views of a healthy 75-year-old woman with a thin posterior mandibular ridge. Note the triangle of bone distal to the last tooth. This was designed by us to place a pin. (*C*) Labial view of the pin placed within the bony triangle. (*D*) Labial view of the second pin placed distolingual. (*E*) Labial view of the 2 pins in place, stabilizing the native collagen membrane. (*F*) Labial view of the composite graft (1:1 proportion of autograft and ABBM) in place. (*G*) Labial view of the next distobuccal pin placement. (*H*) Labial view showing elasticity of the membrane. (*I, J*) Labial view of mesiobuccal pin placement. Note that the membrane is stretched out. (*K*) Labial view of the next step, which is the push-up step. The graft is positioned to the crest. Once the membrane is pushed up, the graft is secured with 2 additional titanium pins. (*L, M*) Labial view of the stretched out and stabilized membrane. Note that the graft is completely immobilized, which is checked using either finger pressure or pressure from an instrument. (*N*) Labial view of flap closure. (*O*) Occlusal view of the regenerated bone. Note the nice wide ridge after uneventful healing at 8 months. (*P*) Occlusal view of 3 implants in place. (*Q*) Periapical radiograph after 5-year follow-up, showing stable bone. ABBM, anorganic bovine bone mineral. (*From* Urban I. Vertical and horizontal ridge augmentation: new perspectives. Batavia (IL): Quintessence; 2017. p. 123; with permission.)

classified as form stable or non–form stable. Form-stable, nonresorbable, titanium-reinforced membranes are considered the gold standard for both vertical and horizontal augmentation.

Although this concept was initially proposed for the regeneration of tissues associated with the periodontium, the proof of principle was soon applied to regenerate edentulous alveolar ridges. This process was first evaluated by Dahlin and colleagues.[4] On histology, it was observed that half of the samples in which GBR was applied with Teflon membranes showed complete bone healing after 3 weeks, whereas the control sites showed no signs of healing after 22 weeks. Posteriorly, the technique was extended to humans and exhaustively evaluated to improve the biomaterials and the technique. Note that, at the time, particulate autogenous bone was the primary source for

scaffolding protected by nonresorbable barrier membranes. Now, developments in material sciences allow clinicians to use bone fillers from other sources (ie, other species or cadavers) and, as aforementioned, resorbable membranes can be used to facilitate and simplify the technique tailored to the clinical needs.

BIOLOGIC PRINCIPLES

Four main principles have been described to achieve successful GBR (**Table 1**).[5]

INDICATIONS/CONTRAINDICATIONS

Indications:
- Fenestration bone defects
- Dehiscence bone defects

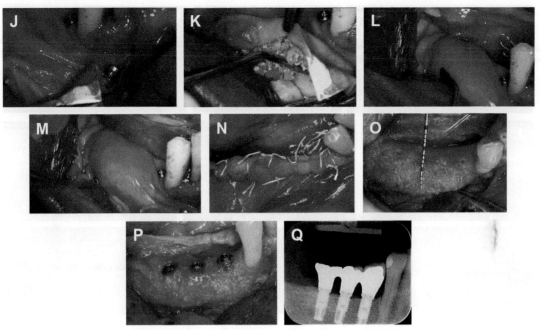

Fig. 1. (*continued*)

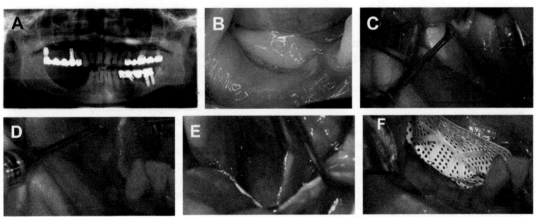

Fig. 2. Step-by-step treatment of a significant vertical defect with placement of implants into regenerated bone. (*A*) Panoramic radiograph showing a vertical defect on the right posterior mandibular defect after implant failure. Note that, on the left side, failing implants were planned to be removed before the regenerative procedure on the right side. (*B*) Labial view of the vertical deficiency of the posterior mandible. (*C–E*) Labial and occlusal views of the modified lingual flap release. Elevation of the retromolar pad (zone I). Careful elevation of the soft tissue located above the superior fibers of the mylohyoid muscle using a blunt instrument (zone II). Semiblunt periosteal release using the back end of a number 15C scalpel blade and blunt stretching of the tissues on the anterior area of the flap (zone III). (*F*) Labial view of the vertical defect. A dense polytetrafluoroethylene (PTFE) membrane was fixed on the lingual side. (*G*) Particulate autogenous bone graft mixed with ABBM is placed on the ridge. (*H*) Buccal view of the dense PTFE-titanium reinforced membrane secured over the graft with titanium tacks. Note that the membrane should not be in contact with the neighboring tooth. (*I*) Vertical flap release (~20 mm). (*J*) The buccal periosteal incision is superficial and the clinician should make certain that only the periosteum is cut and that no incision is made deeper into the tissue. (*K*) Since most patients have "periosteal cross bundles," the flap cannot be advanced as necessary once the periosteal incision has been completed. The dense fibers are gently cut with "sweeping" incisions, using the blade first in a 90-degree angle, like "playing the guitar" as the authors call this motion. (*L*) Then a blunt periosteal instrument should be used in a coronal pushing motion to separate the elastic fibers. This will ensure that the flap will be significantly advanced with less chance of causing injuries to vital anatomical structures. (*M*) Labial view of tension-free double-layer closure of the flap. (*N–P*) Labial and occlusal views of the regenerated bone.

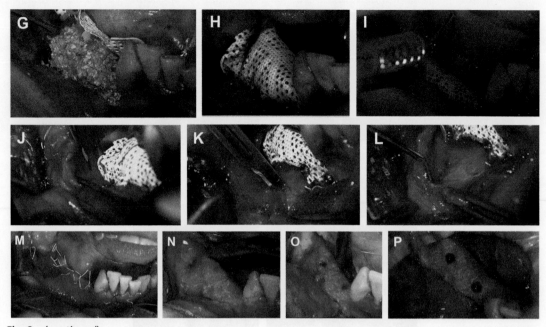

Fig. 2. (*continued*)

- Horizontal bone defect
- Vertical bone defect
- Combined vertical and horizontal bone defects
- Contained 2-wall to 3-wall and circumferential peri-implantitis defect
- Extraction sites with/without immediate implant placement

Contraindications:
- Smoking
- Uncontrolled systemic disorders
- Poor plaque control (>15% full-mouth plaque and bleeding indexes)
- Patient rejection
- Inability to achieve primary wound closure
- Inability to stabilize the bone filler and/or barrier membrane
- Poor clinical skills
- Uncontained peri-implantitis defects

Technique/procedure: vertical and horizontal ridge augmentation.

Preoperative considerations
- Understanding the anatomy
- Understanding the biological principles in order to apply them
- Comprehensive assessment of the area using cone-beam computed tomography
- Evaluation of the feasibility of other less invasive methods (ie, short or narrow dental implants)
- Examine personal oral hygiene measures

Table 1
Principles to achieve successful guided bone regeneration

Principle	Purpose	Outcome
Primary wound closure	Enhance undisturbed healing via tension-free closure	Incision design and subperiosteal scoring incision
Angiogenesis	Provide nutrients and oxygen	Corticotomies
Space creation and maintenance	Provide space and prevent collapse	Intrinsic to membrane/bone filler
Stability of the wound clot	Blood clot formation	Primary wound closure

Data from Wang HL, Boyapati L. "PASS" principles for predictable bone regeneration. Implant Dent 2006;15:8–17.

Table 2
Critical preoperative factors

Critical Factor	Management
Soft tissue phenotype and presence of keratinized mucosa	Consider soft tissue augmentation via incision design. However, the authors do not perform soft tissue grafting before bone grafting, because it might lead to the development of scar tissue
Simultaneous vs staged approach	In cases of vertical ridge augmentation, when <4 mm is needed, a simultaneous approach is suitable. For horizontal ridge augmentation, if primary stability can be achieved, a simultaneous approach can be performed; however, in case of complications, treatment is easier and more successful if surgery does not involve simultaneous implant placement (ie, staged approach)
Implant position	In general, a slightly subcrestal implant position is advocated in regenerated bone
Defect morphology	In general, more favorable outcomes are expected in the presence of a concave topography instead of a convex ridge morphology
Systemic factors and deleterious habits	Smoking should be restricted at least 3 mo before the grafting procedure. Other systemic factors and deleterious habits that can impair wound healing must be further controlled
Active periodontal disease	The periodontal condition must be stable before planning any reconstructive surgery
Nature of the periosteum	If the patient has undergone previous attempts of GBR, the periosteum might be scarred, and this impedes adequate coronal advancement to secure tension-free flap closure

- Evaluate eligibility according to the patient risk profile and deleterious habits (ie, smoking)

CRITICAL PREOPERATIVE FACTORS

Critical preoperative factors are listed in **Table 2**.

Guided Bone Regeneration for Horizontal Ridge Defects

The so called knife-edge ridge, or Cawood and Howell class IV edentulous jaw, represents a unique problem for horizontal augmentation. The necessary height of the ridge is adequate on the lingual/palatal side but the width is insufficient, often making implant placement impossible without prior treatment.[6] The difficulty of using GBR has been that stabilization of the particulate graft is a challenge in such defects when the clinician is not using a form-stable titanium-reinforced

membrane. More recently, clinicians have used non–form-stable collagen membranes to reconstruct severely thin ridges. In most cases, the necessary bone gain was not achieved, and most of the bone growth was obtained apically from the crest.

Sausage-technique surgery has been developed to overcome these challenges.[7] This technique uses a collagen membrane fixated with titanium pins. The aim is to secure bone graft stabilization on the crest so that no migration or collapse of particles occurs. A more rapidly reabsorbing natural collagen membrane and 1:1 mixture of autogenous particulate bone/anorganic bovine bone mineral (ABBM) as grafting material should be selected for horizontal augmentation (**Fig. 1**).[7,8]

Surgical Procedure

1. Safety flap (**Fig. 2**). The safety flap is a full-thickness flap that, depending on the

Table 3
Lingual zones of interest

Zone	Site	Management
First	Retromolar pad	Tunneling and lifting
Second	Molar region	Blunt dissection
Third	Premolar region	Horizontal hockey-stick periosteal incision and blunt tissue advancement

Data from Urban IA, Monje A, Lozada J, et al. Principles for vertical ridge augmentation in the atrophic posterior mandible: a technical review. Int J Periodontics Restorative Dent 2017;37:639–45.

extension, comprises vertical incisions located 2 to 3 teeth beyond the edentulous area. In the posterior mandible, a full-thickness, midcrestal incision is made in the keratinized gingiva with a surgical scalpel (number 15). The distal extension of the crestal incision ends within 2 mm of the retromolar pad. For surgical access, a distal oblique vertical incision is made toward the coronoid process of the mandible. A vertical incision is placed mesiobuccally at least 1 tooth away (preferably 2) from the surgical site. Mesiolingually, a 3-mm to 4-mm incision is made at the mesiolingual line angle of the most distal tooth in front of the defect. Then, periosteal elevators are used to reflect a full-thickness flap beyond the mucogingival junction and at least 5 mm beyond the bone defect.

2. Preparation of the lingual flap. The lingual flap is raised to the mylohyoid line, where attachment of the fibers of the mylohyoid muscle can be identified. Because the mylohyoid attachment is deeper mesially to the region of the second bicuspid, the depth of flap elevation does not follow the location of the muscle.

3. Preparation of the recipient site. Corticotomies are made using a medium-sized round bur to promote bleeding.

4. Trimming of the collagen membrane according to the size and morphology of the defect.

5. Tacking of the membrane using pins. In the case of the posterior mandible, the first pin that should be placed is the crestal pin distal to the last tooth in order to stabilize the membrane and then place the lingual pins.

6. Mixing of the composite autogenous bone previously harvested from the recipient site or other source (ie, mandibular ramus) and the ABBM in 1:1 proportion.

7. Molding of the membrane over the graft material, securing the membrane by tacking it with pins in the mesial and distal areas to achieve total immobilization of the graft beneath the membrane. This molding must be checked using either finger pressure or pressure from an instrument.

8. Tension-free closure, achieved via periosteal scoring incisions at the buccal site of the mandible and modified lingual flap advancement. The rationale for this flap design is based on the location of the attachment of the mylohyoid muscle and also on the protection of vital anatomic landmarks such as the lingual nerve and sublingual artery. There are 3 zones of interest at the lingual site[9] (**Table 3**).

9. Suturing. Horizontal mattress sutures are used, combined with single interrupted sutures using nonresorbable suture material.

POSTPROCEDURE PATIENT CARE

- Chemical plaque control is performed using 0.12% chlorhexidine solution from 24 hours after surgery and until suture removal.
- Antiinflammatory medication such as ibuprofen 200/600 mg 3 times a day for 7 days is provided.
- Antibiotic therapy such as amoxicillin 500 mg 3 times a day for 7 days or clindamycin 600 mg 3 times a day is used in patients allergic to β-lactamases.
- Corticosteroids are not routinely used, because they may decelerate healing and increase the risk of postoperative infection.

POSSIBLE COMPLICATIONS

1. During implant/graft surgery
   - Lack of primary stability caused by insufficient graft maturation or an inadequate drilling sequence.
   - Nerve injury.
2. Early postoperative complications (≤3 weeks)
   - Membrane exposure as a result of inadequate surgical management (insufficient flap release to achieve tension-free closure).
   - Low-grade, medium-grade, or high-grade infection resulting from membrane exposure and/or graft contamination during surgery.
3. Late postoperative complications (>4 weeks)
   - Membrane exposure caused by trauma. This unfortunate event may lead to early

Table 4
Clinical results in the literature

Author	Number of Participants	Follow-up	Type of Augmentation	Type of Membrane	Bone Filler	Bone Gain (mm)	Implant Survival (%)	Peri-implant Marginal Bone Loss
Urban et al,[8] 2014	19	6 mo	VRA	Dense PTFE	AB + ABBM	5.45 ± 1.93	100	NR
Urban et al,[7] 2011	22	8 mo	HRA	Synthetic resorbable membrane	AB ± ABBM	5.56 ± 1.45	100	NR
Urban et al,[3] 2009	35	12–72 mo	VRA	Expanded PTFE	AB + ABBM	5.5 ± 2.29	100	1.4 ± 0.57 mm at 12 mo 1.42 ± 0.1 mm at 72 mo
Urban et al,[10] 2017	16	1–15 y	VRA ± HRA	Dense PTFE and collagen membrane	AB + ABBM	VRA: 5.1 ± 1.8 HRA: 7.0 ± 1.5	100	1.4 ± 1 mm

Abbreviations: HRA, horizontal ridge augmentation; NR, not recorded; VRA, vertical ridge augmentation.

Table 5
Current controversies and future considerations

Clinical Controversies	Future Considerations
Effectiveness of different bone substitutes to achieve ridge augmentation	To examine the different bone substitutes combined or not with autogenous bone
Plausibility of incorporating customized scaffolds according to site morphology	To gain insight to the accuracy of custom-made scaffolds and nonresorbable barrier membranes
Advantages and disadvantages of GBR vs other procedures for tissue reconstruction	To evaluate the clinical, radiographic, and patient-reported outcomes of GBR vs other procedures for tissue reconstruction
Efficacy of biologic agents and platelet-derived aggregates on regenerative outcomes	To evaluate the clinical, radiographic, and patient-reported outcomes of GBR using biologic agents
Radiographic peri-implant marginal bone level and clinical parameters of augmented bone vs implant placed in pristine bone	To compare the clinical and radiographic outcomes of implants placed in augmented vs pristine bone over the long term (>10 y)

membrane removal and less-than-expected bone gain.
4. Late technical and biological complications
   • Peri-implant diseases as a consequence of poor plaque control.

CLINICAL RESULTS IN THE LITERATURE

The results from clinical trials reported in the literature are presented in **Table 4**.

CURRENT CONTROVERSIES/FUTURE CONSIDERATIONS

Current controversies and future considerations are presented in **Table 5**.

SUMMARY

GBR represents a plausible, viable, and effective alternative for the reconstruction of atrophic ridges. Crucial technical aspects, such as the achievement of tension-free flap closure, and stability of the graft and barrier membrane are of paramount importance to secure successful outcomes. The procedure requires great technical expertise and is indicated for low-level patient risk profiles (ie, adequate personal oral hygiene measures and nonsmokers).

REFERENCES

1. Melcher AH. On the repair potential of periodontal tissues. J Periodontol 1976;47:256–60.
2. Schenk RK, Buser D, Hardwick WR, et al. Healing pattern of bone regeneration in membrane-protected defects: a histologic study in the canine mandible. Int J Oral Maxillofac Implants 1994;9:13–29.
3. Urban IA, Jovanovic SA, Lozada JL. Vertical ridge augmentation using guided bone regeneration (GBR) in three clinical scenarios prior to implant placement: a retrospective study of 35 patients 12 to 72 months after loading. Int J Oral Maxillofac Implants 2009;24:502–10.
4. Dahlin C, Linde A, Gottlow J, et al. Healing of bone defects by guided tissue regeneration. Plast Reconstr Surg 1988;81:672–6.
5. Wang HL, Boyapati L. "PASS" principles for predictable bone regeneration. Implant Dent 2006;15:8–17.
6. Proussaefs P, Lozada J. The use of resorbable collagen membrane in conjunction with autogenous bone graft and inorganic bovine mineral for buccal/labial alveolar ridge augmentation: a pilot study. J Prosthet Dent 2003;90:530–8.
7. Urban IA, Nagursky H, Lozada JL. Horizontal ridge augmentation with a resorbable membrane and particulated autogenous bone with or without anorganic bovine bone-derived mineral: a prospective case series in 22 patients. Int J Oral Maxillofac Implants 2011;26:404–14.
8. Urban IA, Lozada JL, Jovanovic SA, et al. Vertical ridge augmentation with titanium-reinforced, dense-PTFE membranes and a combination of particulated autogenous bone and anorganic bovine bone-derived mineral: a prospective case series in 19 patients. Int J Oral Maxillofac Implants 2014;29:185–93.
9. Urban IA, Monje A, Lozada J, et al. Principles for vertical ridge augmentation in the atrophic posterior mandible: a technical review. Int J Periodontics Restorative Dent 2017;37:639–45.
10. Urban IA, Monje A, Lozada JL, et al. Long-term evaluation of peri-implant bone level after reconstruction of severely atrophic edentulous maxilla via vertical and horizontal guided bone regeneration in combination with sinus augmentation: a case series with 1 to 15 years of loading. Clin Implant Dent Relat Res 2017; 19:46–55.

Le Fort I Distraction Osteogenesis of Edentulous Maxillae Combined with Simultaneous Sinus Floor Grafting to Obtain Orthoalveolar Form for Emergence Profile Dental Implant Restorations

Report of Three Patient Treatments Followed for 12 Years

Ole T. Jensen, DDS, MS

KEYWORDS

• Le Fort I distraction • Sinus grafting • Orthoalveolar form • Emergence profile • Dental implants

KEY POINTS

• A moderately atrophic retro-displaced edentulous maxilla can be treated with outpatient Le Fort I (non–down fractured) distraction osteogenesis.
• As in orthognathic surgery, the purpose of distraction is to permit optimal advancement of the maxilla to develop nasolabial support as well as orthoalveolar form for emergence profile implant esthetics.
• However, with the advent of all-on-4 treatment, prosthetic elements more easily and less expensively solve most all esthetic and biomechanical demands.
• The sinus graft can be done at the same time as maxillary jaw distraction provided the sinus membrane is left intact.

A moderately atrophic retro-displaced edentulous maxilla can be treated with outpatient Le Fort I (non–down fractured) distraction osteogenesis.[1] As in orthognathic surgery, the purpose of distraction is to permit optimal advancement of the maxilla to develop nasolabial support as well as *orthoalveolar form* for emergence profile implant esthetics.[2,3] However, with the advent of all-on-4 treatment, prosthetic elements more easily and less expensively solve most all esthetic and biomechanical demands.[4–8] However, younger patients who have substantial remaining bone may not prefer a fixed denture prosthesis.[1] In addition, at some amount of horizontal deficiency, facial bone grafting, such as alveolar split, guided bone regeneration, or block grafts, may be inadequate to gain ideal facial form making the distraction procedure indicated.[9–12] Distractions can move the maxilla forward 15 to 20 mm and down 10 mm, but what is the *minimum* distance where distraction

Department of Oral and Maxillofacial Surgery, University of Utah, School of Dentistry, 530 Wakara Way, Salt Lake City, UT 84108, USA
E-mail address: oletjensen@icloud.com

Oral Maxillofacial Surg Clin N Am 31 (2019) 339–348
https://doi.org/10.1016/j.coms.2018.12.009
1042-3699/19/© 2018 Elsevier Inc. All rights reserved.

might be justified?[13,14] Although this question is one of surgical judgment and requires analysis of several factors, perhaps 10 mm is a good minimum indication in the horizontal dimension, whereas a vertical movement requirement of 5 mm or greater suggests Le Fort I distraction osteogenesis. In addition, consideration for relapse of up to 20% of the distraction must be considered.[15–17]

Alveolar ridge height in the maxilla is often not lost initially because of relative stability of the palatal plate, whereas width deficiency is commonly manifest due to resorption of the facial plate.[18,19] Edentulous maxilla-mandibular alveolar relation becomes a relative telescoping arch discrepancy that if not corrected in the maxilla will make dental implant restorations, nonemergent, ridge-lapped, and off-axis cantilevered as they occlude with the mandibular restoration.[20–22] One additional advantage of the distraction approach is that slight overdistraction permits back-cutting of soft and hard tissue to optimize emergent profile esthetics.[1]

Reported here are late findings of 3 patients who underwent Le Fort I distraction osteogenesis followed by complete arch implant restoration performed more than 10 years ago.

TECHNICAL NOTE

In an outpatient setting under local anesthesia and intravenous sedation, lateral antrostomies for sinus membrane elevation are done bilaterally through limited horizontal vestibular incisions extending from the tuberosity to the bicuspid region. The sinus membrane is elevated from posterior to anterior such that the entire sinus membrane is elevated away from the floor approximately 10 mm. A vertical incision is then made in the midline vestibule to access the anterior nasal spine and nasal septum. The nasal membranes are elevated in the anterior nasal fossa extending laterally to the pyriform rims. Through this access, horizontal osteotomies are made connecting the nasal fossa to the lateral antrostomies bilaterally.

The nasal septum is then freed with an osteotomy, and a limiting vertical osteotomy cut is made in the tuberosity or pterygomaxillary suture bilaterally. The maxilla is mobilized but not down-fractured. Sometimes this may require osteotomy of the lateral nasal wall deep inside the nasal fossa, but in most atrophic maxillae, the wall is thin and can be easily separated by incomplete down-fracture.

Once the maxilla is well mobilized, a 15- to 20-mm distraction bone plate is placed bilaterally with activation arms extending anterior-inferiorly to allow for forward-downward movement of the maxilla (**Fig. 1**). Once the distractors are in place,

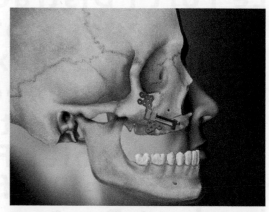

Fig. 1. The atrophic maxilla is commonly retro-displaced several millimeters or more. A horizontal distraction plate is placed bilaterally, intraorally, for forward and downward movement.

the maxilla is distracted about 5 mm to insure mobility and then returned to a minimally distracted state of about a 2-mm bony separation. The final distraction can exceed 15 mm or more (**Fig. 2**). The anterior sinus floor is then grafted with autograft, and the wounds are closed with chromic suture. Conceptually, the jaw not only is being moved into class I jaw relation but also is slightly overdistracted to allow for back-cutting for emergence profile restoration, suggesting ideal regeneration of orthoalveolar form (**Figs. 3–5**).

CASE REPORTS
Patient 1

A 42-year-old woman who had had implant replacement in the lower jaw and an upper denture presented some years later for implant restoration of the upper jaw (**Figs. 6** and **7**). She desired

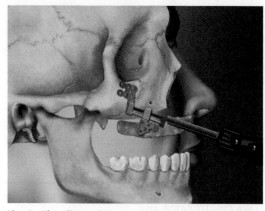

Fig. 2. The distraction proceeds until the facial plate and alveolar crest are displaced to an optimal restorative position.

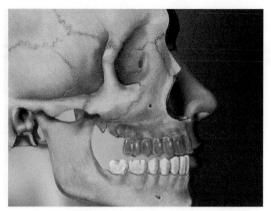

Fig. 3. Once bone healing is complete, usually after 4 months, the distractor plates are removed and a guide stent is used to place implants.

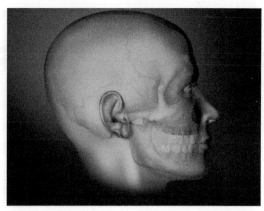

Fig. 5. Orthoalveolar form supports a more ideal dental restoration as well as a nasolabial contour.

natural-appearing teeth and did not want to have "false teeth" or "false gums." The maxilla was approximately 10 mm retro-displaced but was planned for overcorrection of 2 to 3 mm for a 12- to 13-mm distraction. Using 3 incisions as described above, the sinus membranes and nasal mucosa were elevated. The lateral antrostomy was connected to the nasal fossa, and a limiting vertical osteotomy posterior was made through the tuberosity. The distraction devices were then screwed into place with vectors anterior and slightly inferior (**Figs. 8** and **9**). After the distraction devices were placed, the maxilla could be easily advanced and separated vertically. The distraction device was then returned to the starting point. Following sinus grafting using tibia marrow autograft at the anterior sinus floor, the wounds were closed primarily. One week later, distraction commenced at a rate of 1 mm per day for 2 weeks.

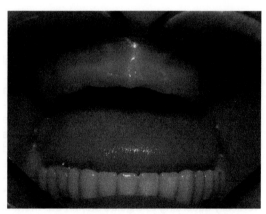

Fig. 6. A 42-year-old woman presents with an edentulous maxilla opposing a mandibular fixed dental implant restoration on tissue level implants.

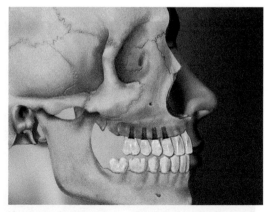

Fig. 4. Implants are generally placed in the first molar, bicuspid(s), and canine sites, 4 on each side, leaving the anterior zone for pontiform restoration using a one-piece ceramo-metal bridge.

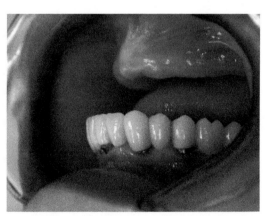

Fig. 7. A lateral view of the maxilla reveals substantial retro-displacement.

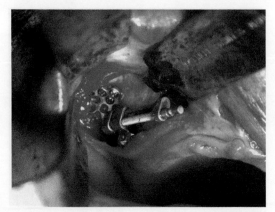

Fig. 8. Using a vestibular incision, the sinus membrane is elevated through a lateral antrostomy window, the Le Fort osteotomy cuts are completed, the sinus floor is grafted with bone from the tibia, and the horizontal distractor is placed on the right side.

The maxilla appeared excessively prominent but was considered optimal by the prosthodontist for both lip support and the gingival emergence strategy (**Figs. 10–12**). The patient was then left to heal for 4 months.

After 4 months, the distraction junction appeared well healed supporting a stable anteriorized maxilla (**Fig. 13**). The distraction devices were then removed; the anterior alveolar segment was back-cut in a scallop pattern to mimic, and approximate emergence profile esthetics was supported by the temporary removable prostheses (**Figs. 14** and **15**). Eight implants were placed vertically according to a guide stent. Four months later, a one-piece fixed porcelain-to-metal bridge was placed (**Figs. 16–18**). Over a period of 12 years, there were no repairs, no loss of implants, or discernible relapse of the advanced maxillary position.

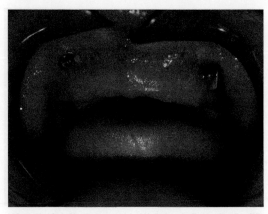

Fig. 10. The distractor activators are left exposed after wound closure.

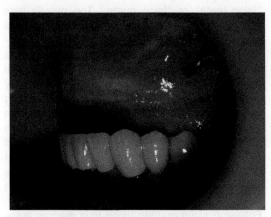

Fig. 11. Three weeks later after 14 days of distraction at a rate of 1 mm per day, the patient presents with marked maxillary displacement.

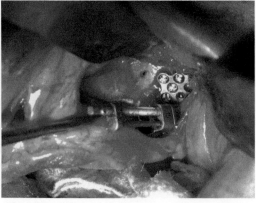

Fig. 9. The distractor is placed in a similar fashion on the left side.

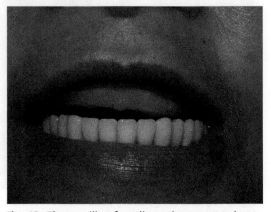

Fig. 12. The maxilla after distraction appears hypertrophic and overly prominent but support of the nasolabial structures appears ideal.

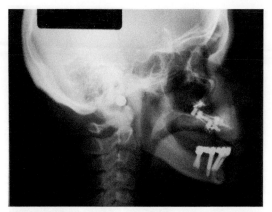

Fig. 13. A postdistraction cephalographic radiograph shows the maxilla has been advanced about 14 mm and brought down vertically 5 mm.

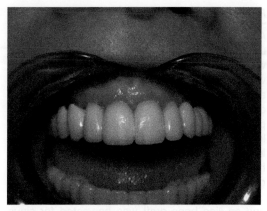

Fig. 16. Several months later after implants have osseointegrated, the final restoration with esthetic gingival emergence is established.

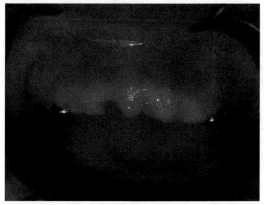

Fig. 14. The anterior alveolar zone is cut back to create a scallop-form anatomy.

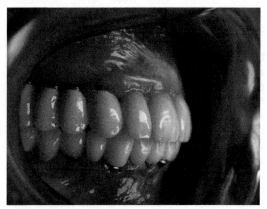

Fig. 17. The left lateral view of the tissue level implant restoration.

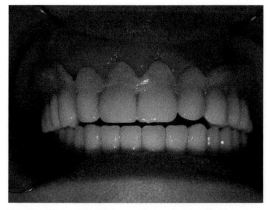

Fig. 15. The removable appliance is modified to support the newly created gingival architecture done at the time of posterior implant placement.

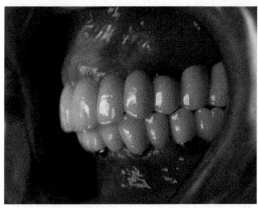

Fig. 18. The right lateral view of the tissue level implant restoration.

Patient 2

A 35-year-old woman presented for extraction of upper remaining teeth due to periodontal disease with significant facial bone loss. Following healing with a denture for more than a year, the maxilla appeared retro-displaced 7 to 8 mm and vertically deficient 2 to 3 mm (**Figs. 19** and **20**). A distraction procedure was elected and planned on a stereolithic model to more accurately place the maxilla into orthoalveolar alignment and provide excess hard and soft tissue from histeogenesis for emergence profile esthetics (**Fig. 21**).

The patient was taken to the operating room, and an iliac bone graft was harvested for sinus floor grafting. The maxilla was freed and down-fractured preserving the sinus and nasal membranes. Following placement of distraction devices, the sinus floors were grafted, and the jaw was placed into a nondistracted position for wound closure. One week later, distraction commenced and continued at a rate of 1 mm per day for 9 days. The net distraction in the horizontal plane appeared to be 8 to 9 mm, and vertical movement was about 3 to 4 mm. There was a notable cant to the maxilla from unequal vertical displacement (**Fig. 22**). The maxilla was left to heal for 4 months, and then the distraction devices were removed in a separate procedure. After 2 more weeks, healing implants were placed posteriorly according to a guide stent, and the anterior alveolar segment was back-cut to provide for emergence profile esthetics (**Figs. 23** and **24**). The patient has remained stable since 2006 without implant loss or jaw relapse with long-term presence of natural-appearing teeth in a patient who displays gingiva upon smiling (**Fig. 25**).

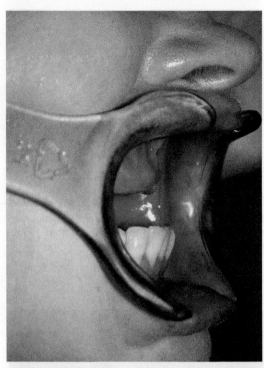

Fig. 20. The facial plate is 7 to 8 mm deficient in the horizontal plane.

Patient 3

A 54-year-old woman presented with an edentulous maxilla that was markedly retro-displaced both horizontally and vertically (**Figs. 26** and **27**). Facially, there was a gross lack of support for the nasolabial structures. The patient had a history of bulimia leading to early loss of teeth and subsequent alveolar atrophy with relative pneumatization of the maxilla. Her desire was to create a

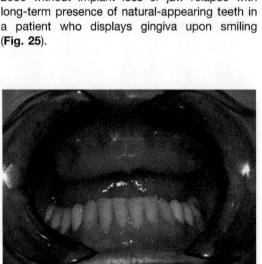

Fig. 19. A 36-year-old woman presents with an edentulous maxilla in retro-displaced position for an ideal restoration.

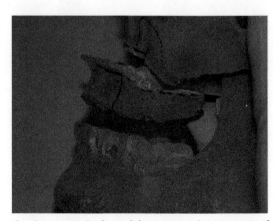

Fig. 21. A medical model suggests the amount of maxillary displacement required to obtain orthoalveolar form.

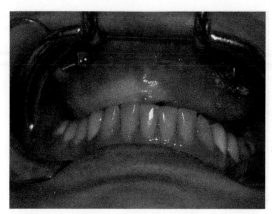

Fig. 22. The maxilla is overdistracted about 8 to 9 mm to provide excess tissue for alveolar-gingival reconstruction.

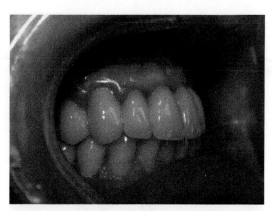

Fig. 25. The gingival projection and idealized labial bone plate create emergence profile esthetics and a natural appearing restoration in a patient with a high smile line.

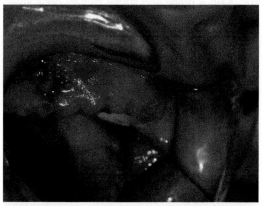

Fig. 23. The day the distractors are removed and implants are placed posteriorly, the soft tissue contours are established.

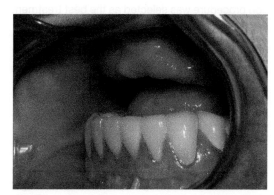

Fig. 26. A 54-year-old woman presented with a markedly retro-displaced maxilla with extensive atrophy anteriorly, but less so in the posterior regions. One of the chief complaints was loss of naso-labial contour esthetics. Left lateral view.

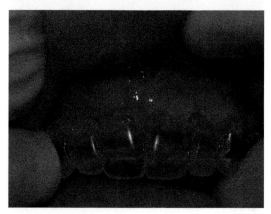

Fig. 24. A dentiform guide is used to confirm cervical contours and papillary positions.

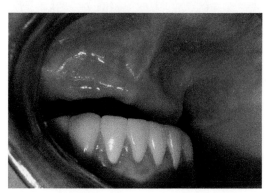

Fig. 27. Right lateral view of resto-displaced maxilla.

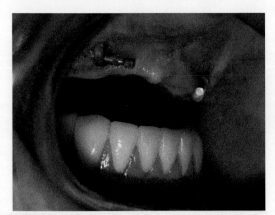

Fig. 28. Frontal view following a 15-mm horizontal distraction and 5-mm vertical displacement of the maxilla.

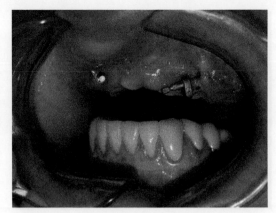

Fig. 30. Left lateral view after a 15-mm distraction.

natural-appearing smile while at the same time augmenting midfacial support. A Le Fort I distraction procedure was selected as the best treatment option. This procedure was accomplished in an office setting under intravenous anesthesia.

Using 3 incisions as described in the technical note above, the maxilla was mobilized and sinus membranes were elevated in preparation for grafting. Distraction devices were placed bilaterally, and then the sinus floors were grafted using tibia plateau autograft. The wounds were then closed, and 1 week later, distraction proceeded at a rate of 1 mm per day for 15 days, the entire length of the 15-mm distractor (**Figs. 28** and **29**). Despite further distraction being required, it was thought that there was enough improvement to not justify repositioning the distraction devices to gain more advancement. After 4 months healing, 8 implants were placed, and soft tissue grafting was done in the anterior for additional support (**Figs. 30** and **31**). The patient was followed for 12 years with minimal peri-implant bone loss evident with the

exception of 2 left-side posterior implants that had lost 3 mm of bone but remained solid and without purulence. An orthopanograph showed stable sinus grafts and stable implant bone levels for the one-piece ceramo-metal restoration 12 years after placement (**Figs. 32** and **33**).

DISCUSSION

The use of modified mandibular distractor plates to move a relatively nonmobilized Le Fort I

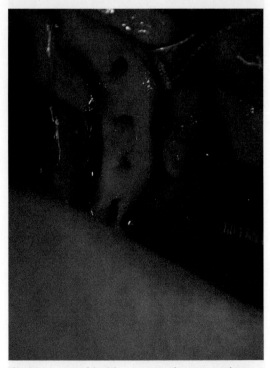

Fig. 31. A crestal incision was used to access the posterior maxilla where, using a guide stent, 4 implants were placed on each side.

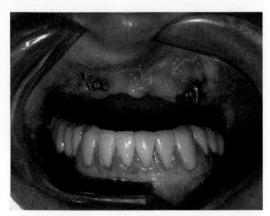

Fig. 29. Right lateral view after a 15-mm distraction.

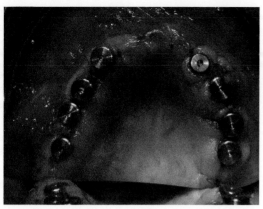

Fig. 32. The posterior implant was placed and gingival bulking done anteriorly.

osteotomy of an atrophic maxilla forward and down leads to highly accurate placement of anterior maxillary bone mass to optimize implant placement for emergence profile esthetics. Furthermore, the advancement of the maxilla leads to improved nasolabial support. However, in general, the procedure should not be done if the alveolar width for implants is inadequate.

In the patients treated, anterior displacement of the maxilla remained stable with little change in dental occlusion because early relapse is somewhat disguised by the delay required in establishing anterior coupling in the final dental restoration, which can approximate 1 year after secession of the distraction procedure.[22] Most relapse from the distraction likely occurred within this first year time period.[22–24] Implant loss did not occur, nor did significant bone loss or gingival dehiscence develop.

Sinus bone graft directed implants remained stable as did bone graft height in the sinus floor after more than 10 years as has been shown in vertical alveolar distraction combined with sinus

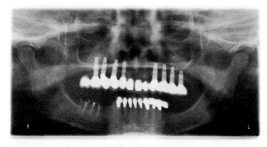

Fig. 33. Twelve years after the distraction procedure, the maxillary jaw position and dental occlusion remained class I. An orthopanograph revealed a stable dental restoration with minimal peri-implant bone loss.

grafting and the posterior sandwich osteotomy combined with sinus floor augmentation.[25,26] Therefore, it appears that sinus membrane elevation for sinus floor grafting done at the same time as distraction is a viable option.

SUMMARY

The combined distraction/sinus graft method, although now superseded by the all-on-4 technique, is still a viable option in select patients for bio-restoration of orthoalveolar form in an effort to provide a natural-appearing dental restoration.

REFERENCES

1. Jensen OT, Leopardi A, Gallegos L. The case for bone graft reconstruction including sinus grafting and distraction osteogenesis for the atrophic edentulous maxilla. J Oral Maxillofac Surg 2004;62: 1423–8.
2. Jensen OT, Ueda M, Laster Z. Distraction osteogenesis. Selected Readings Oral Maxillofac Surg 2002; 10(4):1.
3. Le B, Nielsen B. Esthetic site development. Oral Maxillofac Surg Clin North Am 2015;27(2):283–311.
4. Graves S, Mahler BA, Armellini D, et al. Maxillary all-on-four therapy using angled implants: a 16 month clinical study of 1110 implants in 276 jaws. Oral Maxillofac Surg Clin North Am 2011;23(2):277–87.
5. Jensen OT, Adams MW, Butura C, et al. Maxillary V-4: Four implant treatment for maxillary atrophy with dental implants fixed apically at the vomer-nasal crest, lateral pyriform rim and zygoma for immediate function. Report on 44 patients followed from 1 to 3 years. J Prosthet Dent 2015;114(6): 810–7.
6. Jensen OT, Ringeman JL, Adams MW, et al. Reduced arch length as a factor for 4-implant immediate function in the maxilla: a technical note and report of 39 patients followed for 5 years. J Oral Maxillofac Surg 2016;74(12):2379–84.
7. Malo P, Lopes A, de Araujo Nobre M, et al. Immediate function dental implants inserted with less than 30N cm of torque in full-arch maxillary rehabilitations using All-on-4 concept: retrospective study. Int J Oral Maxillofac Surg 2018;47(8):1079–108.
8. Malo P, Araujo Nobre M, Lopes A, et al. Axial implants in immediate function for partial rehabilitation in the maxilla and mandible: A retrospective clinical study evaluating the long-term outcome (up to 10 years). Implant Dent 2015;24(5):557–64.
9. Jiang X, Zhang Y, Di P, et al. Hard tissue volume stability of guided bone regeneration during the healing stage in the anterior maxilla: a clinical and

radiographic study. Clin Implant Dent Relat Res 2018;20(1):68–75.

10. Chiacpasco M, Zaniboni M. Failures in jaw reconstruction with autogenous onlay bone grafts for pre-implant purposes: incidence, prevention and management of complications. Oral Maxillofac Surg Clin North Am 2011;23:1–15.

11. Farzad M, Mohammadi M. Guided bone regeneration: a literature review. J Oral Health Oral Epidemiol 2012;83:111–22.

12. Jensen OT, Bell W, Cottam J. Osteoperiosteal flaps and local osteotomies for alveolar reconstruction. Oral Maxillofac Surg Clin North Am 2010;22(3):331–46.

13. Malik NA, Kumar VV, Bora P. Lefort I distraction osteogenesis of the edentulous maxilla. Int J Oral Maxillofac Surg 2011;40(4):430–3.

14. Apaydin A, Sermet B, Ureturk S, et al. Correction of malocclusion and oral rehabilitation in a case of amelogenesis imperfecta by insertion of dental implants followed by lefort I distraction osteogenesis of the edentulous atrophic maxilla. BMC Oral Health 2014;14:116.

15. Moran I, Virdee S, Sharp I, et al. Postoperative complications following lefort I maxillary advancement surgery in cleft palate patients: a 5-year retrospective study. Cleft Palate Craniofac J 2018;55(2):231–7.

16. Etti T, Gerlach T, Schusselbauer T, et al. Bone resorption and complications in alveolar distraction osteogenesis. Clin Oral Investig 2010;14(5):481–9.

17. Baek SH, Lee JK, Lee JH, et al. Comparison of treatment outcome and stability between distraction osteogenesis and Lefort I osteotomy in cleft patients with maxillary hypoplasia. J Craniofac Surg 2007;18(5):1209–15.

18. El Nahass H, N Najem S. Anaylsis of the dimensions of the labial bone wall in the anterior maxilla: a cone beam computed tomography study. Clin Oral Implants Res 2015;26(4):57–61.

19. Nevins M, Camelo M, DE Paoli S, et al. A study of the fate of the buccal wall of extraction sockets of teeth with prominent roots. Int J Periodontics Restorative Dent 2006;26(1):19–29.

20. Kuc J, Sierpinskka T, Golebiewska A. Alveolar ridge atrophy related to facial morphology in edentulous patients. Clin Interv Aging 2017;12:1481–94.

21. Monie A, Chan HL, Galindo-Moreno P, et al. Alveolar bone architecture: a systematic review and meta-analysis. J Periodontol 2015;86(11):1231–48.

22. Spielman HP. Influence of the implant position on the aesthetics of the restoration. Pract Periodontics Aesthet Dent 1996;8(9):897–904.

23. Eldho M, Paulose J, Paul ET. Soft tissue changes in cleft lip and palate patients: anterior maxillary distraction versus conventional lefort I osteotomy. J Maxillofac Oral Surg 2013;12(4):429–36.

24. Nevzatoglu S, Kucukkeles N, Guzel Z. Long term stability of intra-oral maxillary distraction in unilateral cleft lip and plate: a case report. Aust Orthod J 2013;29(2):200–8.

25. Boyne PJ, Herford AS. Distraction osteogenesis of the nasal and antral osseous floor to enhance alveolar height. J Oral Maxillofac Surg 2004;672(9 Suppl 2):123–30.

26. Jensen OT, Cottam J. Posterior maxillary sandwich osteotomy combined with sinus grafting with bone morphogenetic protein-2 for alveolar reconstruction for dental implants: report of four cases. Int J Oral Maxillofac Implants 2013;28(6):415–23.

Extra-Long Nasal Wall–Directed Dental Implants for Maxillary Complete Arch Immediate Function: A Pilot Study

Giovanni Nicoli, MD[a], Simone Piva, MD[b],*,
Pietro Ferraris, MD[c], Federico Nicoli, MD, PhD[d,e],
Ole T. Jensen, DDS, MS[f]

KEYWORDS

- Nasal implants • Denture protheses • Zygomatic implants • Pterygoid implants

KEY POINTS

- Complex surgical approach as zygomatic or pterygoid implants could be overcome using a new developed extra-long 24-degree angulated platform.
- One hundred fifteen implants were performed on 33 patients, with a total of 24 patients who received immediate loading.
- There were no complications at follow-up.
- This implant approach with extra-long, angulated "nasal implants" is feasible and safe. The authors' protocol seems to be a viable alternative to the use of the zygomatic implants, potentially increasing patient access to treatment.

INTRODUCTION

Immediate loading of dental implants for complete arch rehabilitation can be done in the maxilla, with the main limitation being inadequate cortical bone to fix implants.[1] Disuse atrophy results in vertical bone loss, leading to deficient horizontal arch-length limiting options for placement of posterior maxillary implants. For this reason, bone augmentation is commonly prescribed, including both sinus floor and alveolar augmentation, followed by delayed implant placement.[2]

In order to provide immediate function and avoid complex bone grafting procedures, zygomatic and pterygoid implants[3] have been advocated. These surgical approaches have some limitations: they may require intravenous or even general anesthesia, are technically challenging, and they can lead to a major complication (ie, oroantral fistula, sinusitis, orbital injury, and implant fracture), which is mainly due to extramaxillary positioning. Computer simulation studies on stress analysis of zygomatic implants have demonstrated a

Disclosure: The authors have nothing to disclose. The study was performed in accordance with the Declaration of Helsinki. Written informed consent was obtained from each patient or their legally authorized representatives before enrollment.
[a] Via Europa, 5/D, Monticelli Brusati, Brescia 25040, Italy; [b] Department of Anesthesia, Critical Care and Emergency, Spedali Civili University Hospital, Piazzale Ospedali Civili, 1, Brescia 25123, Italy; [c] Via Carlo Alberto, 16, Alessandria 15121, Italy; [d] Center for Clinical Ethics, Insubria University, Varese, Italy; [e] Clinical Ethics Services "Teresa Camplani Foundation" Domus Salutis Clinic Brescia, Via Lazzaretto, 3, Brescia 25123, Italy; [f] Department of Oral and Maxillofacial Surgery, University of Utah, School of Dentistry, 530 Wakara Way, Salt Lake City, UT 84108, USA
* Corresponding author.
E-mail address: simone.piva@unibs.it

necessity for bone graft supplementation for severe atrophy.[4] Although not clearly stated in the literature, the zygomatic approach may lead to oroantral communication, presenting as peri-mplantitis. Pterygoid-directed implantation leads to a relatively unfavorable prosthetic position (ie, second and third molar)[3,5] and could result in complications such as bleeding from the pterygoid plexus or implant stability, which is commonly difficult to obtain.[3,6,7] Therefore, to overcome the limitations of zygomatic and pterygoid implants, an extra-long dental implant was developed with an anchorage into cortical bone found at the lateral nasal wall instead of extramaxillary.[6,8] In addition to bicortical anchorage at the residual palatoalveolar ridge and the nasal wall, bone grafting of the sinus floor may help gain osseointegration. The implants are designed for angled placement transsinus with an angled platform, which improves fixation at the alveolar process.

The primary objective of the present study was to test the feasibility of extra-long "nasal implants" for use in maxillary complete arch immediate function.

MATERIALS AND METHODS
Study Design

This prospective observational pilot study was conducted in 2 private clinics from May 2012 to May 2016.

The study was conducted in accordance with the Declaration of Helsinki. Ethical approval for publication of the data was obtained from the local ethics committee (registration number 0/2017). Detailed written and oral information was provided to the patients and family members about the study and written informed consent to participate to the study was obtained. All possible complications of the protocol proposed in the study along with all the surgical alternatives have been largely discussed with patients. The study conforms to CONSORT extension for pilot studies.[9]

Patient Population and Protocol Inclusion Criteria

Patients with complete edentulous maxillae were enrolled in the study if there was less than 5 mm posterior maxillary bone height and the medial maxillary sinus wall was near vertical with the angle of the anterior sinus wall to the sinus floor approximating 90° as viewed by cone beam computed tomography (CBCT).

Patients were excluded if they had significant acute or chronic sinus diseases, periodontal disease, or oral infection. Medical exclusions included pregnancy, insulin-dependent diabetes, patients taking medications or having treatments known to affect bone turnover, or any disease process that effects bone metabolism. Any therapeutic agents or devices known to interfere with or to have an effect on bone induction were not permitted during the study period.

Surgical Procedure

The extra-long implant placement protocol merges 3 different techniques: angulated implant placement,[10] maxillary sinus floor augmentation,[11] and the same criteria for the use of zygomatic implants.[1] A preoperative CBCT was performed using a specific software (Galileo Implants, Sirona) to simulate implant position and measure the distance between the nasal wall and the residual alveolar crest at the approximate second premolar position. The height of the alveolar crest beneath the sinus and the angle of the nasal wall were also determined. Moreover, in the presurgical CBCT, possible nerve anatomic variants were ruled out, in order to avoid a possible nerve complication.[12]

The surgical technique (**Fig. 1**) commenced with a crestal incision made around the arch with a posterior releasing incision at the first molar area. A buccal mucoperiosteal flap reflection exposed the nasal fossa and lateral sinus wall. According to the Bedrossian classification,[13] when the crestal bone was 3 mm or less a sinus floor bone graft was done (**Fig. 2**). A lateral antrostomy window was created for access using a triangle-shaped sinus membrane reflection where the sides of the triangle include the sinus floor and nasal wall to enhance vascularization of the bone graft. The implant osteotomy at the crest was increased to 3.4 mm diameter unless the crestal bone was thin, 1 mm or less, then a 4 mm diameter osteotomy was prepared in order to avoid bone fracture during implant placement. If alveolar crestal bone was greater than 3 mm, bone grafting was not done despite the implants being placed transsinus.[14–16]

Appropriate length implants were determined after measuring the osteotomy.[17] Primary implant stability was assessed by (1) insertion torque, (2) percussion test,[18] and (3) postsurgical CBCT. Two anterior implants were then placed into the premaxilla. A screw-retained acrylic interim denture prosthesis was inserted within 24 hours of implant placement.

Medical management included 2 g of amoxicillin/clavulanic acid given orally 1 hour before surgery and 2% chlorhexidine oral rinse for 30 seconds immediately before surgery. Local anesthesia was administered, associated with

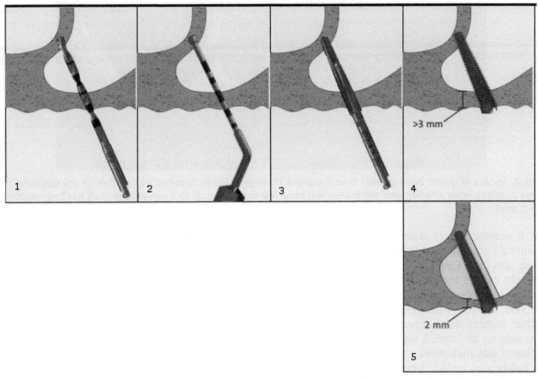

Fig. 1. Nasal implant surgical technique sequence. Illustrations are for a 20 mm implant. (0) Initiate the site preparation with a round burr or equivalent drill. (1) Using the Ø2x24 mm pilot drill, drill through the alveolar, across the sinus, emerging into the nasal cavity. (2) The 24 mm depth gauge can be used to palpate the hole depth for implant selection. (3) Drill to final depth with the D-34TP final drill. (4) Place the implant in accordance with standard implant placement procedures, ensuring the prosthetic axis of the implant is aligned correctly. (5) NB: If the alveolar bone is less than 3 mm thick then bone grafting must be applied.

intravenous sedation when required by the patients. Postoperatively, all patients received 32 mg of methylprednisolone to prevent swelling and 1 g of amoxicillin/clavulanic acid antibiotic taken twice a day for 5 days. Paracetamol (1000 mg) was prescribed for postoperative pain.

Patients were scheduled for check-up examinations and suture removal after 8 days; then, they were seen monthly for 6 months when secondary implant stability was checked by (1) reverse torque test with a removal torque value of 40 Ncm,[19] (2) a percussion test, and (3) a CBCT scan to evaluate the bone growth around the implants.[18] The final prosthesis was then inserted.

Study Materials

In collaboration with the implant manufacturer (Southern Implants), the common distance found between the crestal bone in the region of the second premolar and nasal cortical wall was measured on the CBCT. Based on these data a selection of appropriate length implants was determined. Implants of 20, 22, and 24 mm in length,

each with a 24-degree offset platform in a conical shape with an external hexagon connection, were made (**Fig. 3**).

The sinus floor bone graft material used was xenograft–substitutive bovine bone (Nibec Co., LTD South Korea) mixed with platelet-rich fibrin.[20]

Statistical Analysis

The following variables were recorded in an electronic case report form: age, sex, smoking history, associated comorbidity, and surgery and prosthesis position data; moreover, implant position and length of implants for each patients, as well as any complications, were recorded.

"The primary objectives of the present study were the feasibility and safety of extra-long "nasal implants". Feasibility was tested by the percentage of implant failures; in particular, patients were scheduled for check-up examinations and suture removal after 8 days; then, they were seen monthly during all the study period and secondary implant stability (secondary stability) was checked

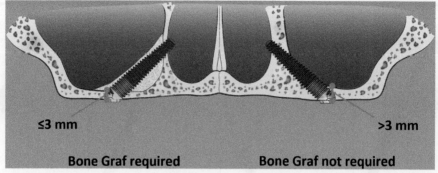

≤3 mm

>3 mm

Bone Graf required

Bone Graf not required

Fig. 2. In case of crestal bone greater than 3 mm the bone graft is not required (right side); on the opposite, in case of severe bone atrophy with residual crestal bone less than or equal to 3 mm a bone graft has been applied (left side).

at 6 months by (1) reverse torque test with a removal torque value of 40 Ncm,[19] (2) a percussion test, and (3) a CBCT scan to evaluate the bone growth around the implants.[18] In case the bone graft was applied to the patients, the bone growth around implant was measured retrospectively. When stability was not reached, the implant was considered as failed, it was removed, and a new attempt was performed.

Safety was tested during the study period (ie, 15–60 months) by monthly clinical evaluation, obtained by (1) any clinical signs of possible complications (presence of headache, sinus congestion, soft tissue, hard tissue, and/or dental implant infection), (2) peri-implant soft tissue conditions including hyperplasia and recession, and (3) in case of clinical sign of sinusitis, CBCT was obtained. If sinusitis developed, the Lund-Mackay staging system was used to grade the Rhinosinusitis.[21] In case of implant failure, the implant was removed and replaced.

We expressed continuous variables as mean (standard deviation, SD) for normal distributed variables or median (interquartile range, IQR) for the non-normal distributed variables. Qualitative variables are expressed as absolute and percent frequencies. The data were analyzed with R 3.2.2.

RESULTS

Thirty-three patients were treated during the study period, of which 24 (72.7%) received immediate loading. Sixteen patients were men, 8 were women, and the mean age was 65 years (9.73 years SD).

In **Table 1**, patient demographic characteristics are represented, along with implant data (including implant length and arch position). The total number of implants placed was 115, ranging from 4 to 6 implants for each patient. Fifty-three implants (46%) were nasal. Two patients smoked more than

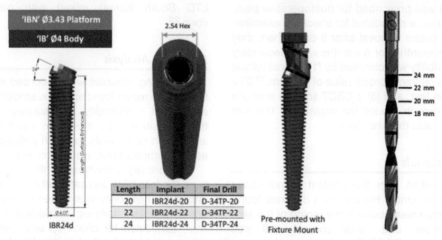

Fig. 3. Nasal implant length and angulation. In the length column, the possible lengths of the implants are represented. In the "Implant" column, "IBR" is the name of the implants, 24d is the degree of the implant platform. In the "Final Drill" column, the specifications of the drill used are represented.

Table 1
Patient's demographic characteristics and implant specifications

Variable	
Age (year), mean (SD)	65 (9.73)
Smokers, number (%)	1 (4%)
Cardiological comorbidity	3 (12.5%)
Male, number (%)	16 (67%)
Type of Implants (diameter [mm]/ length [mm]/ inclination [°])	Number (%)
3.25/10/0	3 (2.6)
3.25/11.5/0	1 (1)
3.25/13/0	5 (4.3)
3.25/13/12	4 (3.5)
40/10/24	1 (1)
40/11/24	2 (1.7)
40/13/12	14 (12)
40/13/24	17 (14.7)
40/15/12	4 (3.5)
40/15/24	17 (14.7)
40/18/12	4 (3.5)
40/18/24	13 (11)
40/20/24	10 (8.8)
40/22/24	4 (3.5)
50/13/12	1 (1)
50/13/24	2 (1.7)
50/15/12	3 (2.6)
50/15/24	2 (1.7)
50/15/36	2 (1.7)
50/18/36	1 (1)
50/18/24	4 (3.5)
60/7/0	1 (1)
Total	115 (100%)
Number of Implants	Number (%)
6	4 (16.7)
5	11 (45.8)
4	9 (37.5)
Implant Position	Total number (%), Nasal number (%)
12 Upper	12 (10.4), 2 (3)
13 Upper	8 (7), 0 (0)
14 Upper	8 (7), 2 (3)
15 Upper	15 (13), 15 (28)
16 Upper	9 (8), 8 (15)
17 Upper	1 (1), 1 (2)
21 Upper	13 (11), 1 (2)
22 Upper	10 (9), 0 (0)
23 Upper	14 (12), 1 (2)
24 Upper	2 (1.7), 1 (2)
25 Upper	18 (15.6), 18 (34)
26 Upper	5 (4.3), 5 (9)
Total	115 (100), 53 (100)

10 cigarettes a day and 3 patients had cardiac comorbidity.

Fourteen patients (58.3%) had sinus floor grafts done (8 bilateral and 6 unilateral). All immediate function implants achieved at least 30 Ncm insertion torque (40 Ncm was achieved in 3 implants and 45 Ncm in 7 implants).

Nine patients (27.3%) were treated with delayed loading, for a total of 29 implants, of which 12 (41.4%) were nasal. All delayed loaded implants osseointegrated and were in prosthetic function within 6 months.

One nasal wall–directed implant (2%) failed during the follow-up period. All the remaining nasal implants (n = 52, 98%) were placed into function.

There were no significant complications at the 6 months or late-term follow-up.

DISCUSSION

The use of extra-long implants seems to be a valid alternative to zygomatic or pterygoid implants. The method results in a slightly increased anterior posterior spread when compared with standard length implants. Also, the technique is less invasive than zygomatic placement and may prove to be better accepted by the patients.

The zygomatic implant, first suggested by Bothur and colleagues,[22] is a technique that could be applied in patients with severe bone atrophy but can lead to oroantral fistula and other complications.[3,17,23] Moreover, the technique is challenging, may require general anesthesia, and has not been fully proved in efficacy over alternative bone augmentation techniques such as the sinus floor bone graft for treating atrophic maxillae.[7] Potential complications include sinusitis (the most common), oronasal fistula, orbital injury, extraoral fistula, and intraoral soft tissue hyperplasia around the implant. Even if the surgeon is experienced and knowledgeable, these complications may occur.[17,24] The complementary technique of pterygoid-directed implantation[25,26] requires only local anesthesia; therefore it may be a more accessible treatment for patients. However, the emergence of the pterygoid implant platform in the second or third molar location renders prosthetic procedures more difficult. Moreover, pterygoid implant placement risks include excessive bleeding and inadequate bone quality or quantity for implant stability.[25,27,28]

Nasal implants may find application in-between the zygomatic and pterygoid implants not only because of anatomic position but also in terms of difficulty of placement. Extra-long implants may increase the available armamentarium for addressing the treatment challenge of severe maxillary atrophy, particularly when there is a short arch-length available for osseointegration.[23,24,28]

The extra-long implant protocol has 2 main advantages: first, it can often be safely applied even in the presence of severe bone atrophy.[17,27]

Second, the nasal implant is less invasive and easier to place than the zygomatic implant.

The nasal implant, where it engages the lateral nasal wall, has been found to be stable over time and to form apparent osseointegration when viewed on CBCT (**Fig. 4**).

From a prosthetic point of view the nasal implant introduces a novelty by its design principle: in addition to increased length (20, 22, 24 mm), the implant platform allows for a more central alveolar position for restoration than alternatives. As shown in **Fig. 5**, the implant platform is in an optimal position when parallel to the residual crestal bone

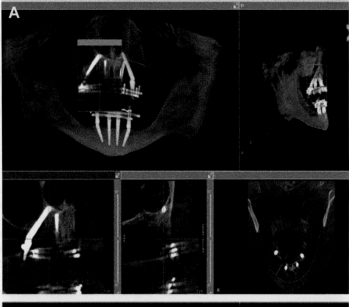
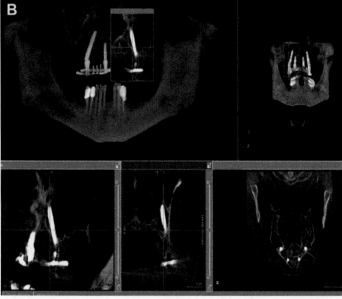

Fig. 4. (*A*) A CBCT performed after 28 months of surgery, in a 48-year-old man who received 6 implants, 2 in position 12, 2 in position 22, and 2 nasal implants in positions 15 and 25. The CBCT shows the transsinus nasal implant with a bicortical anchorage in position 15 in a patient with a crestal bone thickness less than 3 mm, requiring bone graft. (*B*) The CBCT performed after 24 months after surgery, in a 60-year-old woman with 6 implants, 2 of them in position 22, 2 in position 22, and 2 nasal implants in positions 15 and 25. The CBCT shows the transsinus nasal graftless implant with a bicortical anchorage in position 15 in a patient with a crestal bone thickness greater than 3 mm.

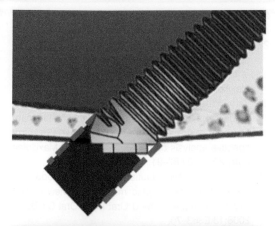

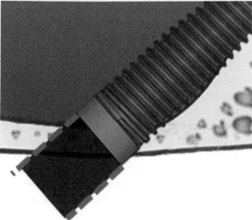

Fig. 5. The optimal position of the nasal implant platform, avoiding the need for an angulated abutment and keeping the platform itself out of the sinus cavity.

avoiding the need for an angulated abutment and keeping the platform itself out of the sinus cavity.

SUMMARY

The use of nasal implants seems to be a safe alternative to zygomatic and pterygoid implants. Extra-long implants placed angulated transsinus into the nasal wall were shown to have a low failure rate with an absence of complications during the study follow-up (16–61 months). The approach adds new armamentarium for addressing moderate to severe maxillary atrophy and enables improved posterior implant position by increasing anterior posterior spread. The use of extra-long implants could potentially increase the number of patients seeking complete arch treatment. Nevertheless, this short-term study requires verification long term to be found comparable to available techniques such as zygomatic and pterygoid implants.

SUPPLEMENTARY DATA

Supplementary data related to this article can be found online at https://doi.org/10.1016/j.coms.2019.01.004

REFERENCES

1. Bedrossian E, Stumpel L, Beckely ML, et al. The zygomatic implant: preliminary data on treatment of severely resorbed maxillae. A clinical report. Int J Oral Maxillofac Implants 2002;17:861–5.
2. Beretta M, Poli PP, Grossi GB, et al. Long-term survival rate of implants placed in conjunction with 246 sinus floor elevation procedures: results of a 15-year retrospective study. J Dent 2015;43:78–86.
3. Davó R, Pons O. Prostheses supported by four immediately loaded zygomatic implants: a 3-year prospective study. Eur J Oral Implantol 2013;6:263–9.
4. Kaman S, Atil F, Tekin U, et al. Stress analysis of zygomatic implants on the augmented maxillary sinus: is it necessary to graft? Implant Dent 2017;26:860–7.
5. Dos Santos PL, Silva GHS, Da Silva Pereira FR, et al. Zygomatic implant subjected to immediate loading for atrophic maxilla rehabilitation. J Craniofac Surg 2016;27:e734–7.
6. Jensen OT, Cottam JR, Ringeman JL, et al. Angled dental implant placement into the vomer/nasal crest of atrophic maxillae for All-on-Four immediate function: a 2-year clinical study of 100 consecutive patients. Int J Oral Maxillofac Implants 2014;29:e30–5.
7. Esposito M, Worthington HV. Interventions for replacing missing teeth: dental implants in zygomatic bone for the rehabilitation of the severely deficient edentulous maxilla. Cochrane Database Syst Rev 2013;(9):CD004151.
8. Jensen OT, Cottam J, Ringeman J, et al. Trans-sinus dental implants, bone morphogenetic protein 2, and immediate function for all-on-4 treatment of severe maxillary atrophy. J Oral Maxillofac Surg 2012;70:141–8.
9. Eldridge SM, Chan CL, Campbell MJ, et al. CONSORT 2010 statement: extension to randomised pilot and feasibility trials. BMJ 2016;355:i5239.
10. Kurtzman G, Dompkowski D, Mahler B, et al. Off-axis implant placement for anatomical considerations using the co-axis implant. Inside Dentistry 2008;4(5). Available at: https://www.aegisdentalnetwork.com/id/2008/05/off-axis-implant-placement-for-anatomical-considerations-using-the-co-axis-implant.
11. Wallace SS, Tarnow DP, Froum SJ, et al. Maxillary sinus elevation by lateral window approach: evolution of technology and technique. J Evid Based Dent Pract 2012;12:161–71.
12. Machado VC, Chrcanovic BR, Felippe MB, et al. Assessment of accessory canals of the canalis

sinuosus: a study of 1000 cone beam computed tomography examinations. Int J Oral Maxillofac Surg 2016;45:1586–91.

13. Bedrossian E, Sullivan RM, Fortin Y, et al. Fixed-prosthetic implant restoration of the edentulous maxilla: a systematic pretreatment evaluation method. J Oral Maxillofac Surg 2008;66:112–22.

14. Abi Najm S, Malis D, El Hage M, et al. Potential adverse events of endosseous dental implants penetrating the maxillary sinus: long-term clinical evaluation. Laryngoscope 2013;123:2958–61.

15. Jung J-H, Choi B-H, Zhu S-J, et al. The effects of exposing dental implants to the maxillary sinus cavity on sinus complications. Oral Surg Oral Med Oral Pathol Oral Radiol Endod 2006;102:602–5.

16. Petruson B. Sinuscopy in patients with titanium implants in the nose and sinuses. Scand J Plast Reconstr Surg Hand Surg 2004;38:86–93.

17. Chrcanovic BR, Abreu MHNG. Survival and complications of zygomatic implants: a systematic review. Oral Maxillofac Surg 2013;17:81–93.

18. Atsumi M, Park S-H, Wang H-L. Methods used to assess implant stability: current status. Int J Oral Maxillofac Implants 2007;22:743–54.

19. Sullivan DY, Sherwood RL, Collins TA, et al. The reverse-torque test: a clinical report. Int J Oral Maxillofac Implants 1996;11:179–85.

20. Ali S, Bakry SA, Abd-Elhakam H. Platelet-rich fibrin in maxillary sinus augmentation: a systematic review. J Oral Implantol 2015;41:746–53.

21. Lund VJ, Mackay IS. Staging in rhinosinusitus. Rhinology 1993;31:183–4.

22. Bothur S, Jonsson G, Sandahl L. Modified technique using multiple zygomatic implants in reconstruction of the atrophic maxilla: a technical note. Int J Oral Maxillofac Implants 2003;18:902–4.

23. Fernández H, Gómez-Delgado A, Trujillo-Saldarriaga S, et al. Zygomatic implants for the management of the severely atrophied maxilla: a retrospective analysis of 244 implants. J Oral Maxillofac Surg 2014;72:887–91.

24. Pi Urgell J, Revilla Gutiérrez V, Gay Escoda CG. Rehabilitation of atrophic maxilla: a review of 101 zygomatic implants. Med Oral Patol Oral Cir Bucal 2008;13:E363–70.

25. Bidra AS, Huynh-Ba G. Implants in the pterygoid region: a systematic review of the literature. Int J Oral Maxillofac Surg 2011;40:773–81.

26. Graves SL. The pterygoid plate implant: a solution for restoring the posterior maxilla. Int J Periodontics Restorative Dent 1994;14:512–23.

27. Curi MM, Cardoso CL, Ribeiro Kde C. Retrospective study of pterygoid implants in the atrophic posterior maxilla: implant and prosthesis survival rates up to 3 years. Int J Oral Maxillofac Implants 2015;30:378–83.

28. Candel E, Peñarrocha D, Peñarrocha M. Rehabilitation of the atrophic posterior maxilla with pterygoid implants: a review. J Oral Implantol 2012;38(Spec No):461–6.